Cancer Hypoxia

This book comprehensively reviews the role of hypoxia in cancer initiation and progression. It explores hypoxia-driven signaling pathways and the immune microenvironment in hypoxic tumors, offering insights into network implications for cancer development and therapy, along with strategies to counter hypoxia-induced immune suppression. Investigating influence of hypoxia on cancer stem cells and cellular stemness, the book highlights its role in maintaining stemness at hypoxic niches and potential therapeutic opportunities. The book, in turn, explores tools and techniques for the detection of hypoxic phenotypes and in vivo models for studying hypoxic cancer, angiogenesis, and vasculature remodeling in hypoxic tumors, discussing innovative drug delivery, and targeting hypoxia-inducible factors. Finally, it outlines clinical applications of hypoxia research in cancer therapy, ranging from advancements in radiation strategies to biomarkers, diagnosis, precision medicine, and future directions in hypoxia-activated prodrug research. This comprehensive resource serves as a valuable reference for researchers, clinicians, and professionals engaged in understanding and combating cancer hypoxia.

Key Features:

- Offers a thorough review of the role of hypoxia in cancer initiation and progression
- Presents complex hypoxia-driven signaling pathways in tumors and their implications for cancer development and therapy
- Role of hypoxia in maintaining stemness within hypoxic niches and potential therapeutic opportunities
- Discusses ways to enhance drug efficacy in hypoxic tumor microenvironments
- Explores therapeutic approaches targeting hypoxic tumor vasculature

Dr Sukhes Mukherjee is working as an Additional Professor in the Biochemistry Department of AIIMS Bhopal, India. He is a committed and hard-working faculty member, involved in teaching and research for the last 18 years, with a very active academic and research career. Dr. Mukherjee has published more than 130 papers in peer-reviewed journals and presented his work at several national and international conferences. He got the best paper award from the "Association of Clinical Biochemists of India" in 2008. He got the international travel fellowship to attend the Neurochemistry conference at Busan, South Korea, in August 2009 and another AACC fellowship in 2011. Dr. Mukherjee was awarded by the International Society for Neurochemistry in 2008 and is a member of the WHO's Who as International Executives. His peers recognize Dr. Mukherjee as a scientific expert who integrates new technologies into everyday clinical practice and finds new areas in biomedical research advancement, particularly in Cancer Biology.

Dr Suman Kumar Ray is working as Research Scientist in the Biochemistry Department of AIIMS Bhopal, India. Dr. Ray is a committed and hard-working researcher who has been involved in research for the last 14 years with a glorious research career. Dr. Ray has published more than

96 papers in peer-reviewed journals and over 18 book chapters and presented his work at several national and international conferences. He is actively associated with national and international Oncology-related associations, like the American Association of Cancer Research. He is an Ambassador of the European Association of Cancer Research. He has given many invited talks at different colleges in India among undergraduate students. Dr. Ray has a vast knowledge of hypoxia-Oncology with several publications by recognition. He is a dedicated researcher and content writer in the field of Oncology. He has also edited two books related to Cancer Hypoxia.

Cancer Hypoxia

Implication in Therapeutics and Precision Oncology

Edited by
Sukhes Mukherjee and Suman Kumar Ray

CRC Press
Taylor & Francis Group
Boca Raton London New York

CRC Press is an imprint of the
Taylor & Francis Group, an **informa** business

Designed cover image: Sukhes Mukherjee and Suman Kumar Ray

First edition published 2026
by CRC Press
2385 NW Executive Center Drive, Suite 320, Boca Raton FL 33431

and by CRC Press
4 Park Square, Milton Park, Abingdon, Oxon, OX14 4RN

CRC Press is an imprint of Taylor & Francis Group, LLC

ISBN: 978-1-032-76180-0 (hbk)
ISBN: 978-1-032-76182-4 (pbk)
ISBN: 978-1-003-47741-9 (ebk)

DOI: 10.1201/9781003477419

Typeset in Times
by KnowledgeWorks Global Ltd.

Contents

About the Editors

Sukhes Mukherjee is a highly esteemed academic and researcher currently serving as Additional Professor in the Department of Biochemistry at AIIMS Bhopal, India. With over 18 years of dedicated experience in teaching and research, he has established himself as a prominent figure in the fields of cancer biology, biochemistry, and molecular biology. His prolific scholarly output includes more than 120 peer-reviewed publications and eight edited books, reflecting his deep engagement with cutting-edge scientific inquiry and his commitment to advancing knowledge in his field. His leadership and expertise are recognized globally, evidenced by his active participation in numerous scientific societies; he is a Fellow of the Linnean Society (UK) and the Royal Society for Medicine, a member of the Royal Society of Biology (UK), a member of the National Academy of Medical Sciences (India), and Clinical Scientist of the American Society of Clinical Pathology, among others. His contributions have been acknowledged through prestigious awards such as the ISSN Award from the International Science and Technology Organization (2023), the Farha Deeba Haq Award from the Indian Academy of Biomedical Sciences (2024), and the Blackbucks Award from Medical Dialogues (2024). Furthermore, his dedication to advancing biomedical sciences, combined with his commitment to education and professional development, positions him as a leading figure in the global scientific community. Dr. Mukherjee's commitment to fostering a vibrant scientific community is evident through his active engagement in organizing conferences, symposiums, and scientific forums that facilitate knowledge dissemination and networking among researchers. Dr. Mukherjee's unwavering commitment to advancing science, fostering collaboration, and mentoring future leaders exemplifies his role as a pioneer in his field. His multifaceted career reflects a blend of scientific rigor, educational passion, and leadership acumen, making him a highly influential figure whose work continues to inspire and shape the future of biomedical sciences worldwide.

Suman Kumar Ray is a highly dedicated and accomplished researcher whose career spans over 15 years of rigorous investigation in the fields of Molecular Biology and Cancer Research. Throughout his esteemed career, he has authored more than 85 peer-reviewed research articles, contributed to several comprehensive book chapters, and presented his groundbreaking work at numerous prestigious national and international conferences, establishing himself as a prominent voice in the oncology community. His expertise in the study of hypoxia and its profound implications in tumor biology has earned him widespread recognition, reflected in his extensive publication record and invitations to deliver lectures at various academic institutions across India. Dr. Ray maintains active and influential affiliations with leading oncology-related organizations, including the American Association for Cancer Research, where he is involved in collaborative research and knowledge dissemination, and he also serves as an ambassador for the European Association for Cancer Research, promoting international cooperation in cancer science. Dr. Ray seamlessly integrates pioneering oncology research with strategic innovation, forging collaborative pathways and advancing scientific frontiers in public health through his dedicated laboratory expertise and visionary leadership. His academic journey is marked by several National Fellowships, which laid the foundation for his innovative research approach and he continues to make significant contributions through his research, editorial work for scientific journals, and content development in oncology. His unwavering commitment to advancing cancer research is complemented by his dedication to mentoring young researchers and engaging in public outreach. Dr. Ray's diverse interests and passions exemplify a well-rounded personality committed to both scientific excellence and personal growth, inspiring colleagues and apprentices alike in the pursuit of knowledge and innovation in cancer research.

1 Hypoxia in Tumor Microenvironment and Cellular Response

Manohar Kugaji
Central Research Laboratory, Maratha Mandal's NGH Institute of Dental Sciences and Research Centre, Bauxite Road, Belagavi, Karnataka, India

Prachi Parvatikar
Department of Biotechnology, School of Applied Sciences and Technology, BLDE (Deemed to be University), Bangaramma Sajjan Campus, Vijaypura, Karnataka, India

INTRODUCTION

A study of occurrence and progression of malignant tumors could be a critical factor in the management of disease condition. Tumor microenvironment (TME) being a major factor in the occurrence and progression of malignant tumors is distinguished by hypoxia, a condition that is frequently encountered in solid malignancies. The key components of the TME are blood vessels, lymphatic vessels, cancer-associated fibroblasts (CAFs), immune cells, and extracellular matrix (ECM) (Balkwill et al. 2012). The diverse physical and functional interactions between these factors and cancer cells result in the clinical outcome.

TME frequently exhibits hypoxic characteristics because of the impact of tumor cells and aberrant vascular structure, particularly in solid tumors (Chen et al. 2022). Tumor cells have adapted to produce energy through hydrolysis in response to the effects of hypoxia. The immunological and metabolic processes of TME are altered by hypoxia, which also results in an upregulation of hypoxia-inducible factor (HIF) expression. The cytotoxic T cells, B cells, and natural killer (NK) cells are inhibited by hypoxia condition. Nevertheless, there is upregulation of marrow-derived suppressor cells and regulatory T cells. The influence of immune system and altered metabolism give tumor cells an optimal environment while impeding the effectiveness of anticancer treatments. Under hypoxic condition, the effect of anti-tumor drugs is decreased by hindering the drug delivery providing ideal surviving conditions for tumor cells (Castells et al. 2012; Khalaf et al. 2021; Seebacher et al. 2021). Due to this reason, the traditional chemotherapy and single dose immunotherapy have limited efficacy in the management of malignant tumors (Sanmamed & Chen 2018, Hegde & Chen 2020).

The primary cause of the hypoxic response is HIFs. Changes that support cancer growth can be promoted by HIF-dependent signaling, which can help cancer and stromal cells adapt and select to the environment. In hypoxic tumor cells, HIF stabilization triggers the expression of target genes that code for proteins that support metastasis (CXCR4, E-cadherin), neo-angiogenesis (VEGF), metabolic modifications, stemness, and epithelial to mesenchymal transition (EMT) (Emami Nejad et al. 2021). Consequently, a deeper comprehension of the hypoxic TME and signaling cascade can provide new avenues for the development of different techniques for the management of hypoxic microenvironment. In this review, the influence of hypoxia on tumor behavior and its correlations with immune cells and cell metabolism are discussed. Additionally, we have provided a summary of

DOI: 10.1201/9781003477419-1

how hypoxia affects drug resistance in tumors and oxidative stress as well as provided the strategies for addressing the hypoxic TME.

HYPOXIA AND METABOLISM

Hypoxia has an effect on TME and its surrounding tissue metabolism. The advancement of TME research has led to the identification of metabolic reprogramming as a characteristic feature of malignant tumors. Tumor cells undergo metabolic modifications and reprogram themselves to continue growing and defy the treatment. Aerobic glycolysis and L-glutamine metabolism are the examples of reprogramming (Schiliro & Firestein 2021). Thus, it is reasonable to conclude that hypoxia prevents tumor cells from undergoing apoptosis by facilitating the metabolic reprogramming.

Glucose metabolism: Low extracellular pH, which is caused by monocarboxylic acid transporter activation, is another feature of solid tumors. The low pH in the ECM results by the accumulation of lactic acid outside the tumor. In addition to preventing lymphocyte proliferation and cytotoxicity, the low pH also increases the invasiveness of tumor cells, impairing the ability of immune effector cells to function in the TME (Chiche et al. 2010; Ward & Thompson 2012; Kobliakov 2018). High rate of glycolysis is commonly found in most of the cancers. Low oxygen levels cause tumor cells to switch from producing metabolic acids through oxidative phosphorylation to glycolysis. Similar to enhanced angiogenesis, these modifications are brought about by transcription induced by HIF-1α, which increases the expression of genes related to glycolysis and glucose transporters (Semenza 2003). The tumor cells produce proteins and lipids by using glycolytic metabolic intermediates. In a hypoxic environment, the metabolic process of aerobic glycolysis helps tumor cells grow and proliferate by weaning them off of oxygen requirement (Rob et al. 2012). Furthermore, there is a tight correlation between the reprogramming of glucose metabolism and the multidrug resistance of tumor cells. Multiple mechanisms were proposed to influence this process, including reduced apoptotic potential, increased activity of the multidrug transporter p-glycoprotein (P-gp), alterations in genes (e.g., p53 mutation), and "ion capture" (Chen et al. 2022).

Galactose metabolism: Under hypoxic conditions, cancer cells typically select an alternate substrate for energy metabolism, such as L-glutamine, instead of glycolysis. According to a research, L-glutamine serves as a substitute energy source for tumor metabolism and is essential for the growth of tumor cells (Yuneva et al. 2007). To make up for the decreased energy output from glycolysis, L-glutamine is first synthesized as glutamate, which is subsequently transformed into α-ketoglutaric acid through transamination and into the tricarboxylic acid cycle for energy metabolism (Zhdanov et al. 2014; Zhang et al. 2017). The much needed nitrogen and carbon source required for tumor cell growth is provided by glutamate. It also facilitates the development of malignant tumors by synthesizing the amino acids and nucleotides (Ko dama et al. 2020). It becomes apparent that L-glutamine can be utilized to produce glutathione, an essential antioxidant that is known to have a role in modulating drug resistance and preventing cancer cells from undergoing apoptosis (Friesen et al. 2004; Matés et al. 2019).

Fatty acid metabolism: Tumor cells are required to produce high level of fatty acids for its rapid proliferation and growth. Pyruvic acid is used during synthesis, which in turn slows down lactic acid synthesis and prevents an excessive build-up of the acid. Tumor cells get their energy from the breakdown of fatty acids, and the free fatty acids in metabolic products function as signal molecules that trigger several signaling pathways (Cheng et al. 2018; Domblides et al. 2018). Previous research indicates a link between β-oxidation and tumor development. Tumors have increased the expression of enzymes such as FASN, ACC, and ACLY which are involved in the fatty acid metabolism (Menendez & Lupu 2007; Pike et al. 2011). It was also shown that lipid metabolism influences T cell longevity, tumor suppression, and the effectiveness of immunotherapy (Xiao et al. 2022).

HYPOXIA AND HYPOXIA-INDUCIBLE FACTORS

The primary cause of the hypoxic response is thought to be HIFs. Changes that support the growth of cancer can be induced by HIF-dependent signaling, which may allow cancer and stromal cells to adapt and select to their environment. HIF-1, HIF-2, and HIF-3 are transcription factors that belong to the HIF family. HIF consists of an oxygen-sensitive α subunit (HIF-1α, HIF-2α, and HIF-3α) and a constitutive β subunit (Vito et al. 2020). Among the HIF-α subunits, HIF-1α and HIF-2α proteins have been investigated the most. The majority of human tissues express HIF-1α (Wiener et al. 1996), whereas less developed tissues and stages, including the developing vascular endothelium or the fetal lung, express HIF-2α and HIF-3α (Flamme et al. 1997; Tian et al. 1997). HIF-1α serves as vital during multiple stages of hypoxia induction (Semenza 2014). Factor inhibiting HIF (FIH) and prolyl-hydroxylases (PHDs) hydroxylate HIF-α proteins in normoxic conditions. In hypoxic conditions when prolyl-hydroxylase (PHD-RRB) activity is inhibited. This prevents HIF-αs from von Hippel-Lindau (VHL) dependent protein degradation. Mitogen-activated protein kinases (MAPKs) phosphorylate HIF-αs, and then the phosphorylated HIF-αs move to the nucleus. HIF-1α and HIF-1β link together in the cell nucleus to produce heterodimers. These heterodimers link with p300/CBP and the hypoxia response element (HRE) and activate HIF target gene to promote HIF expression. Apart from this, in hypoxic conditions, the absence of oxygen molecules hinders the hydroxylation of inhibitor κB kinase (IKK) and encourages the phosphorylation, ubiquitination, and degradation of inhibitor of NFκB (IκB) (Figure 1.1). Thus, NFκB is released and translocates to the nucleus, regulating target gene transcription (D'Ignazio & Rocha 2016). By this they regulate a number of tumor cell biological processes, such as metabolic reprogramming, immunoregulation, angiogenesis, tumor cell invasion, and drug resistance (Qiu et al. 2017; Bosco et al. 2020).

Among them, HIF may suppress the immune response by encouraging immunological checkpoint activation, triggering cytotoxic T cell death, and obstructing phagocytosis, which encourages the growth and development of tumor cells. According to studies, the upregulated immune checkpoint PD-L1 in tumor cells exhibits HIF-1α dependency, encourages cytotoxic T cell destruction, and aids in the immunological evasion of tumor cells (Barsoum et al. 2014; Shen et al. 2022). Similar to this, HIF-1α also affects the expression of CD47 protein on the surface of tumor cells, which inhibits phagocytosis of tumor cells by phosphorylating signal regulatory proteins on the

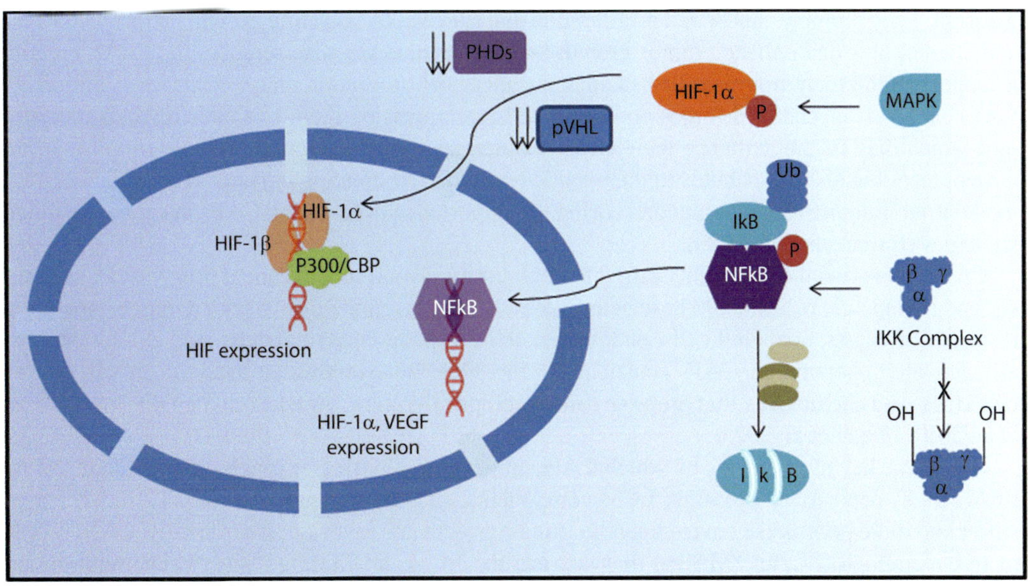

FIGURE 1.1 Schematic diagram illustrating the regulation of hypoxia-inducible factors in hypoxic condition.

surface of macrophages α (SIRP α) (Logtenberg et al. 2020). Recent studies on the CD47 protein have demonstrated that CD47 protein expression also suppresses the activity of NK cells and cytotoxic T cells. Thus, it is anticipated that a number of clinical trials focusing on the CD47 protein will provide anticipated breakthrough in the area of tumor therapy (Samanta et al. 2018; Jia et al. 2021). Furthermore, HIF-1α affects the upregulation of vascular endothelial growth factor (VEGF), which may facilitate immune evasion and metastasis by promoting tumor angiogenesis. HIF-1 not only inhibits the immunological effects in TME but also activates or inhibits the genes of important proteins in the glycolysis pathway to control tumor cell metabolism in a hypoxic environment. Proteins or genes that encode glucose transporters (GLUT1 and GLUT3), hexokinases (HK1 and HK2), lactate dehydrogenase A (LDHA), etc. control the glycolysis pathway and are regulated by HIF-1 (Scarini et al. 2020; Wu et al. 2020; Zhang et al. 2021). Simultaneously, HIF-1 also negatively regulates genes and proteins linked to oxidative phosphorylation. The tumor cells reorganize their glucose metabolism through the differential regulation of proteins or genes related to glycolysis and oxidative phosphorylation by HIF-1. In order to provide a metabolic framework for the development and metastasis of tumor cells, HIF is also engaged in controlling a variety of metabolic pathways, including those involving fatty acids, pentose phosphate, and adenosine (Chen et al. 2022).

The significance of HIF in the development of tumors and its possible mechanism has raised significant concerns among researchers. Future studies in this area should deepen our understanding of hypoxic TME and provide renewed optimism for tumor-targeted therapies (Infantino et al. 2021).

CANCER-ASSOCIATED FIBROBLASTS

CAFs are a diverse group of activated fibroblasts that play a crucial role in the TME. They are considered a major component of the tumor stroma and have significant implications for cancer progression and therapy (Glabman et al. 2022). CAFs are derived from various cell types, including normal fibroblasts, epithelial cells, endothelial cells, cancer stem cells, adipocytes, and pericytes. This diverse origin contributes to their functional heterogeneity, enabling them to perform several pro-tumorigenic roles (Yang et al. 2023), such as ECM remodeling, immunosuppression, and drug resistance.

CAFs interact dynamically with cancer cells, significantly influencing tumor behavior and progression. They promote cancer cell proliferation and survival by secreting growth factors, cytokines, and chemokines that enhance tumor growth and invasion. CAFs also remodel the ECM, creating a supportive microenvironment that facilitates cancer cell migration and metastasis. Additionally, CAFs can exert mechanical forces on cancer cells, compressing them and altering their morphology, which may further enhance their invasive potential. This interaction not only supports tumor development but also contributes to therapeutic resistance by creating barriers to drug delivery and modulating immune responses, underscoring the importance of targeting CAFs in cancer treatment strategies (Barbazan et al. 2023).

CAFs are a crucial component of the TME, playing a pivotal role in cancer progression, metastasis, and therapeutic resistance. These heterogeneous cells originate from various sources, including resident fibroblasts, epithelial cells, endothelial cells, and mesenchymal cells, and exhibit perpetually activated phenotypes. CAFs contribute to the TME by secreting an array of growth factors, cytokines, and chemokines that promote cancer cell proliferation, invasion, and angiogenesis (Xing et al. 2010; Zhang et al. 2023).

One of the key mechanisms by which CAFs influence the TME is through the remodeling of the ECM. CAFs deposit and crosslink ECM components, such as collagen and fibronectin, creating a stiffer and more permissive environment for tumor growth and invasion. Additionally, CAFs secrete matrix metalloproteinases (MMPs) that degrade the ECM, facilitating cancer cell migration and metastasis (Sarkar et al. 2023; Wright et al. 2023). CAFs also play a crucial role in modulating the immune response within the TME. They secrete immunosuppressive cytokines and chemokines that attract and activate immunosuppressive cells, such as regulatory T cells (Tregs) and myeloid-derived suppressor cells (MDSCs). These cells, in turn, inhibit the cytotoxic activity of effector immune cells, such as NK cells and cytotoxic T lymphocytes (CTLs), thereby promoting tumor immune evasion (Zhang et al. 2023).

IMMUNE CELLS

The TME is a complex ecosystem composed of various cell types, including immune cells that interact with and influence tumor progression. Immune cells play a critical role in shaping the TME and determining cancer outcomes (Galli et al. 2020).

T lymphocytes are the most potent mediators of the adaptive anti-tumor immune response. Cytotoxic CD8+ T cells, supported by CD4+ T helper (Th1) cells, generate the final effector mechanism leading to tumor elimination and are associated with a good prognosis. However, the TME often contains an immunosuppressive class of CD4+ T cells known as regulatory T cells (Tregs), which suppress the anti-tumor response (Chew et al. 2012).

Innate immune cells in the TME include macrophages, neutrophils, NK cells, and dendritic cells. Tumor-associated macrophages (TAMs) and MDSCs can promote tumor progression through various suppressive mechanisms. In contrast, NK cells and dendritic cells play an anti-tumor role by secreting cytokines and chemokines (Lu et al. 2023).Tumor-infiltrating dendritic cells can be inhibited by the TME, impairing their ability to mature and present antigens to T cells. Similarly, tumor-infiltrating dendritic cells expressing programmed death receptor-1 (PD-1) mediate immune suppression in the TME. Neutrophils have a dual role in the TME, exhibiting both pro-tumor and anti-tumor functions depending on their phenotype and the cytokines they produce. Increased neutrophil infiltration is associated with poor prognosis in many cancers.

BLOOD VESSEL

The relationship between blood vessels and the TME is critical in understanding cancer progression, treatment efficacy, and metastasis (Hosonuma & Yoshimura 2023). Tumor angiogenesis, the formation of new blood vessels from pre-existing ones, is a hallmark of cancer and is driven by the tumor's need for oxygen and nutrients (Li et al. 2018). However, the blood vessels formed in tumors are often structurally and functionally abnormal compared to normal vasculature. They tend to be disorganized, leaky, and exhibit irregular blood flow, which can lead to areas of hypoxia (low oxygen) and acidosis within the TME (Jiang et al. 2020). This aberrant structure results from a complex interplay of pro-angiogenic factors, such as VEGF, and the tumor's unique biochemical milieu, which includes inflammatory cytokines and ECM components (Ferrara 2004).

The leaky nature of tumor blood vessels not only facilitates the delivery of nutrients but also impacts the efficacy of therapeutic agents. While some drugs can penetrate these leaky vessels, the chaotic blood flow and high interstitial fluid pressure within tumors often hinder effective drug delivery, leading to suboptimal treatment outcomes. Moreover, the compromised integrity of the tumor vasculature can promote metastasis by allowing cancer cells to escape into the bloodstream more easily (Fukumura & Jain 2007; Kobayashi et al. 2014). Circulating tumor cells (CTCs) can lodge in the microvessels of distant organs, further complicating treatment and contributing to the spread of cancer (Tinganelli & Durante 2020).

Additionally, the TME influences the behavior of endothelial cells (Sobierajska et al. 2020), which line the blood vessels. In tumors, these cells often exhibit altered gene expression and reduced adhesion to pericytes, the cells that support and stabilize blood vessels. This instability can lead to increased vessel permeability and fragility, creating a hostile environment that promotes tumor progression and resistance to therapies (Hida et al. 2011; Wragg et al. 2014).

EXTRACELLULAR MATRIX

The TME is composed not only of malignant cells but also of various non-malignant components, including the ECM, which provides structural and biochemical support. Over the years, research has increasingly recognized the ECM's importance in solid tumors, shifting focus from solely tumor cells to the complex interactions within the TME. The ECM is not merely a passive scaffold; it actively regulates intratumoral signaling, cellular behavior, and the overall TME, thereby affecting tumor growth and its response to treatments such as chemotherapy, radiotherapy, and immunotherapy (Henke et al. 2020).

Tumor cells interact with the ECM through integrins and other receptors, which mediate adhesion and signaling. These interactions are crucial for tumor cell survival, migration, and invasion, as they allow cancer cells to exploit the ECM for their advantage (Walker et al. 2018; He et al. 2022). Additionally, the ECM can modulate the immune response within the TME, either facilitating or inhibiting immune cell infiltration and activity, thereby influencing tumor progression and response to therapy (Closset et al. 2023).

LYMPHATIC VESSEL

Lymphatic vessels play a crucial role in the TME, contributing to tumor progression and immunomodulation. Tumor-associated lymphangiogenesis, the expansion of lymphatic vessels in the TME induced by tumor-secreted factors like VEGF-C, facilitates the entry of tumor cells into lymphatic vessels and their subsequent metastasis to lymph nodes. Inhibiting lymphangiogenesis can decrease tumor spread to lymph nodes in animal models (Kataru et al. 2019; He et al. 2021).

Lymphatic vessels also act as immunoregulators in the TME. Tumor-associated lymphatic endothelial cells (LECs) exhibit altered gene expression profiles compared to normal LECs and can upregulate immunosuppressive molecules like PD-L1 to inhibit anti-tumor T cell responses. However, the impact of lymphatic vessels on tumor progression appears to be organ- and context-specific. Depending on the stage of tumor progression and immunological setting, lymphatic vessels can have both positive and negative effects on tumor immunity (Rezzola et al. 2022).

INTERACTION BETWEEN LYMPHATIC VESSELS AND IMMUNE CELLS

Lymphatic vessels connect the primary tumor to lymph nodes, facilitating tumor entry into lymph nodes, systemic circulation, and metastasis. Lymph node metastases provide sites of tumor cell spread, whereas tumor antigen transfer into and presentation in tumor-draining lymph nodes induce activation of tumor-specific T-lymphocyte responses (Vaahtomeri & Alitalo 2020).

Lymphatic vessels have been described as active players in the creation and maintenance of the immunosuppressive TME. Local ablation of lymphatic vessels around tumors resulted in increased peritumoral edema, enhanced inflammatory cell accumulation, increased tumor PD-L1 expression, and decreased accumulation of cytotoxic T cells in the TME. However, enhanced lymphatic drainage of antigens to lymph nodes can also promote CD8+ T cell priming and intratumoral accumulation, leading to rapid cancer clearance (Rezzola et al. 2022).

Hypoxia and HIF have an impact on all non-tumorous cells in the TME. Hypoxia frequently causes their dysregulation, which promotes the growth of cancer: fibroblasts may transform into tumor-prone CAFs, ECM remodeling favors metastases, the vascularization process speeds up the growth of cancer, and anti-tumor immune function generally declines. However, the hypoxic response may also be harmful in terms of tumor development (Petrova et al. 2018). The effect of hypoxia on the components of TME is shown in Table 1.1.

TABLE 1.1
Effect of Hypoxia on the Components of Tumor Microenvironment (TME)

TME Components	Effect of Hypoxic Environment	Tumor Suppression/ Promotion
Cancer-associated fibroblasts (CAFs)	Secretion of cytokines, promoting tumor growth	Promotion
	Deactivation by chronic hypoxia	Suppression
CAF progenitors	Recruitment, activation, and transformation into CAFs	Promotion
Extracellular matrix (ECM)	Increase of ECM deposition (fibrosis) and remodeling	Promotion
	Increase of interaction with cancer cells	Promotion
Blood vessels	Increase in vascularization by HIF-1	Promotion
	Decrease in vascularization by HIF-2	Suppression
Lymphatic vessels	Increase in lymphangiogenesis by HIF-1	Promotion
Macrophage	Recruitment from blood flow	Promotion
	Increase in migratory capacity	Promotion
	M2 polarization	Promotion
Myeloid-derived suppressor cells (MDSCs)	Enhancement of immune-suppressive function	Promotion
	Polarization to M1 type, driven by SIRT1	Suppression
Non-specific CD4+ cells	Differentiation into regulatory T cells and T helpers	Promotion
Regulatory T-cells	Recruitment from blood flow	Promotion
	Enhancement of immune-suppressive function	Promotion
Effector T-cells	Immune checkpoints activation	Promotion
	Repression due to "metabolic competition" for nutrients	Promotion
CD8+ T-cells	Support in proliferation, differentiation, and activation	Suppression

Source: Petrova et al. (2018).

EFFECT OF HYPOXIA ON TUMOR OXIDATIVE STRESS

The primary byproduct of oxidative stress, reactive oxygen species (ROS) have been associated with initiation, progression, and recurrence of tumors. The mitochondria are the source of ROS in tumor cells (Weinberg et al. 2019). The ability of tumor cells to use oxygen is reduced when exposed to hypoxia. As a result, there are more ROS in cells due to a decrease in electron transport efficiency through the mitochondrial complexes in the electron transport chain (ETC) (Guzy et al. 2005; Zhu & Zuo 2013). Interestingly, differing ROS concentrations have distinct effects on the growth of tumor cells. Excessive levels of ROS cause oxidative stress, resulting in proteins and nucleic acids to break down and cause tumor cells to die (Bridge et al. 2014). Low ROS concentrations may facilitate tumor cell growth and metastasis (Liao et al. 2019). Additionally, the level of P-gp in drug resistance may be associated with the concentration of ROS, which impacts the sensitivity and resistance of tumor cells to chemotherapeutic medicines (Galadari et al. 2017).

EFFECT OF HYPOXIA ON DRUG RESISTANCE

Chemotherapy has been the most often used method for cancer treatment. The disruptions in the microenvironment and anoxic metabolic conditions significantly reduce the effectiveness of medications like Bleomycin. This may be the result of the oxygen-dependent chemotherapy medications becoming more active in the presence of oxygen, whereas hypoxia directly reduces the anti-tumor action of oxygen-dependent chemotherapy medications (Minassian et al. 2019). Furthermore, hypoxia impairs the effectiveness of the medications in an indirect manner by disrupting the cell cycle, encouraging DNA repair, and decreasing the potential of p53-mediated apoptosis (Chouaib et al. 2017; Phung et al. 2020). Interestingly, immunotherapy has advanced quickly during the last ten years and yielded noteworthy clinical outcomes. Nonetheless, recent research indicates that hypoxia stimulation severely reduces the efficacy of immunotherapy (Chouaib et al. 2014; Hasmim et al. 2015). Approximately one-third of individuals who responded to immunotherapy developed resistance once more (Hegde & Chen 2020). Tumor cells undergo metabolic alterations driven on by hypoxia, such as low pH, increased ROS, anomalous blood vessel, and proliferating fibrous tissue. These modifications promote the survival of tumor cells, offer benefits against apoptosis, obstruct drug absorption, and encourage the emergence of drug resistance and malignancy (Jain 2014). Additionally, the diffusion of circulating medications may be limited due to the poor vascularization of hypoxic region. Moreover, in hypoxic conditions, HIF-1α promotes the expression of genes involved in multidrug resistance (MDR). The expression of MDR gene products, specifically the drug efflux pump protein ABC transporters, causes cancer cells to discharge intracellular chemotherapeutic medicines, which in turn diminishes the therapeutic effects and increases the drug resistance (Tredan et al. 2007).

The three primary strategies for addressing the problem of drug resistance are early diagnosis, combined ion multidrug therapy and adaptive therapy (Sharma et al. 2022). Effective evaluation molecules may be a useful resource for tracking the early detection and development of malignant tumors. The quantitative monitoring of circulating tumor DNA (ctDNA) would play a significant role in dynamic cancer monitoring and early diagnosis, improving overall survival and directing personalized treatment (Baylin & Jones 2016). By utilizing the findings of computed tomography and positron emission tomography (PET-CT) imaging, the curative effect can be examined. This will help modify the medication regimen to prevent the development of drug resistance and improve the curative outcome (Ansell & Armitage 2012). Additionally, the antibody drug conjugate (ADC) could improve the therapeutic effect by enhancing the local drug concentration (Baah et al. 2021). Currently, multidrug combination therapy remains an effective strategy to address drug resistance. It was found that the combined use of vibostolimab (anti TIGIT humanized IgG1 monoclonal antibody) and pembrolizumab can significantly inhibit the drug resistance and provide the benefits in non-small cell lung cancer (NSCLC) (Attili et al. 2022).

CONCLUSION

Hypoxia is a key feature of solid tumors and is widely engaged in all phases of cancer development. It is widely understood that hypoxia promotes metabolic reprogramming, preventing the tumor cells from going through apoptosis. A deeper comprehension of the hypoxia signaling cascade may lead to novel approaches to target HIFs. This approach may provide greater benefits in the management of hypoxic microenvironment and overcome drug resistance.

REFERENCES

Ansell SM, Armitage JO. Positron emission tomographic scans in lymphoma: Convention and controversy. Mayo Clin Proc (2012) 87(6):571–80. doi: 10.1016/j.mayocp.2012.03.006

Attili I, Passaro A, de Marinis F. Anti-tigit to overcome resistance to immune checkpoint inhibitors in lung cancer: Limits and potentials. Ann Oncol (2022) 33(2):119–22. doi: 10.1016/j.annonc.2021.11.008

Baah S, Laws M, Rahman KM. Antibody-drug conjugates—A tutorial review. Molecules (2021) 26(10):2943. doi: 10.3390/molecules26102943

Balkwill FR, Capasso M, Hagemann T. The tumor microenvironment at a glance. J Cell Sci (2012) 125:5591–96.

Barbazan J, Pérez-González C, Gómez-González M, Dedenon M, Richon S, Latorre E, Serra M, Mariani P, Descroix S, Sens P, Trepat X, Vignjevic DM. Cancer-associated fibroblasts actively compress cancer cells and modulate mechanotransduction. Nat Commun (2023) 14(1):6966. doi: 10.1038/s41467-023-42382-4

Barsoum IB, Smallwood CA, Siemens DR, Graham CH. A mechanism of hypoxia-mediated escape from adaptive immunity in cancer cells. Cancer Res (2014) 74(3):665–74. doi: 10.1158/0008-5472.CAN-13-0992

Baylin SB, Jones PA. Epigenetic determinants of cancer. Cold Spring Harb Perspect Biol (2016) 8(9):a019505. doi: 10.1101/cshperspect.a019505

Bosco MC, D'Orazi G, Del Bufalo D. Targeting hypoxia in tumor: A new promising therapeutic strategy. J Exp Clin Cancer Res (2020) 39(1):8. doi: 10.1186/s13046-019-1517-0

Bridge G, Rashid S, Martin SA. DNA Mismatch repair and oxidative DNA damage: Implications for cancer biology and treatment. Cancers (2014) 6(3):1597–614. doi: 10.3390/cancers6031597

Castells M, Thibault B, Delord J-P, Couderc B. Implication of tumor microenvironment in chemoresistance: Tumor-associated stromal cells protect tumor cells from cell death. Int J Mol Sci (2012) 13(8):9545–71. doi: 10.3390/ijms13089545

Chen G, Wu K, Li H, Xia D, He T. Role of hypoxia in the tumor microenvironment and targeted therapy. Front Oncol (2022) 12:961637.

Cheng C, Geng F, Cheng X, Guo D. Lipid metabolism reprogramming and its potential targets in cancer. Cancer Commun (Lond) (2018) 38(1):27. doi: 10.1186/s40880-018-0301-4

Chew V, Toh HC, Abastado JP. Immune microenvironment in tumor progression: Characteristics and challenges for therapy. J Oncol (2012) 2012:608406. doi: 10.1155/2012/608406

Chiche J, Brahimi-Horn MC, Pouyss´egur J. Tumour hypoxia induces a metabolic shift causing acidosis: A common feature in cancer. J Cell Mol Med (2010) 14(4):771–94. doi: 10.1111/j.1582-4934.2009.00994.x

Chouaib S, Janji B, Tittarelli A, Eggermont A, Thiery JP. Tumor plasticity interferes with anti-tumor immunity. Crit Rev Immunol (2014) 34(2):91–102.

Chouaib S, Noman MZ, Kosmatopoulos K, Curran MA. Hypoxic stress: Obstacles and opportunities for innovative immunotherapy of cancer. Oncogene (2017) 36(4):439–45. doi: 10.1038/onc.2016.225

Closset L, Gultekin O, Salehi S, Sarhan D, Lehti K, Gonzalez-Molina J. The extracellular matrix - immune microenvironment crosstalk in cancer therapy: Challenges and opportunities. Matrix Biol (2023) 121:217–28. doi: 10.1016/j.matbio.2023.07.003

D'Ignazio L, Rocha S. Hypoxia induced NF-kappaB. Cells (2016) 5(1):e10.

Domblides C, Lartigue L, Faustin B. Metabolic stress in the immune function of T cells, macrophages and dendritic cells. Cells (2018) 7(7):68. doi: 10.3390/cells7070068

Emami Nejad A, Najafgholian S, Rostami A, Sistani A, Shojaeifar S, Esparvarinha M, Nedaeinia R, Haghjooy Javanmard S, Taherian M, Ahmadlou M, Salehi R. The role of hypoxia in the tumor microenvironment and development of cancer stem cell: A novel approach to developing treatment. Cancer Cell Int (2021) 21:1–26.

Ferrara N. Vascular endothelial growth factor: Basic science and clinical progress. Endocr Rev (2004) 25(4):581–611. doi: 10.1210/er.2003-0027

Flamme I, Frolich T, Risau W. Molecular mechanisms of vasculogenesis and embryonic angiogenesis. J Cell Physiol (1997) 173(2):206–10.

Friesen C, Kiess Y, Debatin KM. A critical role of glutathione in determining apoptosis sensitivity and resistance in leukemia cells. Cell Death Differ (2004) 11(Suppl 1):S73–85.

Fukumura D, Jain RK (2007). Tumor microvasculature and microenvironment: Targets for anti-angiogenesis and normalization. Microvasc Res 74(2–3):72–84. doi: 10.1016/j.mvr.2007.05.003

Galadari S, Rahman A, Pallichankandy S, Thayyullathil F. Reactive oxygen species and cancer paradox: To promote or to suppress? Free Radic Biol Med (2017) 104:144–64. doi: 10.1016/j.freeradbiomed.2017.01.004

Galli F, Aguilera JV, Palermo B, Markovic SN, Nisticò P, Signore A. Relevance of immune cell and tumor microenvironment imaging in the new era of immunotherapy. J Exp Clin Cancer Res (2020) 39(1):89. doi: 10.1186/s13046-020-01586-y

Glabman RA, Choyke PL, Sato N. Cancer-associated fibroblasts: Tumorigenicity and targeting for cancer therapy. Cancers (2022) 14(16):3906. doi: 10.3390/cancers14163906

Guzy RD, Hoyos B, Robin E, Chen H, Liu L, Mansfield KD, et al. Mitochondrial complex III is required for hypoxia-induced ROS production and cellular oxygen sensing. Cell Metab (2005) 1(6):401–8.

Hasmim M, Messai Y, Ziani L, Thiery J, Bouhris J-H, Noman MZ et al. Critical role of tumor microenvironment in shaping NK cell functions: Implication of hypoxic stress. Front Immunol (2015) 6:482. doi: 10.3389/fimmu.2015.00482

He M, He Q, Cai X, Chen Z, Lao S, Deng H, Liu X, Zheng Y, Liu X, Liu J, Xie Z, Yao M, Liang W, He J. Role of lymphatic endothelial cells in the tumor microenvironment—A narrative review of recent advances. Transl Lung Cancer Res (2021) 10(5):2252–77. doi: 10.21037/tlcr-21-40

He X, Lee B, Jiang Y. Extracellular matrix in cancer progression and therapy. Med Rev (2021) (2022) 2(2): 125–39. doi: 10.1515/mr-2021-0028

Hegde PS, Chen DS. Top 10 challenges in cancer immunotherapy. Immunity (2020) 52(1):17–35. doi: 10.1016/j.immuni.2019.12.011

Henke E, Nandigama R, Ergün S. Extracellular matrix in the tumor microenvironment and its impact on cancer therapy. Front Mol Biosci (2020) 6:160. doi: 10.3389/fmolb.2019.00160

Hida K, Kawamoto T, Ohga N, Akiyama K, Hida Y, Shindoh M. Altered angiogenesis in the tumor microenvironment. Pathol Int (2011) 61(11):630–37. doi: 10.1111/j.1440-1827.2011.02726.x

Hosonuma M, Yoshimura K. Association between pH regulation of the tumor microenvironment and immunological state. Front Oncol (2023) 13:1175563. doi: 10.3389/fonc.2023.1175563

Infantino V, Santarsiero A, Convertini P, Todisco S, Iacobazzi V. Cancer cell metabolism in hypoxia: Role of HIF-1 as key regulator and therapeutic target. Int J Mol Sci (2021) 22(11):5703. doi: 10.3390/ijms22115703

Jain RK. Antiangiogenesis strategies revisited: From starving tumors to all e viatinghypoxia. Cancer Cell (2014) 26(5):605–22. doi: 10.1016/j.ccell.2014.10.006

Jia X, Yan B, Tian X, Liu Q, Jin J, Shi J et al. Cd47/Sirpa pathway mediates cancer immune escape and immunotherapy. Int J Biol Sci (2021) 17(13):3281––87. doi: 10.7150/ijbs.60782

Jiang X, Wang J, Deng X, Xiong F, Zhang S, Gong Z, Li X, Cao K, Deng H, He Y, Liao Q, Xiang B, Zhou M, Guo C, Zeng Z, Li G, Li X, Xiong W. The role of microenvironment in tumor angiogenesis. J Exp Clin Cancer Res (2020) 39(1):204. doi: 10.1186/s13046-020-01709-5

Kataru RP, Ly CL, Shin J, Park HJ, Baik JE, Rehal S, Ortega S, Lyden D, Mehrara BJ. Tumor lymphatic function regulates tumor inflammatory and immunosuppressive microenvironments. Cancer Immun Res (2019) 7(8):1345–58. doi: 10.1158/2326-6066.CIR-18-0337

Khalaf K, Hana D, Chou JT-T, Singh C, Mackiewicz A, Kaczmarek M. Aspects of the tumor microenvironment involved in immune resistance and drug resistance. Front Immunol (2021) 12:656364. doi: 10.3389/fimmu.2021.656364

Kobayashi H, Turkbey B, Watanabe R, Choyke PL. Cancer drug delivery: Considerations in the rational design of nanosized bioconjugates. Bioconjugate Chem (2014) 25(12):2093–2100. doi: 10.1021/bc500481x

Kobliakov AV. Hypoxia and glycolysis as factors determining the malignant phenotype. Tsitologiia (2018) 58(7):499–506.

Ko dama M, Oshikawa K, Shimizu H, Yoshioka S, Takahashi M, Izumi Y et al. A shift in glutamine nitrogen metabolism contributes to the malignant progression of cancer. Nat Commun (2020) 11(1):1320. doi: 10.1038/s41467-020-15136-9

Li T, Kang G, Wang T, Huang H. Tumor angiogenesis and anti-angiogenic gene therapy for cancer. Oncol Lett (2018) 16(1):687–702. doi: 10.3892/ol.2018.8733

Liao Z, Chua D, Tan NS. Reactive oxygen species: A volatile driver of field cancerization and metastasis. Mol Cancer (2019) 18(1):65. doi: 10.1186/s12943-019-0961-y

Logtenberg MEW, Scheeren FA, Schumacher TN. The Cd47-sirpa immune checkpoint. Immunity (2020) 52(5):742–52. doi: 10.1016/j.immuni.2020.04.011

Lu C, Liu Y, Ali NM, Zhang B, Cui X. The role of innate immune cells in the tumor microenvironment and research progress in anti-tumor therapy. Front Immun (2023) 13:1039260. doi: 10.3389/fimmu.2022.1039260

Matés JM, Campos-Sandoval JA, Santos-Jiménez JL, Márquez J. Dysregulation of glutaminase and glutamine synthetase in cancer. Cancer Lett (2019) 467:29–39. doi: 10.1016/j.canlet.2019.09.011

Menendez JA, Lupu R. Fatty acid synthase and the lipogenic phenotype in cancer pathogenesis. Nat Rev Cancer (2007) 7(10):763–77.

Minassian LM, Cotechini T, Huitema E, Graham CH. Hypoxia-induced resistance to chemotherapy in cancer. Adv Exp Med Biol (2019) 1136:123–39.

Petrova V, Annicchiarico-Petruzzelli M, Melino G, Amelio I. The hypoxic tumour microenvironment. Oncogenesis (2018) 7(1):10.

Phung CD, Tran TH, Pham LM, Nguyen HT, Jeong J-H, Yong CS, et al. Current developments in nanotechnology for improved cancer treatment, focusing on tumor hypoxia. J Control Release (2020) 324:413–29. doi: 10.1016/j.jconrel.2020.05.029

Pike LS, Smift AL, Croteau NJ, Ferrick DA, Wu M. Inhibition of fatty acid oxidation by etomoxir impairs NADPH production and increases reactive oxygen species resulting in ATP depletion and cell death in human glioblastoma cells. Biochim Biophys Acta (2011) 1807(6):726–34.

Qiu GZ, Jin M-Z, Dai J-X, Sun W, Feng J-H, Jin W-L. Reprogramming of the tumor in the hypoxic niche: The emerging concept and associated therapeutic strategies. Trends Pharmacol Sci (2017) 38(8). doi: 10.1016/j.tips.2017.05.002

Rezzola S, Sigmund EC, Halin C, Ronca R. The lymphatic vasculature: An active and dynamic player in cancer progression. Med Res Rev (2022) 42(1):576–614. doi: 10.1002/med.21855

Rob A, Cairns I, Harris S. Regulation of cancer cell metabolism. Nat Rev Cancer (2012) 11(2):85–95.

Samanta D, Park Y, Ni X, Li H, Zahnow CA, Gabrielson E et al. Chemotherapy induces enrichment of Cd47/Cd73/Pdl1 immune evasive triple-negative breast cancer cells. Proc Natl Acad Sci USA (2018) 115(6):E1239–E48. doi: 10.1073/pnas.1718197115

Sanmamed MF, Chen L. A paradigm shift in cancer immunotherapy: From enhancement to normalization. Cell (2018) 175(2):313–26. doi: 10.1016/j.cell.2018.09.035

Sarkar M, Nguyen T, Gundre E, Ogunlusi O, El-Sobky M, Giri B, Sarkar TR. Cancer-associated fibroblasts: The chief architect in the tumor microenvironment. Front Cell Dev Biol (2023) 11:1089068. doi: 10.3389/fcell.2023.1089068

Scarini J, Rosa L, Souza R, Egal E, Tincani A, Martins A, et al. Gene and immunohistochemical expression of HIF-1a, GLUT-1, FASN, and adipophilin in carcinoma ex pleomorphic adenoma development. Oral Dis (2020) 26(6):1190–1199. doi: 10.1111/odi.13332

Schiliro C, Firestein BL. Mechanisms of metabolic reprogramming in cancer cells supporting enhanced growth and proliferation. Cells (2021) 10(5):1056.

Seebacher NA, Krchniakova M, Stacy AE, Skoda J, Jansson PJ. Tumour microenvironment stress promotes the development of drug resistance. Antioxidants (2021) 10(11):1801. doi: 10.3390/antiox10111801

Semenza GL. Targeting HIF-1 for cancer therapy. Nat Rev Cancer (2003) 3(10):721–32. doi:10.1038/nrc1187

Semenza GL. Oxygen sensing, hypoxia-inducible factors, and disease pathophysiology. Annu Rev Pathol (2014) 9:47–71.

Sharma M, Bakshi AK, Mittapelly N, Gautam S, Marwaha D, Rai N, et al. Recent updates on innovative approaches to overcome drug resistance for better outcomes in cancer. J Control Release (2022) 346: 43–70. doi: 10.1016/j.jconrel.2022.04.007

Shen DD, Bi Y-P, Pang J-R, Zhao L-J, Zhao L-F, Gao Y, et al. Generation, secretion and degradation of cancer immunotherapy target pd-L1. Cell Mol Life Sci CMLS (2022) 79(8):413. doi: 10.1007/s00018-022-04431-x

Sobierajska K, Ciszewski WM, Sacewicz-Hofman I, Niewiarowska J. Endothelial cells in the tumor microenvironment. Adv Exp Med Biol (2020) 1234:71–86. doi: 10.1007/978-3-030-37184-5_6

Tian H, McKnight SL, Russell DW. Endothelial PAS domain protein 1 (EPAS1), a transcription factor selectively expressed in endothelial cells. Genes Dev (1997) 11(1):72–82.

Tinganelli W, Durante M (2020). Tumor hypoxia and circulating tumor cells. Int J Mol Sci 21(24):9592. doi: 10.3390/ijms21249592

Tredan O, Galmarini CM, Patel K, Tannock IF. Drug resistance and the solid tumor microenvironment. J Natl Cancer Inst (2007) 99(19):1441–54.

Vaahtomeri K, Alitalo K. Lymphatic vessels in tumor dissemination versus immunotherapy. Cancer Res (2020) 80(17):3463–65. doi: 10.1158/0008-5472.CAN-20-0156

Vito A, El-Sayes N, Mossman K. Hypoxia-driven immune escape in the tumor microenvironment. Cells (2020) 9(4):992. doi: 10.3390/cells9040992

Walker C, Mojares E, Del Río Hernández A. Role of extracellular matrix in development and cancer progression. Int J Mol Sci (2018) 19(10):3028. doi: 10.3390/ijms19103028

Ward PS, Thompson CB. Metabolic reprogramming: A cancer hallmark even Warburg did not anticipate. Cancer Cell. 2012; 21(3):297–308. doi: 10.1016/j.ccr.2012.02.014

Weinberg F, Ramnath N, Nagrath D. Reactive oxygen species in the tumor microenvironment: An overview. Cancers (2019) 11(8):1191. doi: 10.3390/cancers11081191

Wiener CM, Booth G, Semenza GL. In vivo expression of mRNAs encoding hypoxia-inducible factor 1. Biochem Biophys Res Commun (1996) 225(2):485–88

Wragg JW, Durant S, McGettrick HM, Sample KM, Egginton S, Bicknell R. Shear stress regulated gene expression and angiogenesis in vascular endothelium. Microcirculation (New York, N.Y.: 1994) (2014) 21(4):290–300. doi: 10.1111/micc.12119

Wright K, Ly T, Kriet M, Czirok A, Thomas SM. Cancer-associated fibroblasts: Master tumor microenvironment modifiers. Cancers (2023) 15(6):1899. doi: 10.3390/cancers15061899

Wu Z, Wu J, Zhao Q, Fu S, Jin J. Emerging roles of aerobic glycolysis in breast cancer. Clin Trans Oncol (2020) 22(5):631–46. doi: 10.1007/s12094-019-02187-8

Xiao L, Ma X, Ye L, Su P, Xiong W, Bi E et al. Il-9/Stat3/Fatty acid oxidation-mediated lipid peroxidation contributes to Tc9 cell longevity and enhanced antitumor activity. J Clin Invest (2022) 132(7):e153247. doi: 10.1172/JCI153247

Xing F, Saidou J, Watabe K (2010). Cancer associated fibroblasts (CAFs) in tumor microenvironment. Front Biosci (Landmark Ed) 15(1):166–79. doi: 10.2741/3613

Yang D, Liu J, Qian H, Zhuang Q. Cancer-associated fibroblasts: From basic science to anticancer therapy. Exp Mol Med (2023) 55(7):1322–32. doi: 10.1038/s12276-023-01013-0

Yuneva M, Zamboni N, Oefner P, Sachidanandam R, Lazebnik Y. Deficiency in glutamine but not glucose induces MYC-dependent apoptosis in human cells. J Cell Biol (2007) 178(1):93–105.

Zhang C, Fei Y, Wang H, Hu S, Liu C, Hu R, Du Q. CAFs orchestrates tumor immune microenvironment-A new target in cancer therapy? Front Pharmacol (2023a) 14:1113378. doi: 10.3389/fphar.2023.1113378

Zhang H, Yue X, Chen Z, Liu C, Wu W, Zhang N, Liu Z, Yang L, Jiang Q, Cheng Q, Luo P, Liu G (2023b). Define cancer-associated fibroblasts (CAFs) in the tumor microenvironment: New opportunities in cancer immunotherapy and advances in clinical trials. Mol Cancer 22(1):159. doi: 10.1186/s12943-023-01860-5

Zhang J, Pavlova NN, Thompson CB. Cancer cell metabolism: The essential role of the nonessential amino acid, glutamine. EMBO J (2017) 36(10):1302–15. doi: 10.15252/embj.201696151

Zhang J, Zhang Y, Mo F, Patel G, Butterworth K, Shao C, et al. The roles of HIF-1a in radiosensitivity and radiation-induced bystander effects under hypoxia. Front Cell Dev Biol (2021) 9:637454. doi: 10.3389/fcell.2021.637454

Zhdanov AV, Waters AHC, Golubeva AV, Dmitriev RI, Papkovsky DB. Availability of the key metabolic substrates dictates the respiratory response of cancer cells to the mitochondrial uncoupling. BiochimBiophys Acta (2014) 1837(1):51–62. doi: 10.1016/j.bbabio.2013.07.008

Zhu X, Zuo L. Characterization of oxygen radical formation mechanism at early cardiac ischemia. Cell Death Dis (2013) 4:e787. doi: 10.1038/cddis.2013.313

2 Role of Hypoxia in Cancer Progression and Its Significance

Avani Kulkarni and Sukhes Mukherjee
Department of Biochemistry, All India Institute of Medical Sciences, Bhopal, Madhya Pradesh, India

INTRODUCTION

Cancer has become a feared disease and has garnered global attention with 20 million new year cases and 9.7 million deaths due to cancer, as per reports in 2022 (1). Cancer is notorious for its ability to arise from practically any part of the body following aberrant genetic mutation and replication and its propensity to invade and destroy the preexisting cellular architecture and to spread to other organ systems in a process called metastasis. The growth of normal cells is strictly governed by cellular growth factors and regulatory signals. The loss of certain regulatory factors or the upregulation of cellular growth factors forms the basis of the pathophysiology of various malignancies and therein lies the understanding of the role of hypoxia in the grand scheme of events. This is also accompanied by various changes in the local microenvironment that facilitate the growth of the tumor, ranging from redirection of blood vessel growth resulting in abnormal angiogenesis to immune modulation wherein the neoplastic cells evade immune surveillance.

Hypoxia is defined as a state of inadequate oxygenation. While the cause can be multifactorial, broadly it can be due to disrupted oxygen delivery or increased demand. Oxygen is essential for the holistic functioning of any body, starting from the process of respiration, right down to the level of aerobic metabolism. This process is regulated by various physiological means and also at the biochemical level. Hypoxia in cancer is of special significance primarily because of the metabolic reprogramming that occurs in the setting of tumors. The growth of the cells that happens in an unregulated format far exceeds the ability of the local vasculature to keep up which results in the development of hypoxia. This also results in the development of abnormal angiogenesis that contributes to the hypoxic environment of the tumor.

Hypoxia is considered one of the hallmarks of neoplasia (2). Hypoxia plays a central role in the progression of cancer and the resistance it develops to various therapeutic modalities. Solid tumors are the most common types of tumors encountered in clinical practice. Many compensatory mechanisms exist at different levels to allow the cells to function in a hypoxic environment. These compensatory mechanisms have profound effects on the way the tumor progresses. Hypoxia works through mediators like hypoxia-inducible factors (HIFs). This leads to the activation of several transcriptional factors that result in several metabolic changes and alterations in the cellular biochemical functioning. Hypoxic zones are frequently observed throughout the tissue in solid tumors as a result of necrosis and disrupted vascular architecture. Compared to normal tissues, these hypoxic conditions exhibit spatial and temporal fluctuations, resulting in transient hypoxia cycling that markedly increases HIF protein activity. The degree of hypoxia is highly correlated with aggressive tumor behavior, treatment resistance, and a poor prognosis for patients. Nonetheless, there is still much to learn about the precise function of hypoxia and HIF proteins in tumor biology.

Hypoxia has important implications in treatment and overall progression and prognosis in a clinical setting, showing consistently that intra-tumoral hypoxia leads to poor disease outcomes in

DOI: 10.1201/9781003477419-2

multiple solid tumors (3). Hypoxia results in the activation of a cascade of cellular signaling pathways, primarily governed by HIF which is also in constant cross-talk with other cellular pathways of metabolism and growth resulting in the development of more resilient neoplastic cells (4).

HYPOXIA IN CANCER-DEVELOPMENT AND PROGRESSION

Tumors need a constant oxygen supply for proliferation, but when they outgrow their blood supply, these neoplastic cells adapt by developing strategies to survive in a hypoxic environment. There are alterations in cellular metabolism that further promote its survival in the hypoxic environment. Additionally, HIF proteins activate genes involved in angiogenesis, the formation of new blood vessels, to compensate for the lack of oxygen. The blood supply of tumors is characterized by abnormal vasculature, including tortuous and leaky vessels. This results in heterogeneous oxygen delivery, leading to hypoxic regions within the tumor. Some studies have found that hypoxia can be used as a therapeutic target. Understanding the complex interactions between the blood supply feeding the tumor and the tumor itself holds the key to making headways in the treatment of cancer.

A good blood supply to the tissue ensures adequate delivery of nutrients and oxygen and also means efficient extraction of waste products from the cellular milieu. However, in the setting of a malignant environment, the vascular endothelial cells are exposed to toxic metabolites and a locally acidified tumor microenvironment that modify the local vasculature to suit its environment leading to a dysregulated vasculature. The setting of a dysregulated, haywire vasculature provides a fertile ground for hypoxia to develop in the local tissue environment (5). Neoplastic cells proliferate at very high rates resulting in the formation of a disorganized tumor with insufficient vasculature that further exacerbates the hypoxia. This results in the expression of angiogenic factors that in turn lead to the development of dysfunctional vasculature, resulting in a vicious cycle (6). Chronic hypoxia develops in the tumor microenvironment as the distance of the cells increases from the source of blood. The diffusion of oxygen decreases. Hypoxia usually begins to develop at a distance greater than 200μM from a functional blood supply as per Folkman's theory (4).

The development of hypoxia in the tumor microenvironment can be summarized to be because of the following reasons:

1. Carcinogenic factors like drugs/carcinogens and microbes.
2. Tumor microenvironment remodeling leading to vascular deformation due to pressure effects.
3. Increased metabolism in the tumor microenvironment due to high cell turnover.
4. Dysfunctional angiogenesis.
5. Folkman's distance effect on the cells.

Broadly speaking, two kinds of hypoxic cells make up the solid tumor microenvironment, namely transient hypoxic cells and chronic hypoxic cells, while some tumors may contain both (2). The transient hypoxic cells are found close to the functional vasculature where the hypoxic microenvironment is short-lived. Among the chronic hypoxic cells, different cell populations make up the tumor population; the first type of cells, if left in the tumor microenvironment, are unable to survive the hypoxic conditions and undergo cell death. These cells are considered the primary source of central necrosis in solid tumors. The second type of chronic hypoxic cells is viable in the hypoxic microenvironment of the solid tumor and develops cellular mechanisms due to genetic alterations that respond to the hypoxic environment. These cells are responsible for the development of cellular drug resistance and radio-resistance (7) (Figure 2.1).

Hypoxia damages the cellular genome and drives carcinogenesis. It was found that the gene mutation frequencies increased by two- to five-fold in in-vivo and in-vitro cancer models exposed to hypoxia (8). By aiding in the reprogramming process, hypoxia signaling preserves stem cell self-renewal. This is of special importance concerning cancer stem cells (CSCs). Cancer stem cells, a subpopulation of cancer cells thought to be responsible for tumor initiation and recurrence, are often found in hypoxic niches. Targeting the blood supply of tumors has become a key strategy in cancer

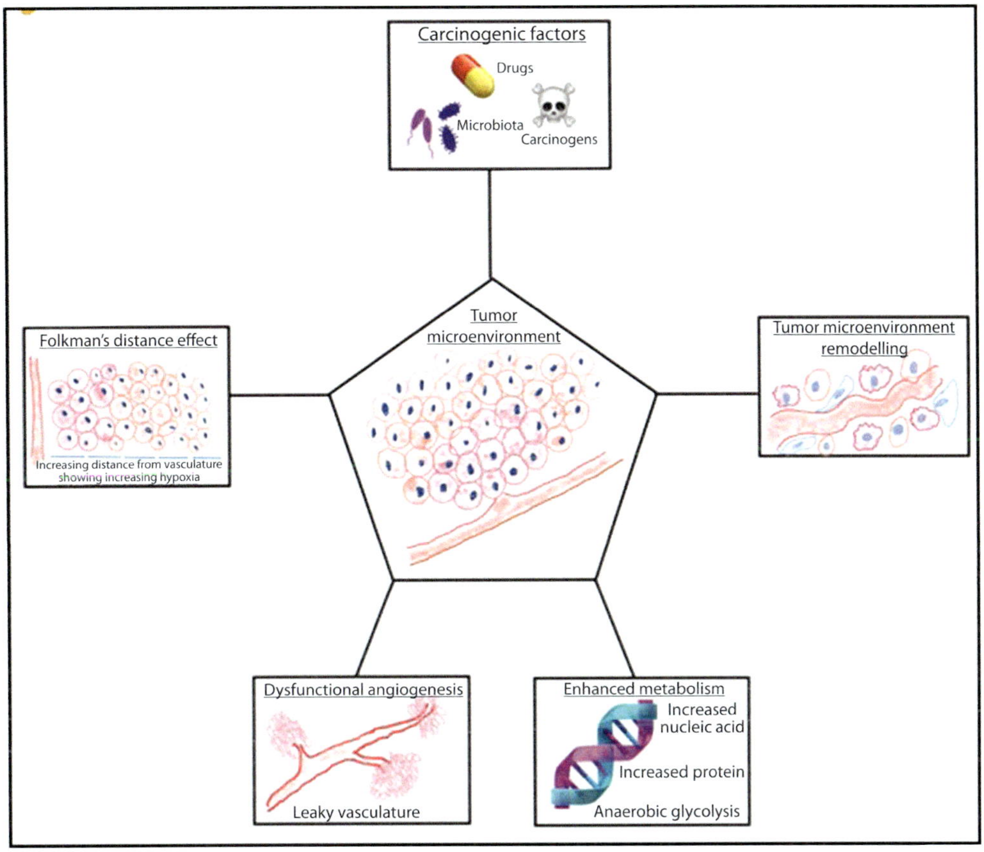

FIGURE 2.1 A summary of how various factors contribute to the development of the tumor microenvironment. There are five main factors: (1) carcinogenic factors, (2) tumor microenvironment remodeling, (3) increased metabolism, (4) dysfunctional angiogenesis, and (5) Folkman's distance effect.

therapy. Anti-angiogenic drugs, such as bevacizumab, aim to normalize tumor vasculature and improve oxygen delivery. However, these therapies can also lead to increased hypoxia, promoting the selection of more aggressive cancer cells. These stem cells have the potential to develop into a tumor at novel sites by metastasis. Under hypoxic conditions, two main things happen (9):

a. Cellular genomic damage
b. Formation of reactive oxygen species

This results in the better survival of CSCs and the formation of more resistant CSCs giving rise to novel cancer cell variants with more aggressive potential to metastasize and grow.

The way hypoxia affects gene repair is of special importance. DNA damage repair checkpoints like ataxia-telangiectasia mutated (ATM) and ATM and RAD3-related (ATR) checkpoints are primarily affected under the direct influence of hypoxia. Hypoxia activates the above checkpoints. Through a complex series of phosphorylation and dephosphorylation of various intermediates leading to inactivation of cell cycle progression pathways, leads to hypoxia-induced apoptosis of the cells. Persistent hypoxia enhances DNA misreplication and DNA strand breaks resulting in the development of mutations (10). The other well-known method of regulating DNA repair is through non-homologous end-joining (NHEJ), homologous recombination (HR), and mismatch repair (MMR). It has been observed that hypoxic conditions directly affect the HR and MMR DNA repair pathways but the NHEJ is relatively spared. This malfunction leads to the development of mutations and dinucleotide repeat instability and this results in cell transformation and contributes to carcinogenesis (11).

So far, we have discussed the effect of hypoxia on the cells and its genome, and how hypoxia develops in the tumor microenvironment setting. As the phrase "survival of the fittest" goes, neoplastic cells in the tumor microenvironment rewire their cellular metabolism and cell cycle progression through the interplay and activation of different transcription factors (3). The most significant effects of hypoxia are mediated through HIFs. HIFs reprogram all aspects of the cell's metabolic activity and this is one of the major reasons why the neoplastic cells can survive the tumor microenvironment. HIFs are heterodimeric proteins with an oxygen-sensitive HIF-1α, HIF-2α, or HIF-3α subunit and a constitutively expressed HIF-1β subunit (also known as ARNT) (12). HIF-1α is expressed in all body tissues and HIF-2α and HIF-3α are expressed only in specific tissues. HIF-1β is expressed in all mammalian cells under normoxic conditions (13). HIF-1α is an oxygen-labile protein and is stabilized in response to hypoxia, iron chelators, and divalent cations (14). Moreover, elevated HIF-1α protein levels can be found in normoxic conditions if the intracellular concentrations of ROS are elevated (15). The hypoxia response elements (HRE) in the promoter region of the target gene respond to the HIF accumulated under hypoxic conditions and reduce cellular oxygen consumption (16). Numerous cell signaling pathways, including PI3K-mTOR, JAK-STAT3, NF-κB, mitogen-activated protein kinase (MAPK), Wnt/β-catenin, Notch, and cancer suppressor gene deletion, including p53, phosphatase, and tensin homolog (PTEN), as well as IDH1-R132H-FAT1-ROS-HIF-1α (17–23), regulate HIFs.

HYPOXIA AND ITS SIGNIFICANCE IN CANCER PROGRESSION

Tumor cells that are susceptible to hypoxia are eliminated by hypoxic environments, and the remaining tumor cells undergo molecular changes to adjust to the reduced oxygen environments. These survivor cells are more resistant to the difficult microenvironment that the tumor presents. HIFs affect the tumor mechanics by affecting four primary functions (Figure 2.2):

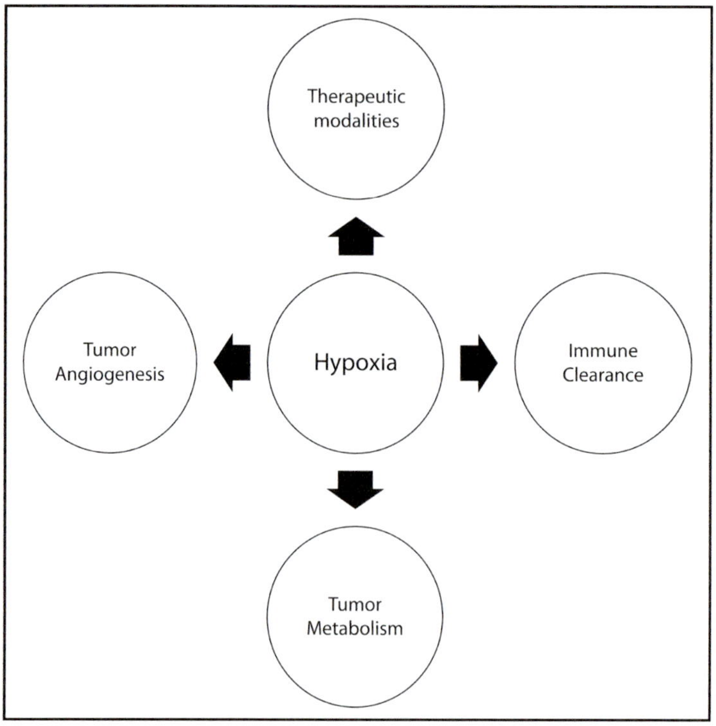

FIGURE 2.2 The effect of hypoxia can be broadly be studied under four headings, namely tumor metabolism, tumor angiogenesis, immune clearance, and therapeutic modalities.

1. Tumor metabolism
2. Tumor angiogenesis
3. Tumor response to immune clearance and other
4. Tumor response to therapeutic modalities (chemotherapy and radiotherapy)

HYPOXIA AND TUMOR METABOLISM WITH RESPECT TO DEVELOPMENT AND PROGRESSION

Glycolysis

The primary source of energy for the cells is adenosine triphosphate (ATP) and owing to the high cell metabolic activity, the neoplastic cells have a very high requirement of this energy currency. The cancer cells increase glucose uptake to keep up with the energy demand and increase their dependence on the glycolytic pathway through the well-known phenomenon "Warburg Phenomenon" (24). HIF-1α is one of the key players in the activation of Warburg metabolism in the tumor, following HIF-1α activation of glycolysis regulators like phosphoglycerate mutase 1 (PGAM1), pyruvate kinase M (PKM), recombinant phosphoglycerate kinase 1 (PGK1), lactate dehydrogenase A (LDHA), lactate dehydrogenase C (LDHC), and lactate dehydrogenase-5 (LDH-5) (25). The other key mechanism of note is the promotion of MYC target gene and further adds to the constitutive expression of LDHA (26). Additionally, pyruvate dehydrogenase (PDH) is rendered inactive by HIF-1α, as it triggers the activation of pyruvate dehydrogenase kinase 1 (PDK1). As a result, pyruvate cannot enter the tricarboxylic acid cycle because PDK1 is unable to convert it into acetyl-CoA. As previously discussed, this results in the accumulation of lactate, which inhibits the generation of hypoxic ROS and increases intracellular adenosine triphosphate (ATP) levels, so sparing these cells from hypoxia-induced death (27).

Lipid Metabolism

Malignant tumors have an advantage over healthy ones due to the altered lipid metabolism, which promotes the production of signaling molecules, energy storage, membrane formation, and fatty acid oxidation (FAO). It contributes significantly to the synthesis of ATP as well. The induction of sterol regulatory element-binding protein (SREBP)-1 is facilitated by HIF-1. This is a major transcriptory regulator of the fatty acid synthase (FASN) gene (28). This promotes de novo lipid synthesis and increases overall cell survival. To avoid hypoxia-induced apoptosis, inhibition of acetyl-CoA carboxylase (ACC1) and adenosine triphosphate citrate lyase (ACLY) raises the level of α-ketoglutarate by lowering the activity and level of ETS translocation variant (ETV4). The spread of cancer is also facilitated by the lipid catabolic metabolism. The primary enzymes involved in lipid catabolism in tumor cells under hypoxic settings are carnitine palmitoyl transferase 1 (CPT1), phospholipase A2 (PLA2), and phospholipase D (PLD).

Protein Metabolism

The α-ketoglutarate dehydrogenase (αKGDH) complex of mitochondrial enzymes is significantly less active when HIF-1 is activated. This complex of enzymes stops α-ketoglutarate (α-KG), a consequence of the metabolic conversion of glutamine to succinate, from oxidizing. HIF-1α decreases granzyme B, TNF-α, and IFN-γ production in CD8+, CD4+ T, and NK cells isocitrate dehydrogenase (IDH) then reductively carboxylates this isocitrate to citrate (29). Fatty acid production is increased by HIF, which encourages the conversion of glutamine-derived citrate to cytoplasmic acetyl-CoA. This serves as an important link between protein and lipid metabolism.

TUMOR HYPOXIA AND ANGIOGENESIS

HIFs activate multiple angiogenic growth factors that contribute to the growth of intra-tumoral blood vessels like vascular endothelial growth factors (VEGF), stromal-derived factor 1 (SDF1), stem cell factor (KIT Ligand), placental growth factor, angiopoeitin2, angiopoietin-like 4, and other factors (30). Hypoxia also increases hyaluronic acid synthesis and hyaluronidase activity, which may encourage angiogenesis as a compensatory mechanism for hypoxia. Hyaluronic acid is a major component of the vascular basement membrane (31). It is important to understand that this neo-angiogenesis does not mean enhanced tumor blood supply. Tumor angiogenesis does not always equate to the tumor blood supply, though, because of the immature neovascularization's discontinuous basement membrane, which permits extravasation of proteins and plasma, increased intra-tumor interstitial pressure, persistent vascular collapse, and inadequate nutrition delivery (32). As a result, even in tumors with high vascular densities, the neointima that develops is usually poorly formed, making it less effective in delivering oxygen, and nutrients, and has clinical relevance in understanding the drug delivery hindrance it poses (Figure 2.3).

TUMOR HYPOXIA AND ITS ROLE IN IMMUNE TOLERANCE

HIF-1α has been shown to increase the expression of programmed cell death ligand-1 (PD-L1) in neoplastic cells (33). Hypoxia, through HIF, affects both innate and adaptive immunity. This has been used as a means for developing immunotherapeutic agents that can act on the tumor more effectively.

T-Cells

Hypoxia induces molecular expression changes that enhance the cytotoxic differentiation and lytic functions of killer T-cells against the neoplastic targets. HIF-1α promotes the

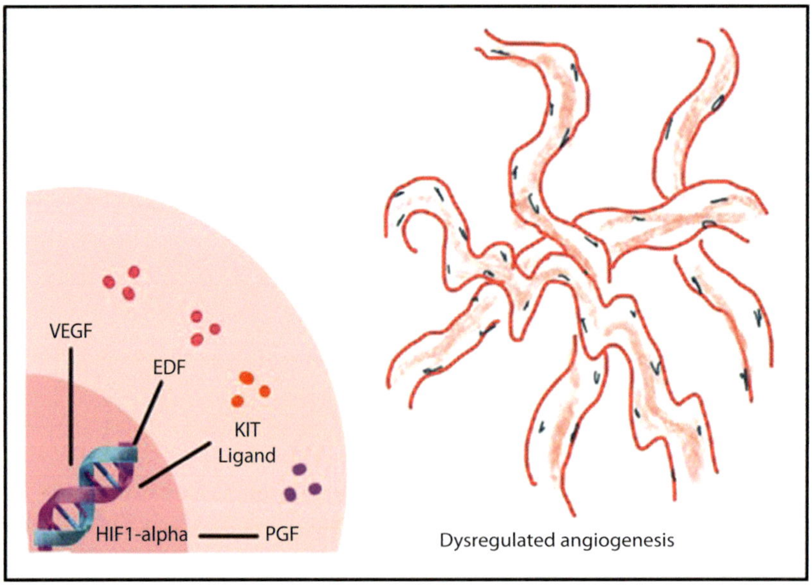

FIGURE 2.3 Role of hypoxia in dysregulated angiogenesis.

accumulation and anticancer action of CD8+ tumor-infiltrating lymphocytes (TILs) (34). HIF-1α also improves the ability of CD8+ cells to infiltrate the microenvironment by its effect on increasing VEGF-A levels. However, it has also been seen that hypoxia attenuates the T-cell function by reducing the levels of IFN-γ, IL-2, and NK group 2 member D (NKG2D). It is also observed that T-cell proliferations are strongly correlated with oxygen concentrations and are therefore suppressed under hypoxic conditions likely due to hypoxia-associated changes in Ca^{+2} channels (35). HIF-1α reduces the production of granzyme B, TNFα, and interferon-gamma in CD4+ and CD8+ T-cells. This results in the development of resistance to PD1 and PD-L1 inhibition and a reduction in T-cell-mediated toxicity. Prolonged exposure to hypoxia increases mitochondrial stress which further impairs anti-PD-1 activity raises ROS levels in T-cells and causes mitochondrial dysfunction.

B-Cells

Hypoxia impairs B-cell proliferation and also alters B-cell metabolism. The results are disruption of the formation of high-affinity IgG antibody production and sustained hypoxia impairs B-cell clonal expansion. By stimulating VEGF to promote the development of lymphatic and endothelial vessels, improve DC maturation, and improve antigen presentation, HIF activation in B-cells regulates immunological responses. There have been reports of B-cells causing cancer. Hypoxia stimulates HIF-1α and triggers autocrine transforming growth factor-beta (TGF-β) signaling, which in turn supports the survival and proliferation of B-cells and encourages the recurrence of cancer by activating myofibroblasts, inducing CXCL13, and recruiting B lymphocytes (36).

Macrophages

Hypoxia, HIF-1α, and tumor secretion of multiple chemokines facilitate cancer-associated macrophage (TAM) recruitment to the TME. Hypoxia-induced HIF-1α is linked to a better prognosis for cancer and facilitates TAM adaptability to the hypoxic environment. The hypoxic environment causes macrophages to express more inducible nitric oxide synthase (iNOS) and raises HIF-1α levels. This quickly inhibits T-cell proliferation by forming peroxynitrite through NO (37).

NK Cells

NK cells are bone marrow-derived and account for 10–18% of peripheral blood mononuclear lymphocytes. NK cells can kill various cancer targets, including cancer cells with low expression MHC-I. Some cancer cells secrete chemokines to recruit NK cells. Activated autophagy in hypoxic cancer cells selectively degrades the pro-apoptotic NK-derived serine protease GZMB/granzyme B, leading to the suppression of NK-mediated target cell apoptosis (38).

Neutrophils

Neutrophils are the major players in the innate immune system. Neutrophil infiltration is uncommon in normal tissues. In a hypoxic environment, neutrophils reduce glycogen recycling, leading to impaired functions, and consume extracellular proteins to promote their own central carbon metabolism to maintain their functions. Infiltrating neutrophils in the TME, known as tumor-associated neutrophils (TANs), promote cancer growth and are strongly associated with poor prognosis (39). Elimination of neutrophil infiltration leads to cancer regression and prolonged survival outcomes.

Myeloid-Derived Suppressor Cells

Cancer cells in hypoxic areas express various cytokines, such as chemokine (C-C motif) ligand 26, G-CSF, and IL-6, to recruit MDSCs. MDSCs enhance the evasion of cancer cells from immune surveillance and promote cancer drug resistance. Inhibiting the infiltration of MDSCs improves anti-tumor effects (40).

Innate Lymphocytes

Innate lymphocytes (ILCs) consist of NK cells ILC1, ILC2, and ILC3 and are involved in the immune response to viruses, bacteria, parasites, and transformed cells. Specific changes in cancer cytokines alter ILC composition in cancers by inducing plasticity and altering ILC functions. Administration of hypoxic ILC2 resulted in a higher cancer volume, suggesting that hypoxia-exposed ILC2 enhanced the progression of pancreatic cancer cells. These outcomes were attributed to the conversion of ILC2 to ILCregs under hypoxic conditions, which inhibited T-cell infiltration and IFN-γ expression by secreting IL-10 (41) (Figure 2.4; Table 2.1).

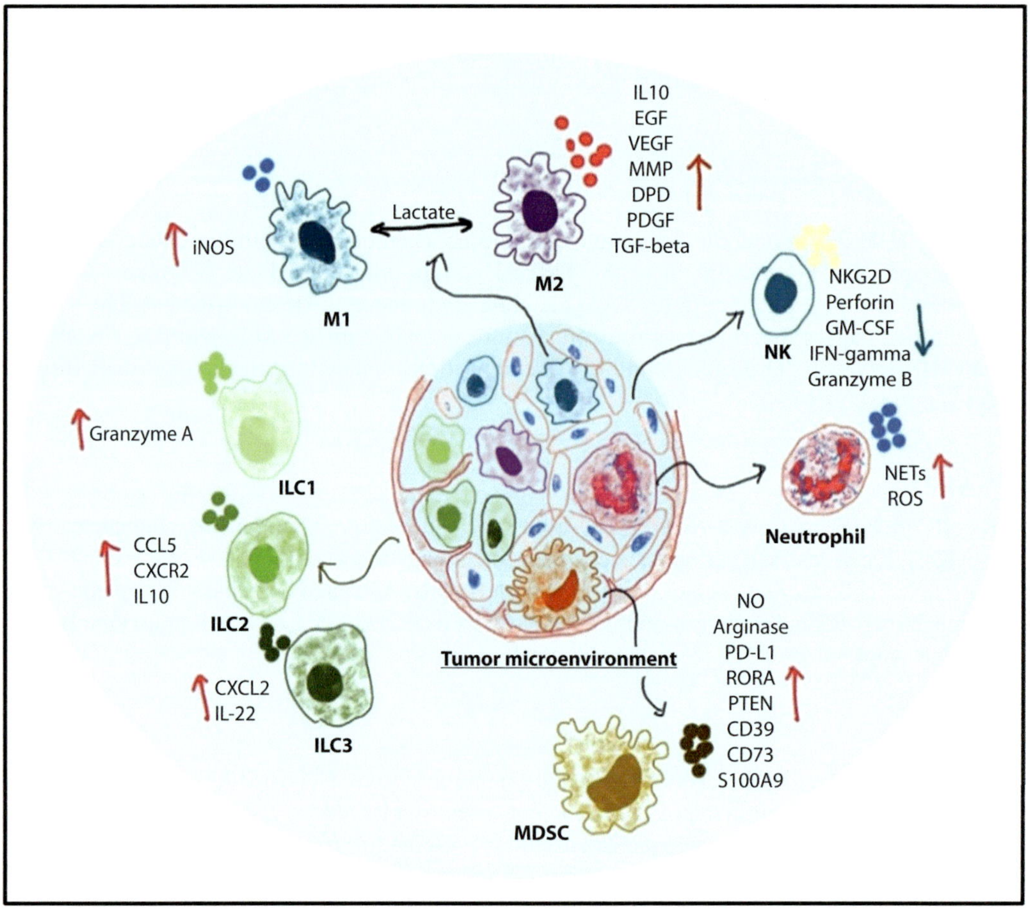

FIGURE 2.4 A figure depicting the various cytokines that are at play in the tumor microenvironment.

TABLE 2.1
A Summary of the Ongoing Clinical Trials That Target Hypoxia or Downstream Hypoxia Factors (42)

Drug	Target	Cancer Type	Status	Clinical Trials	Intervention/Treatment	FDA Approval
[F 18]HX4	Hypoxia regions	Head and neck cancer Lung cancer Hepatocellular carcinoma Rectal cancer Cervical cancer	Phase 2	NCT01075399	Intravenous injection	Yes
F 18 ([A18 F] FMISO)	Hypoxia regions	Cervical adenocarcinoma Hepatocellular carcinoma Glioblastoma Brain métastasés from breast cancer	Phase 2	NCT00559377 NCT02471313 NCT00902577 NCT01985971 NCT02695628	Intravenous injection	Yes
[18 F]EF5	Hypoxia regions	Squamous cell carcinoma of the head and neck	Phase 2	N CT01774760	Intravenous injection	Yes
Digoxin	HIF-1α	Breast cancer	Phase 2	N CT01763931	Oral	Yes
Bevacizumab Tarceva Cisplatin	EGFR	Head and neck cancer	Phase 1	NCT00140556	Intravenous infusion	Yes
Topotecan Cisplatin Bevacizumab	VEGF	Cervical cancer	Phase 2	NCT00548418	Intravenous infusion	Yes
Erlotinib (Tarceva/ OSI-774)	EGFR	Carcinoma, non-small-cell lung	Phase 2	NCT00983307	Oral	Yes
B KM 120/ Buparlisib	PI3K	Carcinoma, non-small-cell lung	Phase 1	NCT02128724	Oral	Yes
Avastin (bevacizumab) Docetaxel	HIF/VEGF/VEGFR	Breast cancer	Phase 2	NCT00559754	Intravenous infusion	Yes
Clostridium novyi-NT spores	Anaerobic bacteria	Solid tumor malignancies	Phase 1	NCT01924689	Intra-tumoral injection	–
TH-302	Hypoxia regions	Pancreatic adenocarcinoma Soft tissue sarcoma	Phase 3	NCT01746979 NCT01440088	Intravenous infusion	Yes

(Continued)

TABLE 2.1 *(Continued)*
A Summary of the Ongoing Clinical Trials That Target Hypoxia or Downstream Hypoxia Factors (42)

Drug	Target	Cancer Type	Status	Clinical Trials	Intervention/Treatment	FDA Approval
Bevacizumab irinotecan	HIF-2α	Glioblastoma	Phase 2	NCT00381797	Intravenous infusion	Yes
	VEGF	Medulloblastoma		NCT02076152		
		Ependymoma				
Melatonin	HIF-1α	Oral squamous cell carcinoma	Phase 3	NCT04137627	Oral	Yes
Everolimus (RAD001)	mTOR	Renal cell carcinoma	Phase 4	NCT01206764	Oral	Yes
Cetuximab	EGFR	Squamous cell carcinoma of the head and neck	Phase 2	NCT01104922	Intravenous infusion	Yes
Tivozanib	HIF-1/2	Renal cell carcinoma	Phase 2	NCT01297244	Oral	Yes
Pazopanib	HIF	Melanoma	Phase 2	NCT01107665	Intravenous infusion	Yes
Paclitaxel						
PT2385	HIF-2α	Glioblastoma	Phase 2	NCT03216499	Oral	Yes
Dinitrobenzamide(CB1954)	Hypoxia regions	Prostate cancer	Phase 1	NCT04374240	Intra-prostatlc injection	–
Mitomycin C	Hypoxia regions	Squamous cell carcinoma of the head and neck	–	NCT02352792	Intravenous infusion	Yes
Porfimycin	Hypoxia regions	Head and neck cancer	Phase 3	NCT00002507	Intravenous injection	–
Apaziquone	Hypoxia regions	Bladder cancer	Phase 3	NCT00461591	Intravesical	–
Tirapazamine	Hypoxia regions	Cervical cancer	Phase 2	NCT00003369	Intravenous infusion	–
		Head and neck squamous cell carcinoma	Phase 3	NCT00174837		
		Small-cell lung cancer	Phase 2	NCT00066742		
Nlmorazole	Hypoxia regions	Head and neck squamous cell carcinoma	Phase 3	NCT01950689	Oral	–
Topotecan	HIF-1α	Small-cell lung cancer	Phase 2	NCT00698516	Oral	Yes
		Non-small-cell lung cancer	Phase 3	NCT00390806		
		Ovarian cancer	Phase 2	NCT00317772		
Belzutifan (MK-6482/ PT2977)	HIF-2α	Clear cell renal cell carcinoma	Phase 1	NCT04846920 NCT04994522	Oral	Yes

TUMOR HYPOXIA AND ITS ROLE IN AFFECTING THERAPEUTIC MODALITIES

Chemotherapy

Hypoxia increases the tolerance of the neoplastic cells to the drug toxicity. It induces the expression of drug-resistance genes in the cancer cells, increases chemotherapeutic drug efflux, and reduces intracellular drug concentrations. Once they are combined with anticancer drugs, P-glycoprotein (PGP), known as multidrug resistance protein 1 (MDR1), and breast cancer resistance protein (BCRP) are ATP-binding cassette (ABC) transporters and energy-dependent drug excretion pumps that can pump drugs out of the cell by providing energy through ATP. The intracellular concentration of drugs continues to decrease, which weakens their cytotoxic effects until they are dissipated, and drug resistance occurs. ROS generated under hypoxic conditions induce PGP and BCRP expression through HIF-1α and increase cancer cell drug resistance (43). HIF-1α enhances the inactivation of chemotherapeutic drugs and reduces their cytotoxic effects. Cytidine deaminase (CDD), an important metabolic enzyme involved in drug resistance development in cancer cells, is derived from cancer cells or bacteria within cancer cells (44). The mechanism of hypoxia-enhanced chemoresistance can be summarized as follows: increased PGP expression and excretion of drugs from the cells via PGP and BRCA channels. HIF-1α also enhances the activity of pyruvate kinase muscle 1 (PKM1), olfactomedin 4 (OLFM4) (chemotherapeutic resistance genes) enhances mitochondrial oxidative phosphorylation (OXPHOS) that further promotes PGP expression. Under hypoxic conditions, there is enhanced autophagy that inhibits the chemotherapy-induced cell death pathway which in turn helps in resisting chemotherapy-induced cell toxicity. HIF-2 upregulation promotes the ability of hypoxic cancer cells to resist drug toxicity by activating the TGF-alpha/EGFR pathway and COX-2 (Figure 2.5).

Radiotherapy

Radiotherapy directly destroys macromolecule fixation and leads to DNA damage through the generation of free radicals, such as hydroxyl (OH•) and hydrogen (H•) radicals, by ionizing radiation (IR), a process known as "oxygen fixation theory". The damage caused by radiotherapy is

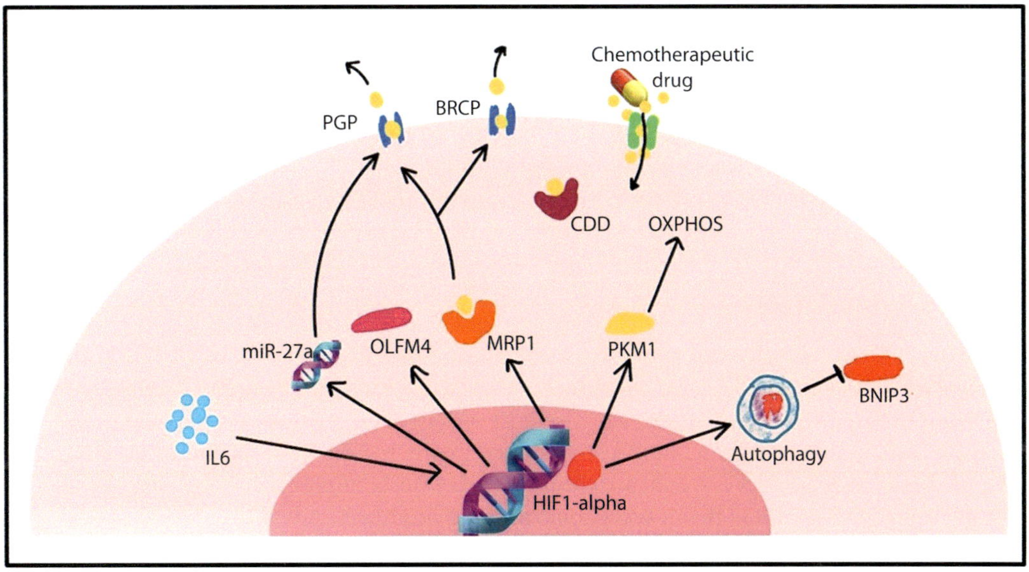

FIGURE 2.5 A summary of how HIF-1α affects the chemotherapeutic agents.

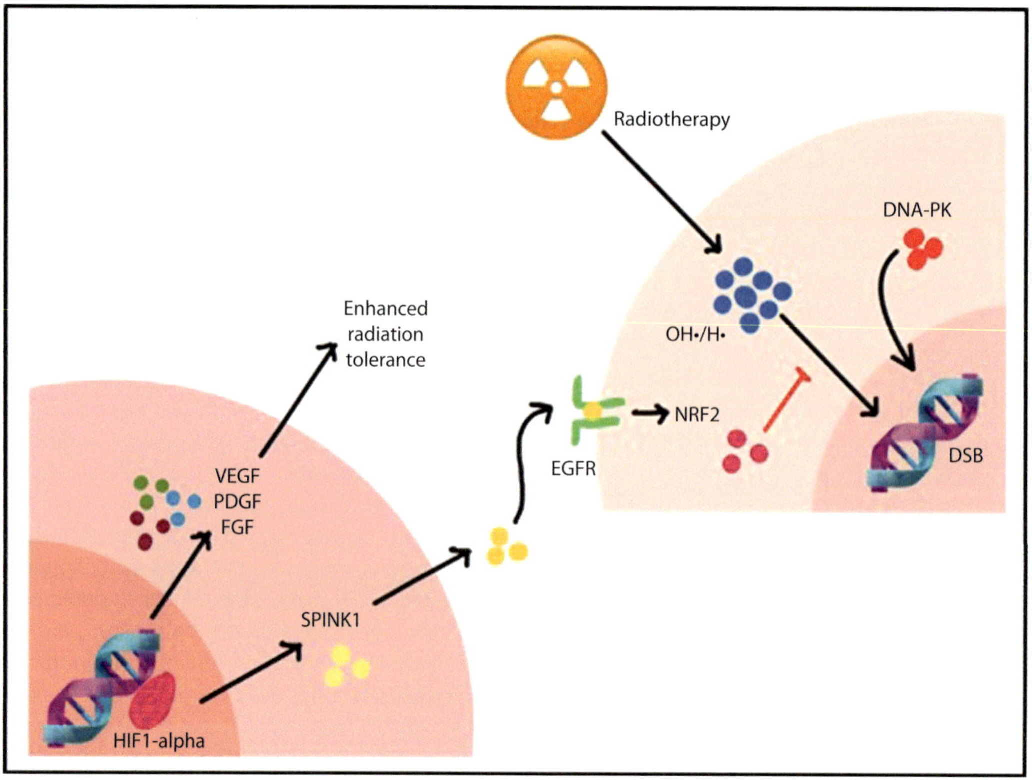

FIGURE 2.6 Summary of the effect of hypoxia on radiotherapy.

permanent and irreversible. Hypoxia reduces the effectiveness of radiotherapy and free radicals become unstable, leading to a limited extent of their damage, and most of the damage can be easily repaired. Classical in-vitro and in-vivo experiments have shown that at O_2 (pO_2) partial pressures below 10 mmHg, tumor cells can acquire radiobiologic hypoxia and thus become relatively resistant to radiotherapy. HIF-1α stimulates DNA-dependent protein kinase (DNA-PK) expression and repairs DNA DSB caused by IR (45). Radiation upregulates HIF-1 expression and enhances its activity in cancer cells. Elevated HIF-1α levels confer radio-resistance via various pro-cancer mechanisms. HIF-1α promotes ATP metabolism and p53 activation and stimulates EC survival, thereby mediating the ultimate cancer radiation responses. The radiosensitivity of hypoxic cancer cells was shown to be significantly increased after reoxygenation (Figure 2.6).

Nano Application Therapy

Nanoparticles are characterized by small sizes, large surface areas, high bioavailability, and good biocompatibility and have great potential for safely and efficiently transporting external oxygen to the hypoxic TME (46). Nanoparticles can also host various drugs, such as oxygenating agents, chemotherapeutic agents, and immune-boosting drugs, improving the anticancer effects. Manganese dioxide-based nanocarriers can enhance the anticancer effects of piggyback paclitaxel by alleviating the degree of hypoxia in the in-situ glioma microenvironment. Advances in nanotechnology to improve the hypoxic TME, or to combine chemotherapy, radiotherapy, and immunotherapy, have achieved satisfactory outcomes, compared to traditional treatments, and may become a treatment measure with great potential in the future (47).

Biotherapy

Accumulating evidence suggests that microbiota play an important role in cancer by damaging cellular DNA, inducing transformation, activating and altering stromal cell components in the TME, and influencing cellular metabolism. Recent research has demonstrated that a combination of live bacteria and treatment modalities such as surgery, chemotherapy, and radiotherapy can produce good clinical outcomes. Certain bacteria have the potential to gravitate to the hypoxic core of cancer cells and can spread and proliferate. Spores of the anaerobic bacterium *Clostridium novyi-NT* were used to treat the transplanted tumors in mice. In several mouse models including colorectal cancer, biliary cancer, melanoma, and squamous cell carcinoma, this bacterium was found to significantly improve the efficacy of radiotherapy (48). The use of the attenuated pathogenic anaerobe *Salmonella* VNP20009 to target the cancer hypoxic region, equipped with photosensitizers and bromodomain and extra terminal domain (BET) protein inhibitors with mitochondrial targeting properties improved the heat elimination abilities of photothermal therapy (PTT) and significantly inhibited the expressions of PD-L1 in cancer cells, thereby enhancing and maintaining a durable immune response (49). Maximizing the use of live bacteria under hypoxic conditions has the potential to be a therapeutic modality for the treatment of cancer.

CONCLUSION

Hypoxia plays a central role in cancer progression, metastasis, and resistance to therapy. The dynamic interplay between tumor hypoxia, metabolic reprogramming, angiogenesis, immunomodulation, and treatment outcomes underlines the complexity of tumor biology. The field requires further research to unravel the molecular mechanism underlying hypoxia's impact on tumors and identify targets that can be used for developing cost-effective and efficacious therapeutic modalities and improve the clinical outcomes of even devastating cancers. Hypoxia is a critical factor in the development and progression of cancer. The hallmark of hypoxia is the creation of a microenvironment that perpetuates genomic instability and triggers the development of metabolic and biochemical changes to suit the microenvironment. This enables the cancer cells to proliferate despite the hostile conditions.

Understanding the role of hypoxia in tumor biology provides valuable insight for developing more effective strategies. Research can help in finding a breakthrough in achieving better clinical outcomes with solid tumors and help in the advancement of tumor biology.

CONSENT FOR PUBLICATION

Not applicable.

FUNDING

None.

CONFLICT OF INTEREST

The authors declare no conflict of interest, financial or otherwise.

REFERENCES

1. https://www.who.int/news/item/01-02-2024-global-cancer-burden-growing–amidst-mounting-need-for-services
2. Bristow RG, Hill RP. Hypoxia and metabolism. Hypoxia, DNA repair and genetic instability. *Nat Rev Cancer.* 2008;8:180–192. doi: 10.1038/nrc2344.
3. Gray LH, et al. The concentration of oxygen dissolved in tissues at the time of irradiation is a factor in radiotherapy. *Br J Radio.* 1953;26:638–648. doi: 10.1259/0007-1285-26-312-638.

4. Sebestyén A, Kopper L, Dankó T, Tímár J. Hypoxia signaling in cancer: From basics to clinical practice. *Pathol Oncol Res*. 2021;27:1609802. doi: 10.3389/pore.2021.1609802.
5. Auerbach W, Auerbach R. Angiogenesis inhibition: A review. *Pharm Ther*. 1994;63:265–311. doi: 10.1016/0163-7258(94)90027-2.
6. Nagy JA, et al. Heterogeneity of the tumor vasculature. *Semin Thromb Hemost*. 2010;36:321–331. doi: 10.1055/s-0030-1253454.
7. Ludwig C. Drug resistance of hypoxic tumour cells in vitro. *Cancer Treat Rev*. 1984;11(Suppl A): 173–178. doi: 10.1016/0305-7372(84)90057-4.
8. Papp-Szabó E, Josephy PD, Coomber BL. Microenvironmental influences on mutagenesis in mammary epithelial cells. *Int J Cancer*. 2005;116:679–685. doi: 10.1002/ijc.21088.
9. Tuy K, Rickenbacker L, Hjelmeland AB. Reactive oxygen species produced by altered tumor metabolism impacts cancer stem cell maintenance. *Redox Biol*. 2021;44:101953. doi: 10.1016/j.redox.2021.101953.
10. Koritzinsky M, et al. Gene expression during acute and prolonged hypoxia is regulated by distinct mechanisms of translational control. *EMBO J*. 2006;25:1114–1125. doi: 10.1038/sj.emboj.7600998.
11. Chan N, Bristow RG. "Contextual" synthetic lethality and/or loss of heterozygosity: Tumor hypoxia and modification of DNA repair. *Clin Cancer Res*. 2010;16:4553–4560. doi: 10.1158/1078-0432.CCR-10-0527.
12. Huang D, Li C, Zhang H. Hypoxia and cancer cell metabolism. *Acta Biochim Biophys Sin (Shanghai)*. 2014;46(3):214–219. doi: 10.1093/abbs/gmt148.
13. Brahimi-Horn C, Berra E, Pouysségur J. Hypoxia: The tumor's gateway to progression along the angiogenic pathway. *Trends Cell Biol*. 2001;11:S32–S36. doi: 10.1016/S0962-8924(01)82185-1.
14. Chong TW, et al. A mycobacterial iron chelator, desferri-exochelin, induces hypoxia-inducible factors 1 and 2, NIP3, and vascular endothelial growth factor in cancer cell lines. *Cancer Res*. 2002;62:6924–6927.
15. Park J-H, et al. Gastric epithelial reactive oxygen species prevent normoxic degradation of hypoxia-inducible factor-1alpha in gastric cancer cells. *Clin Cancer Res*. 2003;9:433–440.
16. Schofield CJ, Ratcliffe PJ. Oxygen sensing by HIF hydroxylases. *Nat Rev Mol Cell Biol*. 2004;5: 343–354. doi: 10.1038/nrm1366.
17. Nakamura H, et al. TCR engagement increases hypoxia-inducible factor-1 alpha protein synthesis via rapamycin-sensitive pathway under hypoxic conditions in human peripheral T cells. *J Immunol*. 2005;174:7592–7599. doi: 10.4049/jimmunol.174.12.7592.
18. LaGory EL, Giaccia AJ. The ever-expanding role of HIF in tumour and stromal biology. *Nat Cell Biol*. 2016;18:356–365. doi: 10.1038/ncb3330.
19. Bollinger T, et al. Transcription regulates HIF-1α expression in CD4(+) T cells. *Immunol Cell Biol*. 2016;94:109–113.
20. Wan J, Wu W. Hyperthermia induced HIF-1a expression of lung cancer through AKT and ERK signaling pathways. *J Exp Clin Cancer Res*. 2016;35:119. doi: 10.1186/s13046-016-0399-7.
21. Li Y, et al. Expression of Notch-Hif-1α signaling pathway in liver regeneration of rats. *J Int Med Res*. 2020;48:300060520943790.
22. Ravi R, et al. Regulation of tumor angiogenesis by p53-induced degradation of hypoxia-inducible factor 1alpha. *Genes Dev*. 2000;14:34–44. doi: 10.1101/gad.14.1.34.
23. Li L-C, Zhang M, Feng Y-K, Wang X-J. IDH1-R132H suppresses glioblastoma malignancy through FAT1-ROS-HIF-1α signaling. *Neurol India*. 2020;68:1050–1058.
24. Vander Heiden MG, Cantley LC, Thompson CB. Understanding the Warburg effect: The metabolic requirements of cell proliferation. *Science*. 2009;324:1029–1033. doi: 10.1126/science.1160809.
25. Pouysségur J, et al. 'Warburg effect' controls tumor growth, bacterial, viral infections, and immunity – Genetic deconstruction and therapeutic perspectives. *Semin Cancer Biol*. 2022;86:334–346. doi: 10.1016/j.semcancer.2022.07.004.
26. Hoefflin R, et al. HIF-1α and HIF-2α differently regulate tumour development and inflammation of clear cell renal cell carcinoma in mice. *Nat Commun*. 2020;11:4111. doi: 10.1038/s41467-020-17873-3.
27. Faubert B, et al. Lactate metabolism in human lung tumors. *Cell*. 2017;171:358–371.e9. doi: 10.1016/j.cell.2017.09.019.
28. Furuta E, et al. Fatty acid synthase gene is up-regulated by hypoxia via activation of Akt and sterol regulatory element binding protein-1. *Cancer Res*. 2008;68:1003–1011. doi: 10.1158/0008-5472.CAN-07-2489.
29. Sun RC, Denko NC. Hypoxic regulation of glutamine metabolism through HIF1 and SIAH2 supports lipid synthesis that is necessary for tumor growth. *Cell Metab*. 2014;19:285–292. doi: 10.1016/j.cmet.2013.11.022.

30. Du R, et al. HIF-1α induces the recruitment of bone marrow-derived vascular modulatory cells to regulate tumor angiogenesis and invasion. *Cancer Cell*. 2008;13(3):206–220. doi: 10.1016/j.ccr.2008.01.034.
31. Gao F, et al. Hypoxia-induced alterations in hyaluronan and hyaluronidase. *Adv Exp Med Biol*. 2005;566:249–256. doi: 10.1007/0-387-26206-7_33.
32. Duffy JP, Eibl G, Reber HA, Hines OJ. Influence of hypoxia and neoangiogenesis on the growth of pancreatic cancer. *Mol Cancer*. 2003;2:12. doi: 10.1186/1476-4598-2-12.
33. Ding X-C, et al. The relationship between expression of PD-L1 and HIF-1α in glioma cells under hypoxia. *J Hematol Oncol*. 2021;14:92. doi: 10.1186/s13045-021-01102-5.
34. Lee JH, Elly C, Park Y, Liu Y-C. E3 ubiquitin ligase VHL regulates hypoxia-inducible factor-1α to maintain regulatory T cell stability and suppressive capacity. *Immunity*. 2015;42:1062–1074. doi: 10.1016/j.immuni.2015.05.016.
35. Robbins JR, et al. Hypoxia modulates early events in T cell receptor-mediated activation in human T lymphocytes via Kv1.3 channels. *J Physiol*. 2005;564:131–143. doi: 10.1113/jphysiol.2004.081893.
36. Sander S, et al. Synergy between PI3K signaling and MYC in Burkitt lymphomagenesis. *Cancer Cell*. 2012;22:167–179. doi: 10.1016/j.ccr.2012.06.012.
37. Doedens AL, et al. Macrophage expression of hypoxia-inducible factor-1 alpha suppresses T-cell function and promotes tumor progression. *Cancer Res*. 2010;70:7465–7475. doi: 10.1158/0008-5472.CAN-10-1439.
38. Viry E, et al. Autophagic degradation of GZMB/granzyme B: A new mechanism of hypoxic tumor cell escape from natural killer cell-mediated lysis. *Autophagy*. 2014;10:173–175. doi: 10.4161/auto.26924.
39. Gentles AJ, et al. The prognostic landscape of genes and infiltrating immune cells across human cancers. *Nat Med*. 2015;21:938–945. doi: 10.1038/nm.3909.
40. Horikawa N, et al. Anti-VEGF therapy resistance in ovarian cancer is caused by GM-CSF-induced myeloid-derived suppressor cell recruitment. *Br J Cancer*. 2020;122:778–788. doi: 10.1038/s41416-019-0725-x.
41. Ye L, et al. Hypoxia-reprogrammed regulatory group 2 innate lymphoid cells promote immunosuppression in pancreatic cancer. *EBioMedicine*. 2022;79:104016. doi: 10.1016/j.ebiom.2022.104016.
42. Chen Z, Han F, Du Y, Shi H, Zhou W. Hypoxic microenvironment in cancer: Molecular mechanisms and therapeutic interventions. *Signal Transduct Target Ther*. 2023 Feb 17;8(1):70. doi: 10.1038/s41392-023-01332-8.
43. Sakata K, et al. Hypoxia-induced drug resistance: Comparison to P-glycoprotein-associated drug resistance. *Br J Cancer*. 1991;64:809–814. doi: 10.1038/bjc.1991.405.
44. Geller LT, et al. Potential role of intratumor bacteria in mediating tumor resistance to the chemotherapeutic drug gemcitabine. *Science*. 2017;357:1156–1160. doi: 10.1126/science.aah5043.
45. Um JH, et al. Association of DNA-dependent protein kinase with hypoxia inducible factor-1 and its implication in resistance to anticancer drugs in hypoxic tumor cells. *Exp Mol Med*. 2004;36:233–242. doi: 10.1038/emm.2004.32.
46. Zhang C, Pu K. Molecular and nanoengineering approaches towards activatable cancer immunotherapy. *Chem Soc Rev*. 2020;49:4234–4253. doi: 10.1039/C9CS00773C.
47. Wang Y, et al. CXCR4-guided liposomes regulating hypoxic and immunosuppressive microenvironment for sorafenib-resistant tumor treatment. *Bioact Mater*. 2022;17:147–161. doi: 10.1016/j.bioactmat.2022.01.003.
48. Bettegowda C, et al. Overcoming the hypoxic barrier to radiation therapy with anaerobic bacteria. *Proc Natl Acad Sci USA*. 2003;100:15083–15088. doi: 10.1073/pnas.2036598100.
49. Chen W, et al. Dual drugs decorated bacteria irradiate deep hypoxic tumor and arouse strong immune responses. *Biomaterials*. 2022;286:121582. doi: 10.1016/j.biomaterials.2022.121582.

3 Unraveling Intricate Hypoxia Signaling Networks and Implications for Cancer Development and Therapy

Suman Kumar Ray and Sukhes Mukherjee
Department of Biochemistry, All India Institute of Medical Sciences, Bhopal, Madhya Pradesh, India

INTRODUCTION

Aerobic metabolism in human cells cannot take place without oxygen. Consequently, hypoxia is common in cancer, lung disorders, acute and chronic vascular diseases, and other similar conditions (1). Rapidly, reproducing cells use the available oxygen at the periphery of a tumor, which is 70–150 μm distant from the tumor blood arteries. This inhibits the diffusion of oxygen into the deep layers of the tumor, leading to an oxygen tension below 10 mmHg, which is called tumor hypoxia (2). The root of most solid tumors is located in this hostile microenvironment, which is caused by vascular malformation (3).

Solid tumors stand out from normal tissues due to their abnormal vascular network structure, which prevents the tumor from receiving oxygen and nutrients it needs to thrive (4). In most cases, there are two ways to categorize hypoxia in solid tumors: acute and chronic. Differences in hypoxia-related responses between the two subtypes may influence tumor growth and therapeutic efficacy. Multiple methods, including a high metabolic rate, are employed by tumor cells to generate hypoxia, according to six studies (5) and rapid oxygen consumption (6), which destroys oxygen delivery owing to endothelial dysfunction or other impacts on blood vessels (7). A persistent hypoxic environment speeds up tumor growth, makes tumors more invasive, and encourages tumor spread via activating the signaling cascade of hypoxia-inducible factors (HIFs) (Figures 3.1 and 3.2) (8). Scientists have grown cancer cells in both normal and hypoxic conditions and discovered that the former greatly increases cell proliferation, invasion, and metastasis compared to the latter (9).

Both in the laboratory and in the clinic, people have been trying to find ways to combat tumor hypoxia for over a hundred years (10). In order to hinder tumor progression and treatment resistance, it is crucial to create medicines that target the hypoxic environment and enhance intratumoral oxygenation. Inhibitors of hypoxia-related pathways, including HIFs and mTOR, have been created to target hypoxic cells (11).

Supplemental hyperoxia therapy is one method that researchers have developed to alleviate the hypoxic tumor environment and increase tumor oxygenation. An intervention to alleviate tissue hypoxia in critically ill patients, oxygen therapy is among the most commonly utilized therapies in modern medicine (12).

 DOI: 10.1201/9781003477419-3

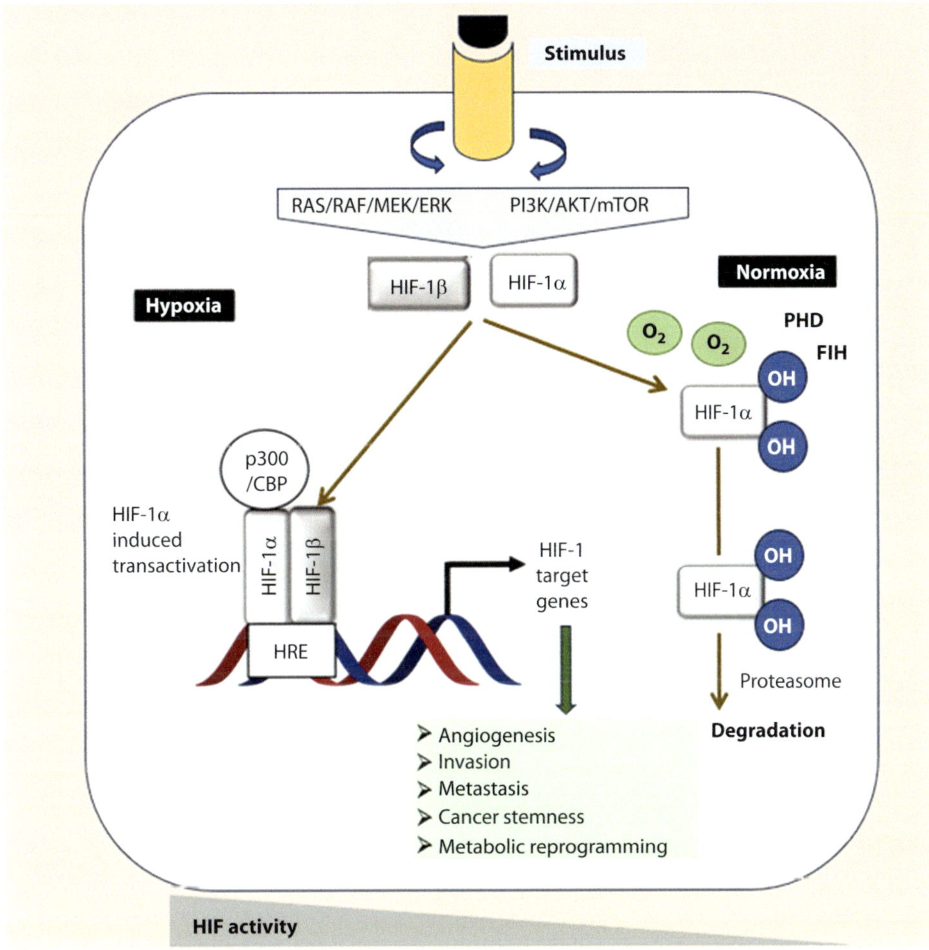

FIGURE 3.1 Role of HIFs in cancer development and progression.

TUMOR HYPOXIA

When oxygen (O_2) levels are too low, it hinders biological processes, a condition known as tissue hypoxia (13). Hypoxia can be caused by several factors. These include (1) low O_2 partial pressure (O_2 tension) in arterial blood, which can be caused by pulmonary diseases or high altitude (hypoxemic hypoxia), (2) reduced blood O_2 carrying capacity, which can be caused by anemia, methemoglobin formation, or carbon monoxide poisoning (anemic hypoxia), (3) reduced tissue perfusion, either generalized or localized (circulatory or ischemic hypoxia), (4) deterioration of the diffusion geometry, such as increased diffusion distances or concurrent versus countercurrent blood flow within microvessels (diffusional hypoxia), (5) intoxication of cells, such as cyanide poisoning (histotoxic or cytotoxic hypoxia). Unless the system controlling blood flow fails to meet the increased O_2 demand of the tissue in question, hypoxia will not typically occur as a result of increases in tissue O_2 consumption because of finely tuned regulatory systems. When discussing hypoxia, most biochemists will use the term "O_2-limited electron transport" (14). By reducing or eliminating O_2 partial pressures below critical thresholds, hypoxia limits or eliminates the function of organs, tissues, or cells, according to physiologists and clinicians. In the absence of oxygen, a condition known as anoxia is defined as an oxygen partial pressure of zero millimeters of mercury (mmHg) in the tissue (15). Declining diffusion geometry, serious structural abnormalities of tumor microvessels

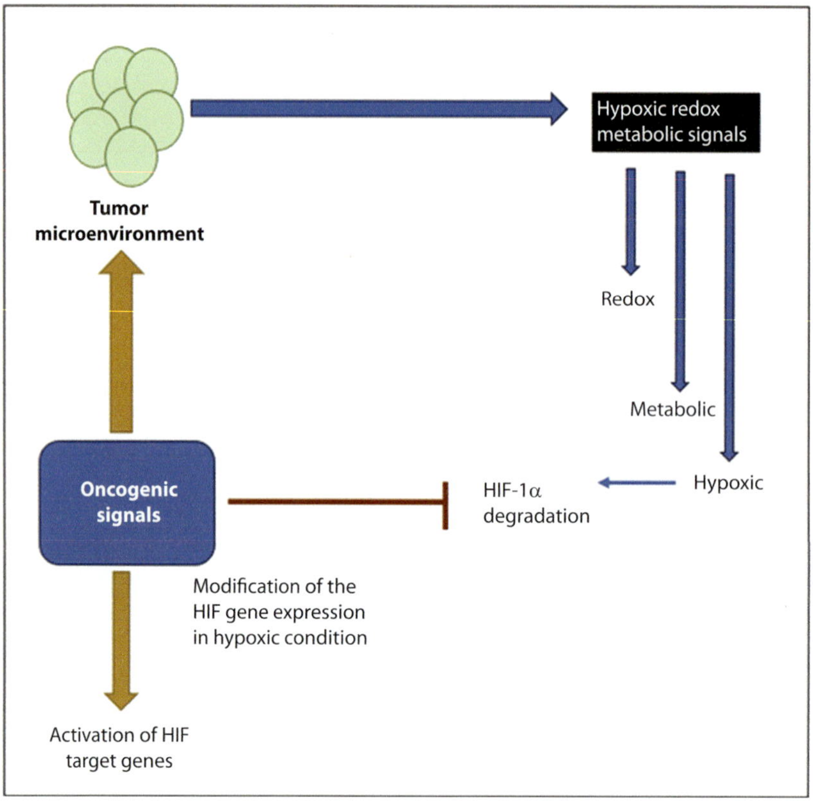

FIGURE 3.2 HIFs and different cellular oncogenic signaling that helps to modify the HIFs gene expression in hypoxic condition.

and disrupted microcirculation can limit or eliminate oxygen delivery to respiring neoplastic and stromal cells in solid tumors (16). Furthermore, the ability of the blood to carry O_2 is diminished by anemia and the production of methemoglobin or carboxyhemoglobin. Consequently, solid tumors can have either acute or chronic regions with oxygen partial pressures that are extremely low, if not nil. Microregions with negligible or nonexistent O_2 partial pressures can be found in close proximity to areas with normal O_2 partial pressures, and their distribution within the tumor mass is quite uneven. When compared to healthy tissue, neoplastic tissue is unable to perform its original physiological roles. Areas of necrosis, which are frequently visible in tumor tissue under a microscope, suggest the loss of critical cellular functions; however, functional impairments cannot be used to characterize tumor hypoxia (17, 18).

HYPOXIC SIGNALING IN THE PRIMARY TUMOR MICROENVIRONMENT

The capacity of cancer cells to proliferate and persist within the initial tumor setting, spread to and penetrate the stroma of neighboring tissues, invade blood and lymphatic arteries both intravasally and extravasally, and eventually colonize target organs is an essential component of the dynamic and intricate process known as metastasis (19).

Stromal cells inside the tumor microenvironment (TME) influence tumor progression and metastasis via several pathways, in addition to genetic and epigenetic processes that occur during the formation of malignant tumors (20). Hypoxia, also known as low oxygen tension, is a newly recognized molecular characteristic of the TME that controls the ability of tumor and stromal cells to metastasize.

A notable aspect of the TME is hypoxia, which results from an imbalance between the delivery and consumption of oxygen (21). The aberrant vasculature that forms in solid tumors as a consequence of an imbalance between pro- and antiangiogenic signals hinders oxygen supply.

Hypoxic areas develop within the TME because proliferating tumor cells and invading immune cells need oxygen at high rates (22). The molecular level response to hypoxia is the stabilization of HIF-1 and HIF-2. These transcription factors aid cells in responding to hypoxic stress by regulating processes such as angiogenesis, invasion, migration, glycolytic metabolism, and erythropoiesis (23). From a clinical standpoint, several solid tumor types have been linked to HIF-1 and HIF-2, which in turn are linked to metastasis and poor patient survival (24). It has been shown that HIF and its downstream targets play a significant role in metastasis (25). Additionally, HIF signaling is essential and sufficient to enhance the metastatic capacity of tumor cells.

ROLE OF HYPOXIA IN TUMOR PROGRESSION

Hypoxia is a reality for many cancers, and this is mostly because tumor cells express HIF. Research into the process of erythropoietin (EPO) gene regulation led to the accidental discovery of HIF (19, 20). HIF-1 is an isoform that includes a beta subunit (HIF-1β, also known as aryl hydrocarbon nuclear transporter, or ARNT) and one of three alpha subunits (HIF-1α, HIF-2α, or HIF-3α). According to research, HIF-1α is seen as a transcriptional regulator that controls how tumor cells react to low oxygen levels (26). In order to study the relationship between intracellular O_2 concentration and HIF-1 expression, Jiang and his colleagues (1996) subjected human cervical cancer HeLa cells to different concentrations of O_2. The amounts of HIF-1α and HIF-1β proteins, as well as the HIF-1 DNA-binding activity of cells, grew exponentially as the O_2 concentration decreased (27).

The uncommon autosomal dominant genetic condition known as Von Hippel-Lindau (VHL) syndrome is brought about by harmful variations in the VHL gene. About 70% of people who have VHL will have renal cell carcinoma (RCC) at some point in their lives (28). The VHL protein can ubiquitinate the HIF-α component in an oxygen-dependent way, leading to the proteolysis of HIF, because it is an E3 ubiquitin ligase.

Mutations in the VHL gene cause RCC to develop by stabilizing HIF subunits and constitutively activating transcriptional pathways regulated by HIF (29, 30). One of the fundamental drivers of renal carcinogenesis and metastasis in VHL-deficient renal clear cell carcinoma is the abnormal activation of Akt, also known as protein kinase B, PKB, in a manner that is both HIF independent and prolyl hydroxylation dependent (31). Ubiquitin-specific protease 22 (USP22) has the ability to stabilize HIF1α and increase stemness and glycolysis in hypoxia-induced hepatocellular carcinoma (HCC) (32). Because VHL does not degrade it, HIF-α accumulates when oxygen levels decrease. A protein called asparagine hydroxylase (FIH), which affects the C-terminal domain (C-TAD) of the HIF-1α protein, regulates the activation capacity of HIF-α.

To activate HIF-1α c-TAD activity, it is essential and sufficient to inhibit FIH activity in hypoxia (33). An inhibitor of DNA binding protein 2 (ID2) destabilizes the VHL complex in hypoxic brain tumor cells, which stops HIF-2α from being degraded by ubiquitin-mediated proteasomal degradation (34). Vascular endothelial growth factor (VEGF) activation is another outcome of hypoxia-induced HIF-1 overexpression. The presence of VEFG mRNA may be a marker of hypoxia, as demonstrated by Chiarotto's use of varied oxygen concentrations to confirm the overexpression of VEFG mRNA in three cervical cancer cell lines. In addition, Takahiro and colleagues showed that hypoxia induced the initial production of HIF-1α in metastatic lymph nodes, which in turn caused a surge in VEFG-A expression and a subsequent increase in VEFG-C expression. Hypoxia is a primary inducer of VEFG gene transcription, and that most human cancer cell types highly express VEFG (35, 36). Characteristics of solid TMEs include low oxygen levels, inadequate blood flow, and unchecked cell proliferation (37). Rapid DNA repair, immune response modulation, angiogenesis, metastasis, and metabolic program rewiring are all necessary for cancer cells to continue growing and surviving (38) (Table 3.1).

TABLE 3.1
Different Cellular Activity in the Hypoxic Tumor Microenvironment (39, 40)

Tumor Hypoxia	Different Cellular Activity in the Hypoxic Tumor Microenvironment
Tumor hypoxia induces abnormal cell metabolism	• The role of oxygen in cell metabolism is crucial, as cancer cells live in nutrient- and oxygen-deficient environments due to rapid tumor growth. • To maintain proliferation, cancer cells reconnect their metabolic pathways, known as the Warburg effect, mediated by HIF-1. • Mutations in gene regulatory networks can drive the heterogeneous behavior of cancer metabolism. • Oxygen, glucose, and glutamine in the TME are considered the main nutrients that promote cell growth. • Hypoxia can provide energy to tumor cells by activating transcriptional programs that induce glucose uptake and glycolysis. • Tumor cells adaptively turn to androgen/androgen receptor-independent pathways to survive and grow, resulting in therapeutic resistance. • Hypoxia supports macropinocytosis-mediated cancer metabolic reprogramming through the HIF/EHD2 pathway and uses extracellular proteins as a nutrient for survival. • Mitochondria are the energy reservoir in organisms, and HIF-1 regulates metabolic pathways that influence mitochondrial viability. • Inhibition of phospholipase C under hypoxia promotes the metabolic process of cancer cells, reduces the formation of mitochondrial ROS, and converts tumor bioenergy into glycolysis.
Tumor hypoxia promotes angiogenesis	• In 1971, Professor Folkman proposed the theory that tumor growth and metastasis depend on neovascularization, leading to the development of antiangiogenic antitumor drugs. • The mechanism of angiogenesis is complex, with over 40 molecules playing key roles in vascular recruitment. • Most studies focus on HIF and VEGF and their receptors. In the hypoxic environment of the tumor mass, the HIF-1 dimeric complex remains stable and activates the expression of numerous genes responsible for the angiogenesis process. • HIF-1-induced proteins include VEGF, which promotes vascular permeability, and basic fibroblast growth factor (bFGF), which promotes endothelial cell growth. • Due to the essential function of angiogenesis in tumor development, the development of antiangiogenic drugs has been put on the agenda. • Commonly used antiangiogenic drugs include bevacizumab, ramucirumab, and olaratumab. • Traditional angiogenesis inhibitors mainly block VEGF signaling and prune tumor vessels. • However, the expected antiangiogenic therapy has not been achieved due to their less effectiveness against tumors with alternate blood supply sources.
Tumor hypoxia promotes metastasis	• Hypoxia is linked to metastasis, but its impact on metastasis progression is controversial. • Epithelial-mesenchymal transition (EMT) is a key process in cancer cell colonization from the primary tumor to distant organs. • Hypoxia triggers EMT by regulating HIFs, which directly regulate EMT-related proteins like zinc finger E-box binding homeobox 1, Snail, and Twist. HIF can also modulate microRNA (miRNA) to promote cellular EMT. • Studies have reported downregulation of Drosha and Dicer, key enzymes involved in miRNA biogenesis. • HIF-1α downregulates Dicer expression by promoting ubiquitination of the E3 ligase parkin, inhibiting tumor suppressors like let-7 and microRNA-200B. • Hypoxia can promote EMT in tumor-bearing mice by downregulating miRNA expression. • Recent studies have shown that CSN8, the smallest subunit of the COP9 signalosome, is a key regulator of hypoxia-induced EMT and dormancy, enhancing colon cancer cells' invasion and metastatic abilities.

TABLE 3.1 *(Continued)*

Different Cellular Activity in the Hypoxic Tumor Microenvironment (39, 40)

Tumor Hypoxia	Different Cellular Activity in the Hypoxic Tumor Microenvironment
Tumor hypoxia accelerates DNA damage repair	• Cancer therapies often cause DNA damage, but cancer cells can activate repair mechanisms and signaling pathways to overcome this damage. • These repaired cells become more resistant to standard treatment. • The success of cancer treatment is limited by insufficient DNA damage during treatment and rapid DNA repair after treatment. • The ATM and RAD3-related (ATR)/Chk1 and ataxia-telangiectasia mutation (ATM)/Chk2 signaling pathways play key roles in the DNA damage response. • After DNA damage, tumor hypoxia can drive DNA repair, allowing tumor cells to continue growing and causing resistance to antitumor therapy. • The antiangiogenic agent cediranib inhibits the expression of the homology-directed DNA repair factor BRCA1/2 and RAD51 recombinase, promoting the sensitivity of the poly (ADP-ribose) polymerase (PARP) inhibitor olaparib. • Combination treatment with drugs inhibiting HDR can modulate DNA repair, potentially enabling the development of combination therapies aiming to exploit DNA repair defects in cancer cells.
Tumor hypoxia promotes immune escape	• Hypoxia can directly affect the biology of infiltrating immune cells and the response to therapy in tumors. • It can upregulate the expression of various cellular immune checkpoints, such as PD-L1, and maintain the function of myeloid-derived suppressor cells (MDSCs), which have immunosuppressive activity. • Targeting HIF-1α with drugs or genes can inhibit PD-L1 expression in the TME and enhance interferon production by T cells. • HIFs can also switch tumor-associated macrophages (TAMs) from an antitumorigenic (M1-like) phenotype to a protumorigenic (M2-like) phenotype. • The effects of hypoxia on T cells are controversial. Some studies suggest that O2 is required for T-cell activation and the development of effector functions, and that HIF-1α acts as a negative regulator of T-cell responses. • For example, tumor hypoxia activates the γδT-cell protein kinase A pathway, resulting in the inhibition of the activating receptor natural killer cell group 2D (NKG2D). • Alleviating tumor hypoxia enhances the expression of NKG2D and enhances the antitumor function of γδT cells. • However, some studies have reported that HIF-1α signaling increases T-cell function, such as the production of 2-hydroxyglutarate (2-HG) and VEGF-A production by tumor cells.
Immune evasion	• Tumors can survive if they can evade immune attack, and immune suppression is crucial for tumor control. • However, tumor cells use complex mechanisms that prevent the immune system from responding effectively, limiting the efficacy of single-agent immunotherapy. • Understanding the mechanisms that coordinate immunosuppression in the tumor microenvironment (TME) is an active area of investigation. • Hypoxia is implicated as a factor driving the immunosuppressive TME, as it promotes resistance to cytotoxic CD8+ T cell (CTL)-mediated killing, HIF signaling, and NK cell-mediated lysis. • Hypoxic cancer cells also secrete chemokines and cytokines to recruit immunosuppressive regulatory T cells (Tregs) and myeloid-derived suppressor cells (MDSCs) to the TME.

(Continued)

TABLE 3.1 *(Continued)*
Different Cellular Activity in the Hypoxic Tumor Microenvironment (39, 40)

Tumor Hypoxia	Different Cellular Activity in the Hypoxic Tumor Microenvironment
Invasion	• Tumor cells invade tissue parenchyma to initiate the metastatic cascade. • They alter cell adhesion molecules, upregulate extracellular proteases, and recruit macrophages, fibroblasts, and mesenchymal stem cells for invasion. • Hypoxia activates promigratory and invasive tumor cell phenotypes through various mechanisms. • Hypoxia induces epithelial plasticity and a migratory phenotype through regulating epithelial to mesenchymal transcription factors. • HIF signaling also enhances invasion of the surrounding ECM by upregulating proteolytic enzymes. • HIF signaling also induces the expression of chemokines and cytokines, recruiting macrophages and mesenchymal stem cells for invasion.
Cancer stem cell phenotype	• Cancer stem cells (CSCs) are a small fraction of tumor cells with enhanced tumor-initiating potential, self-renewal, and differentiation into multiple cell types. • They are hypothesized to be responsible for metastases derived from primary CSCs that regain their regenerative potential at metastatic sites. • The expression of adult stem cell markers in patient primary tumors is associated with poor prognosis and metastasis. • Recent studies have begun to define niches and signaling pathways that select and maintain the CSC phenotype. • Hypoxia is an important microenvironmental factor that selects for the CSC phenotype, supporting the generation and maintenance of CSCs through HIF-dependent activation of genes that drive self-renewal.
Intravasation and extravasation	• HIF plays a crucial role in tumor cell intravasation and extravasation from the vasculature. • It releases factors that modulate endothelial cell-endothelial cell and tumor cell-tumor cell interactions. • HIF upregulates angiopoietin-like 4 (ANGPTL4), disrupting endothelial cell-endothelial cell interactions and allowing tumor cell passage through blood vessels. • It also strengthens tumor cell-endothelial cell interactions through the activation of L1 cell adhesion molecule (L1CAM). • HIF also activates genes controlling vascular permeability, such as VEGF, angiopoietin 2, MMPs, and UPAR. • In the endothelium, HIF signaling increases cell adhesion, coagulation, and endothelial permeability. • Recent studies suggest that HIF-1 contributes to metastatic spread by modulating lymphatics.

TARGET THERAPEUTICS BASED ON HYPOXIA

The regular progression of life's activities is guaranteed by oxygen balance. Hypoxia modulates the expression of numerous genes that have important implications in the pathophysiology of numerous human disorders (41). The hypoxia pathway is thought to revolve around HIF-1. Researchers have exerted significant effort to intervene at each step of the hypoxia signaling pathway in order to create target treatments for tumor hypoxia (Figure 3.3). Among HIF several roles in the hypoxic milieu of tumors include facilitating angiogenesis through increased VEGF expression and improving glucose metabolism. Inflammation, anaerobic glycolysis, and abnormally high levels of angiogenesis all contribute to neoplastic disorders and carcinogenesis (42). A cascade of tumor-initiating activities is set in motion when the stably generated HIF successively activates the downstream target

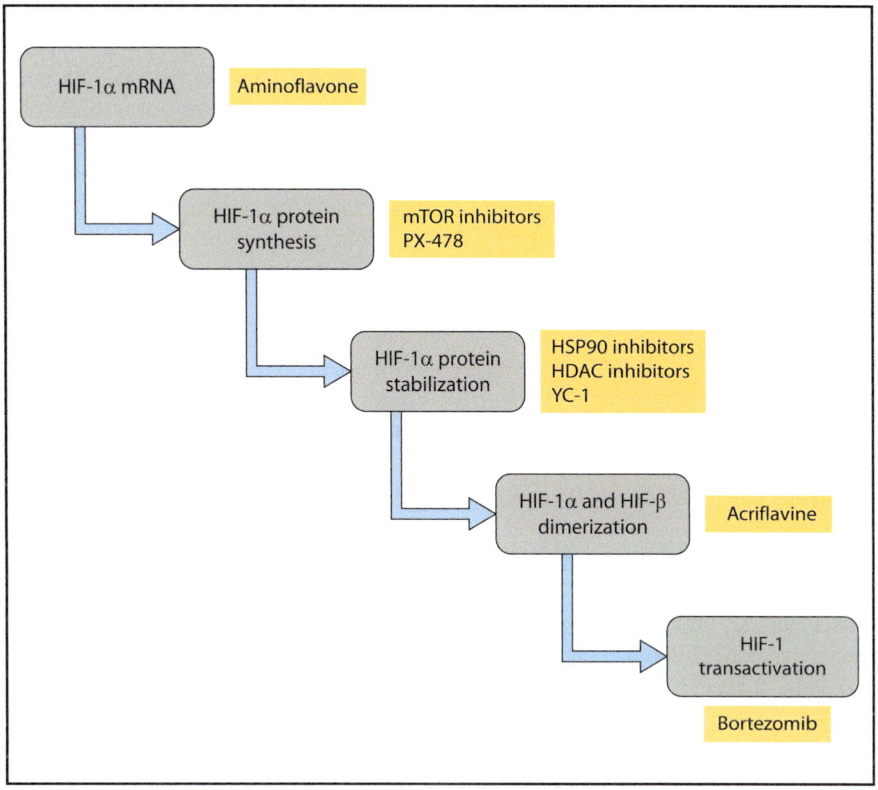

FIGURE 3.3 Molecular mechanism of HIF-1 targeting drugs.

genes. For this reason, HIF is one of the targets for tumor therapy (43). However, its functions in various tumor types can be different. The EGLN/HIF axis, for instance, promotes carcinogenesis in RCC (44), but the converse is true for other cancers.

One of the most prevalent forms of kidney cancer is ccRCC. Inactivation of the pVHL tumor suppressor gene is an important step in ccRCC (45). Stabilizing HIF-1α and HIF-2α occurs when pVHL is inactivated. Hence, anti-caking compounds for HIF-2α have been the subject of multiple investigations. In human ccRCC cells, the small-molecule inhibitor PT2399 blocks carcinogenesis in 56% of its congeners and dissociates HIF-2 (46).

Both in vivo and in vitro tests demonstrate the anticancer efficacy of topotecan, an HIF-1α inhibitor (47), and it is useful for treating ovarian cancer and SCLC, among other cancers. The proteasome inhibitor bortezomib (PS-341), which is used to reduce HIF-1α activity, does so by preventing the recruitment of P300 coactivators (48) items. While Bortezomib was found to change tumor sensitivity to hypoxia, it was ineffective in metastatic colon cancer in a phase II experiment (49).

Bortezomib significantly reduces VEFG synthesis by as much as 90%, according to in vivo studies conducted on mice carrying xenografts. One possible explanation for this result is that the therapy reduces HIF-1 transcriptional activity (50). The potential clinical advantage of RO7070179, an additional HIF-1α inhibitor, was demonstrated in a phase Ib clinical trial by its ability to decrease the level of HIF-1α mRNA in patients with HCC (51). Advanced colorectal cancer (CRC) and gastric cancer (GC) were treated with the anticancer medicine oxaliplatin (52).

Oxaliplatin has been tested in many clinical trials when combined with different medications (53). According to certain research, oxaliplatin is more effective in treating CRC when it induces HIF-1α breakdown (54). An other tactic is to control HIF-1 ubiquitination. One potential pharmacological target is the regulation of deubiquitinases (DUBs), which are enzymes that can deubiquitinate substrates (55). Normoxically, these medications have little to no effect, but they can bioreduce hypoxically to create cell-toxic metabolites called hypoxia-activated prodrugs (HAPs) (56).

A HAP called evofosfamide (TH-302) inhibits the progression of neuroendocrine prostate cancer (NEPC) tumors (57, 58). There have been a number of studies looking into the effectiveness of TH-302 in combination with other treatments for cancer. Results from a phase II study in patients with advanced pancreatic cancer demonstrated that there was a statistically significant improvement in progression-free survival and tumor response when the combination of gemcitabine and TH-302 was administered. The combination of hypoxia-targeted treatment and checkpoint inhibition is more effective than either approach alone in controlling tumor progression in a transgenic mice model of adenocarcinoma (59). Combination therapy with doxorubicin was found to be more effective than other first-line treatments in another phase II trial of patients with advanced soft tissue sarcoma, and TH-302 was found to not cause any damage to the liver, kidneys, or heart (60).

In a number of malignancies, members of the ErbB receptor tyrosine kinase family are thought to be oncogenes (61). Another HAP, tarloxotinib, works by blocking the activation of four different ErbB family members. *In vitro* studies with cancer cells taken from patients show that it suppresses signaling and cell proliferation, and in several xenograft models with mice, it slows tumor growth (62).

CONCLUDING REMARKS

Hypoxia is a fundamental physiological difference between tumor cells and normal cells, with the ability to survive under hypoxic conditions being a key difference. Hypoxia is a crucial microenvironmental factor that contributes to metastatic tumor progression at primary and distant tissue sites. The role of oxygen sensors, such as proline hydroxylase, is also important, as they may be targets for oncogenes and anticancer drugs. Additionally, proteins like fibronectin and heterogeneous nuclear ribonucleoprotein (hnRNP) interact with VHL, which might also be important in the response to hypoxia. Further research is needed to determine the ratio of pro-survival and apoptotic pathways activated by cancer cells in response to hypoxia and how these are regulated. The process involves the activation of a complex transcriptome, which includes pathways downstream of HIF-1α and other signaling pathways. Understanding how cells sense hypoxia and activate these pathways is crucial, as well as the integration of these pathways.

Modulation of the HIF signaling pathway in tumor cells has begun to reveal the diverse mechanisms by which HIF signaling promotes metastatic progression. Recent studies indicate that HIF signaling can be activated within tumor stromal cells through various mechanisms, including hypoxia and secreted factors produced by tumor cells. However, the role of HIF signaling within individual stromal cell populations remains largely unexplored. Tumor cells must adapt to tissue-specific barriers to colonization and exploit survival signals. Hypoxia is a key barrier to successful metastatic colonization of breast and colon cancer cells in the liver, and hematopoietic stem cells reside within hypoxic niches in the bone marrow. Hypoxia and HIF signaling couple metastasis with immune evasion, with hypoxic tumor cells upregulating the expression of EMT transcription factors Zebl and Snail. Clinical studies have shown a correlation between the expression of EMT transcription factors and the expression of immunosuppressive checkpoint inhibitors and infiltrating Tregs. A variety of HIF inhibitors and other agents targeting the hypoxic signaling pathway are in preclinical and clinical development for cancer. Understanding the mechanisms by which hypoxia modulates tumor growth and identifying tissue- and cell-specific response patterns is essential for developing effective treatments. Evaluating the efficacy of these agents in immune-competent preclinical models and clinical studies is essential to understand the impact of HIF inhibition on tumor progression.

CONSENT FOR PUBLICATION

Not applicable.

FUNDING

None.

CONFLICT OF INTEREST

The authors declare no conflict of interest, financial or otherwise.

ACKNOWLEDGMENTS

Declared none.

REFERENCES

1. Harris AL. Hypoxia—a key regulatory factor in tumour growth. Nat Rev Cancer. 2002;2(1):38–47.
2. Bennewith KL, Dedhar S. Targeting hypoxic tumour cells to overcome metastasis. BMC Cancer. 2011;11:504.
3. Dewhirst MW, Secomb TW. Transport of drugs from blood vessels to tumour tissue. Nat Rev Cancer. 2017;17(12):738–750.
4. Zhang M, Ye JJ, Xia Y, et al. Platelet-mimicking biotaxis targeting vasculature-disrupted tumors for cascade amplification of hypoxia-sensitive therapy. ACS Nano. 2019;13(12):14230–14240.
5. Dang CV. Links between metabolism and cancer. Genes Dev. 2012;26(9):877–890.
6. Yang J, Staples O, Thomas LW, et al. Human CHCHD4 mitochondrial proteins regulate cellular oxygen consumption rate and metabolism and provide a critical role in hypoxia signaling and tumor progression. J Clin Invest. 2012;122(2):600–611.
7. Skuli N, Liu L, Runge A, et al. Endothelial deletion of hypoxiainducible factor-2alpha (HIF-2alpha) alters vascular function and tumor angiogenesis. Blood. 2009;114(2):469–477.
8. LaGory EL, Giaccia AJ. The ever-expanding role of HIF in tumour and stromal biology. Nat Cell Biol. 2016;18(4):356–365.
9. Wang P, Wan W, Xiong S, et al. HIF1α regulates glioma chemosensitivity through the transformation between differentiation and dedifferentiation in various oxygen levels. Sci Rep. 2017;7(1):7965.
10. Vilaplana-Lopera N, Besh M, Moon EJ. Targeting hypoxia: revival of old remedies. Biomolecules. 2021;11(11):1604.
11. Jing X, Yang F, Shao C, et al. Role of hypoxia in cancer therapy by regulating the tumor microenvironment. Mol Cancer. 2019,18(1):157.
12. Hochberg CH, Semler MW, Brower RG. Oxygen toxicity in critically ill adults. Am J Respir Crit Care Med. 2021;204(6):632–641.
13. Ray SK, Mukherjee S. Imitating hypoxia and tumor microenvironment with immune evasion by employing three dimensional in vitro cellular models: impressive tool in drug discovery. Recent Pat Anticancer Drug Discov. 2022;17(1):80–91.
14. Boyer PD, Chance B, Ernster L, Mitchell P, Racker E, Slater EC. Oxidative phosphorylation and photophosphorylation. Annu Rev Biochem. 1977;46:955–1026.
15. Ortiz-Prado E, Dunn JF, Vasconez J, Castillo D, Viscor G. Partial pressure of oxygen in the human body: a general review. Am J Blood Res. 2019;15(1):1–14.
16. Kizaka-Kondoh S, Inoue M, Harada H, Hiraoka M. Tumor hypoxia: a target for selective cancer therapy. Cancer Sci. 2003;94(12):1021–1028.
17. Höckel M, Vaupel P. Tumor hypoxia: definitions and current clinical, biologic, and molecular aspects. J Natl Cancer Inst. 2001;93(4):266–276.
18. Lee SY, Ju MK, Jeon HM, Jeong EK, Lee YJ, Kim CH, Park HG, Han SI, Kang HS. Regulation of tumor progression by programmed necrosis. Oxid Med Cell Longev. 2018;2018:3537471.
19. Obenauf AC, Massague J. Surviving at a distance: organ specific metastasis. Trends Cancer. 2015;1:76–91.
20. Hanahan D, Coussens LM. Accessories to the crime: functions of cells recruited to the tumor microenvironment. Cancer Cell. 2012;21:309–322.
21. Mukherjee S, Ray SK. Targeting tumor hypoxia and hypoxia-inducible factors (HIFs) for the treatment of cancer—a story of transcription factors with novel approach in molecular medicine. Curr Mol Med. 2022;22(4):285–286.

22. Brown JM, Giaccia AJ. The unique physiology of solid tumors: opportunities (and problems) for cancer therapy. Cancer Res. 1998;58:1408–1416.
23. Semenza GL. Hypoxia-inducible factors in physiology and medicine. Cell. 2012;148:399–408.
24. Luan Y, et al. Clinicopathological and prognostic significance of HIF-1alpha and HIF-2alpha expression in small cell lung cancer. Pathol Res Pract. 2013;209:184–189.
25. Hiraga T, et al. Hypoxia and hypoxia-inducible factor-1 expression enhance osteolytic bone metastases of breast cancer. Cancer Res. 2007;67:4157–4163.
26. Blouw B, Song H, Tihan T, et al. The hypoxic response of tumors is dependent on their microenvironment. Cancer Cell. 2003;4(2):133–146.
27. Jiang BH, Semenza GL, Bauer C, Marti HH. Hypoxia-inducible factor 1 levels vary exponentially over a physiologically relevant range of O2 tension. Am J Physiol. 1996;271(4):C1172–C1180. Pt 1.
28. Zhang Z, Wang Y, Yang W, Liu T, Wang C, Huang C, Xu Y, Chen X, Zhou J, Wang Y, Zhou X, Gong Y, Gong K. Metabolomic landscape of renal cell carcinoma in von Hippel-Lindau syndrome in a Chinese cohort. iScience. 2024;27(7):110357. doi: 10.1016/j.isci.2024.110357. PMID: 39055909; PMCID: PMC11269943.
29. Jonasch E, Donskov F, Iliopoulos O, et al. Belzutifan for renal cell carcinoma in von Hippel-Lindau disease. N Engl J Med. 2021;385(22):2036–2046.
30. Krishnan B, Rose TL, Kardos J, Milowsky MI, Kim WY. Intrinsic genomic differences between African American and White patients with clear cell renal cell carcinoma. JAMA Oncol. 2016;2(5):664–667.
31. Guo J, Chakraborty AA, Liu P, et al. pVHL suppresses kinase activity of Akt in a proline-hydroxylation-dependent manner. Science. 2016;353(6302):929–932.
32. Ling S, Shan Q, Zhan Q, et al. USP22 promotes hypoxia-induced hepatocellular carcinoma stemness by a HIF1α/USP22 positive feedback loop upon TP53 inactivation. Gut. 2020;69(7):1322–1334.
33. Sim J, Cowburn AS, Palazon A, et al. The factor inhibiting HIF asparaginyl hydroxylase regulates oxidative metabolism and accelerates metabolic adaptation to hypoxia. Cell Metab. 2018;27(4):898–913.
34. Lee SB, Frattini V, Bansal M, et al. An ID2-dependent mechanism for VHL inactivation in cancer. Nature. 2016;529(7585):172–177.
35. Kato I, Nishinaka Y, Nakamura M, et al. Hypoxic adaptation of leukemic cells infiltrating the CNS affords a therapeutic strategy targeting VEGFA. Blood. 2017;129(23):3126–3129.
36. Nakajima T, Anayama T, Koike T, et al. Endobronchial ultrasound Doppler image features correlate with mRNA expression of HIF1-α and VEGF-C in patients with non-small-cell lung cancer. J Thorac Oncol. 2012;7(11):1661–1667.
37. Sun H, Meng Q, Shi C, et al. Hypoxia-inducible exosomes facilitate liver-tropic premetastatic niche in colorectal cancer. Hepatology. 2021;74(5):2633–2651.
38. Schiliro C, Firestein BL. Mechanisms of metabolic reprogramming in cancer cells supporting enhanced growth and proliferation. Cells. 2021;10(5):1056.
39. Zhuang Y, Liu K, He Q, Gu X, Jiang C, Wu J. Hypoxia signaling in cancer: implications for therapeutic interventions. MedComm (2020). 2023;4(1):e203.
40. Rankin EB, Nam JM, Giaccia AJ. Hypoxia: signaling the metastatic cascade. Trends Cancer. 2016;2(6):295–304.
41. Choudhry H, Harris AL. Advances in hypoxia-inducible factor biology. Cell Metab. 2018;27:281–298.
42. Ajith TA. Current insights and future perspectives of hypoxia-inducible factor targeted therapy in cancer. J Basic Clin Physiol Pharm. 2018;30:11–18.
43. Li T, et al. Epigenetic crosstalk between hypoxia and tumor driven by HIF regulation. J Exp Clin Cancer Res. 2020;39:224.
44. Huang Y, Lin D, Taniguchi CM. Hypoxia inducible factor (HIF) in the tumor microenvironment: friend or foe? Sci. China Life Sci. 2017;60:1114–1124.
45. Choueiri TK, Kaelin WG Jr. Targeting the HIF2-VEGF axis in renal cell carcinoma. Nat Med. 2020;26:1519–1530.
46. Cho H, et al. On-target efficacy of a HIF-2alpha antagonist in preclinical kidney cancer models. Nature. 2016;539:107–111.
47. Beppu K, et al. Topotecan blocks hypoxia-inducible factor-1alpha and vascular endothelial growth factor expression induced by insulin-like growth factor-I in neuroblastoma cells. Cancer Res. 2005;65:4775–4781.
48. Shin DH, et al. Bortezomib inhibits tumor adaptation to hypoxia by stimulating the FIH-mediated repression of hypoxia-inducible factor-1. Blood. 2008;111:3131–3136.
49. Mackay H, et al. A phase II trial with pharmacodynamic endpoints of the proteasome inhibitor bortezomib in patients with metastatic colorectal cancer. Clin Cancer Res. 2005;11:5526–5533.

50. Birle DC, Hedley DW. Suppression of the hypoxia-inducible factor-1 response in cervical carcinoma xenografts by proteasome inhibitors. Cancer Res. 2007;67:1735–1743.
51. Wu J, et al. Evaluation of a locked nucleic acid form of antisense oligo targeting HIF-1alpha in advanced hepatocellular carcinoma. World J. Clin. Oncol. 2019;10:149–160.
52. Wang D, Lippard SJ. Cellular processing of platinum anticancer drugs. Nat Rev Drug Disco. 2005;4:307–320.
53. Boku N, et al. Safety and efficacy of nivolumab in combination with S-1/capecitabine plus oxaliplatin in patients with previously untreated, unresectable, advanced, or recurrent gastric/gastroesophageal junction cancer: interim results of a randomized, phase II trial (ATTRACTION-4). Ann Oncol. 2019;30:250–258.
54. Wei TT, et al. Metabolic targeting of HIF-1alpha potentiates the therapeutic efficacy of oxaliplatin in colorectal cancer. Oncogene. 2020;39:414–427.
55. Mennerich D, Kubaichuk K, Kietzmann T. DUBs, hypoxia, and cancer. Trends Cancer. 2019;5:632–653.
56. Wilson WR, Hay MP. Targeting hypoxia in cancer therapy. Nat Rev Cancer. 2011;11:393–410.
57. Li Y, Zhao L, Li XF. The hypoxia-activated prodrug TH-302: exploiting hypoxia in cancer therapy. Front. Pharm. 2021;12:636892.
58. Guo H, et al. ONECUT2 is a driver of neuroendocrine prostate cancer. Nat Commun. 2019;10:278.
59. Jayaprakash P, et al. Targeted hypoxia reduction restores T cell infiltration and sensitizes prostate cancer to immunotherapy. J Clin Invest. 2018;128:5137–5149.
60. Chawla SP, et al. Phase II study of the safety and antitumor activity of the hypoxia-activated prodrug TH-302 in combination with doxorubicin in patients with advanced soft tissue sarcoma. J Clin Oncol. 2014;32:3299–3306.
61. Wang Z. ErbB receptors and cancer. Methods Mol Biol. 2017;1652:3–35.
62. Estrada-Bernal A et al. Tarloxotinib is a hypoxia-activated Pan-HER kinase inhibitor active against a broad range of HER-family oncogenes. Clin Cancer Res. 2021;27:1463–1475.

4 Strategies to Target Hypoxia-Induced Immune Suppression and Immune Escape Mechanisms

Pramedha Kamplikar, Sukhes Mukherjee, and Jagat R Kanwar
Department of Biochemistry, All India Institute of Medical Sciences, Bhopal, M.P., India

INTRODUCTION

The absence of oxygen in the tumor microenvironment (TME), or hypoxia, plays a significant role in developing immune escape and suppression mechanisms that help cancer cells elude the body's defense (Figure 4.1). Tumor cells adapt to this hostile hypoxic environment and acquire an aggressive phenotype, enabling them to survive and proliferate despite the challenges posed by limited oxygen and nutrients.[1]

An essential modulator of the cellular response to hypoxic stress is the transcription factor hypoxia-inducible factor 1 (HIF-1), which controls a gene expression program that alters anaerobic metabolism, angiogenesis, invasion, and survival.[2] These adaptations can enhance the ability of cancer cells to circumvent host immune responses, such as by upregulating the expression of immune checkpoint proteins that inhibit T-cell activation or by promoting the recruitment and activation of immunosuppressive cell types like myeloid-derived suppressor cells (MDSCs) and regulatory T cells.[3] Therapeutic approaches that disrupt the hypoxic TME modulate the activity of HIFs or directly target the immune evasion pathways employed by hypoxic tumor cells may hold promise.[4]

This hypoxic condition significantly impacts cellular behavior, gene expression, and metabolic pathways. HIFs are key transcription factors activated under low oxygen conditions, orchestrating a wide array of adaptive responses that facilitate tumor survival, angiogenesis, metabolic reprogramming, and immune evasion.[5]

Recent advances in the TME have shed light on the critical role that hypoxia plays in modulating immune responses.[6] Hypoxia, which arises due to the rapid proliferation of tumor cells outpacing their blood supply, leads to a series of molecular events that promote tumor survival and progression. Central to these events are the HIFs, which regulate the expression of numerous genes involved in angiogenesis, metabolism, cell survival, and immune modulation.[7] By orchestrating these processes, hypoxia not only enhances the adaptability of tumor cells but also creates a hostile environment for immune effector cells, thereby facilitating immune escape.[4]

One of the primary consequences of hypoxia within the TME is the metabolic reprogramming of both tumor and immune cells. Tumor cells under hypoxic conditions shift their metabolism from oxidative phosphorylation to glycolysis, leading to the accumulation of lactate and acidification of the TME.[8] This acidic environment impairs the function of immune cells such as cytotoxic T lymphocytes (CTLs), and natural killer (NK) cells that are critical for anti-tumor immunity. Moreover, the immune response may be further suppressed by hypoxia-induced metabolic alterations that promote regulatory T cells (Tregs) and MDSCs as well as inhibit dendritic cell (DC) function.[9] Hypoxia-induced immune suppression and immune escape are formidable barriers to effective cancer treatment.[10]

DOI: 10.1201/9781003477419-4

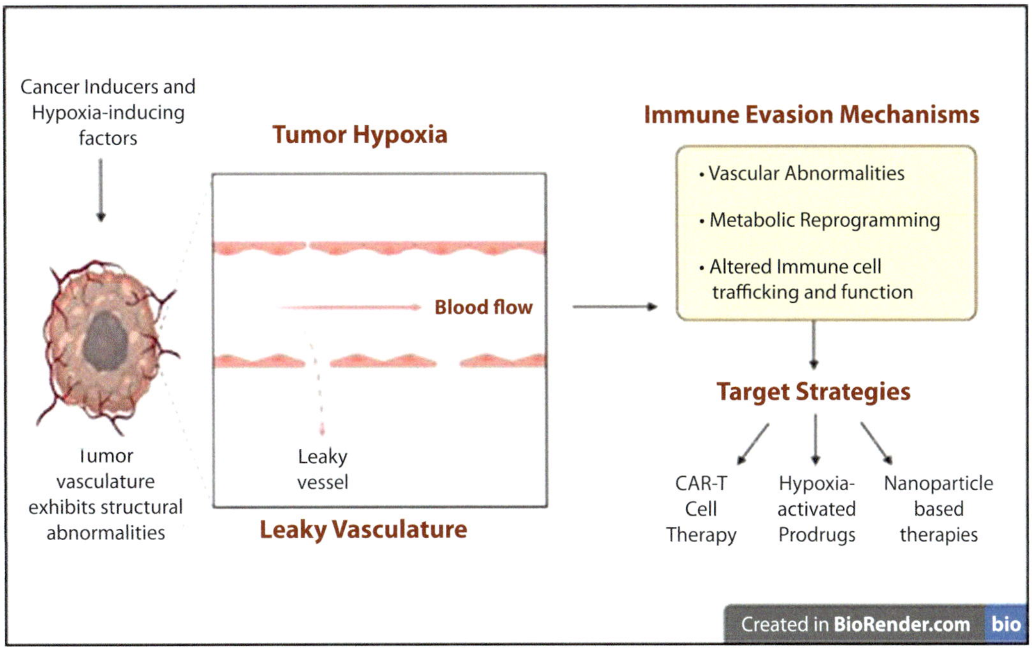

FIGURE 4.1 Hypoxia-inducing factors contribute to the development of hypoxic tumors, which in turn activate immune evasion mechanisms. To counteract this, strategies such as CAR-T cell therapy, hypoxia-activated prodrugs, and nanoparticle-based therapies have been developed to target these resistant tumors.

Beyond metabolic alterations, hypoxia also influences the expression of immune checkpoint molecules. Hypoxia can upregulate the expression of programmed death-ligand 1 (PD-L1) on tumor cells through HIF-1α, thereby inhibiting the activity of PD-1-expressing T cells.[3] The identification of this hypoxia-driven pathway has paved the way for combining immune checkpoint inhibitors (ICIs) with therapies targeting hypoxia signaling to enhance the overall efficacy of cancer immunotherapy.[11]

Approaches such as HIF inhibitors, metabolic modulators, and vascular normalization agents are being investigated for their potential to reprogram the hypoxic TME and restore effective anti-tumor immunity.[12] Clinical trials are increasingly focusing on combination therapies that integrate these hypoxia-targeting strategies with existing immunotherapies. The goal is to create a more favorable environment for immune cells to function optimally, thereby improving patient responses and outcomes. As we continue to unravel the complexities of hypoxia-induced immune modulation, these integrated approaches hold promise for more effective cancer treatments in the future (Figure 4.2).

MECHANISMS OF HYPOXIA–INDUCED IMMUNE SUPPRESSION

HIFs are key regulators of the cellular response to low oxygen levels.[13] HIF-1α and HIF-2α, the primary isoforms, are stabilized under hypoxic conditions and drive the transcription of genes that promote survival and adaptation. In immune cells, HIFs influence various functions, such as proliferation, differentiation, and cytokine production.[14] HIF-1α enhances the glycolytic activity of T cells and macrophages crucial for their activation and function under hypoxia. However, this metabolic shift can also lead to an immunosuppressive environment, particularly within tumors, where HIF-mediated pathways support the recruitment and activity of regulatory T cells (Tregs) and MDSCs, both of which inhibit effective anti-tumor immune responses.[15]

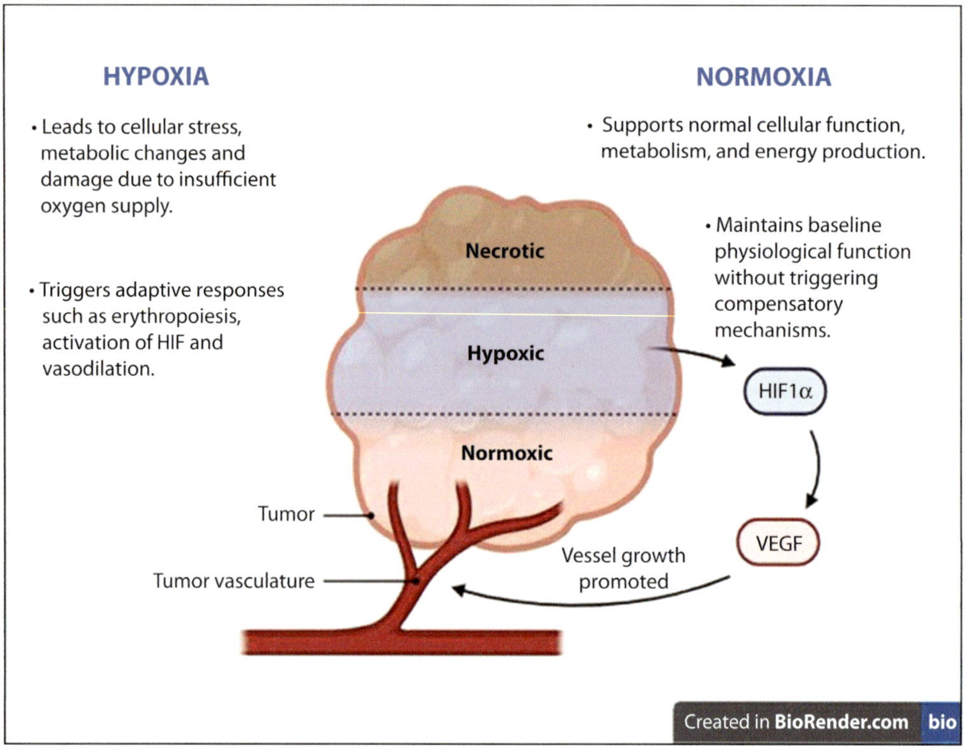

FIGURE 4.2 Diagram illustrating differences between hypoxia and normoxia conditions in a tumor microenvironment. Hypoxia triggers activation of HIF-1α that leads to the activation of vascular endothelial growth factor (VEGF). VEGF promotes blood vessel formation to combat hypoxia condition by carrying more oxygen supply to meet the deficit demands in tumor regions.

Metabolic reprogramming is a key aspect of hypoxia-induced immune suppression.[2] This altered metabolic state can impair the function of effector T cells and NK cells, reducing their cytotoxic activity and ability to control tumor growth. Additionally, hypoxia-induced metabolic changes can enhance the immunosuppressive properties of Tregs and MDSCs. For example, increased glycolysis and lactate production can promote the expression of immunosuppressive molecules like PD-L1 on cancer cells and immune cells, further dampening the immune response.[16]

The TME is a critical context in which hypoxia-induced immune suppression is prominently observed. Tumors often outgrow their blood supply, creating regions of low oxygen that are highly immunosuppressive. Hypoxia within the TME promotes the expression of various immunosuppressive factors, including VEGF, adenosine, and transforming growth factor-beta (TGF-β), which collectively inhibit the function of effector immune cells and support the survival of immunosuppressive cells.[17] The hypoxic TME also fosters the formation of a physical barrier through extracellular matrix remodeling, hindering the infiltration and function of anti-tumor immune cells. Consequently, hypoxia within the TME not only supports tumor survival and progression but also poses a significant challenge to immunotherapeutic interventions.[18]

Inhibitors of HIFs, glycolysis, and other metabolic pathways are being explored to restore effective immune responses. Additionally, strategies to modulate the hypoxic TME, such as improving tumor oxygenation or blocking the recruitment and function of Tregs and MDSCs, are under investigation.[26] Understanding the precise mechanisms of hypoxia-induced immune suppression will be crucial for developing these therapeutic strategies and improving outcomes for patients (Table 4.1).

TABLE 4.1
Mechanism to Target Immune Suppression in TME

Mechanism	Description	Immune Cells Affected	Reference
HIF-1α stabilization	Hypoxia-inducible factor 1-alpha (HIF-1α) is stabilized under low oxygen conditions, leading to the transcription of genes that suppress immune responses.	T cells, myeloid cells	19
Adenosine accumulation	Hypoxia leads to the accumulation of extracellular adenosine, which binds to A2A receptors on immune cells, inhibiting their activity.	T cells, NK cells, myeloid cells	20
VEGF production	Hypoxia induces vascular endothelial growth factor (VEGF) production, which can contribute to immune evasion by promoting an immunosuppressive microenvironment.	Dendritic cells, T cells	21
PD-L1 upregulation	Hypoxia can increase the expression of programmed death-ligand 1 (PD-L1) on tumor cells, leading to the inhibition of T-cell activity.	T cells	22
Lactic acid production	Hypoxia induces glycolysis and lactic acid production, which can suppress the function of immune cells such as T cells and NK cells.	T cells, NK cells	23
Recruitment of regulatory T cells (Tregs)	Hypoxic conditions promote the recruitment and function of Tregs, which are known to suppress anti-tumor immune responses.	T cells	24
Myeloid-derived suppressor cells (MDSCs)	Hypoxia promotes the accumulation and activation of MDSCs, which suppress T-cell responses and promote tumor growth.	T cells, myeloid cells	25
Inhibition of dendritic cell maturation	Hypoxia inhibits the maturation of dendritic cells, leading to reduced antigen presentation and weakened immune responses.	Dendritic cells	21
Indoleamine 2,3-dioxygenase (IDO) activity	Hypoxia can induce IDO, which catabolizes tryptophan, leading to immune suppression by inhibiting T cell proliferation.	T cells	25
Increased tumor-associated macrophages (TAMs)	Hypoxia increases the recruitment and polarization of TAMs toward an M2 phenotype, which supports tumor growth and immune suppression.	Macrophages, T cells	8

METABOLIC REPROGRAMMING

Metabolic reprogramming is a critical mechanism by which hypoxia induces immune suppression. Under low oxygen conditions, immune cells shift from oxidative phosphorylation to anaerobic glycolysis to meet their energy demands, resulting in the accumulation of metabolic byproducts that significantly impacts the function and phenotype of various immune cells.[27] Effector T cells and NK cells experience reduced cytotoxicity due to the hypoxia-induced glycolytic shift. This diminished function is partly due to the acidification of the TME caused by lactate accumulation, which impairs the ability to effectively target and kill tumor cells.[28]

Moreover, metabolic alterations brought on by hypoxia amplify the immunosuppressive capabilities of MDSCs and regulatory T cells (Tregs). These cells are very immunosuppressive because they flourish in an environment that is hypoxic and favors glycolysis. Tregs, under hypoxic conditions, increase their expression of immunosuppressive molecules such as Cytotoxic T-lymphocyte associated protein-4 (CTLA-4) and PD-1, which further inhibit effector T-cell function.[29] MDSCs, on the other hand, upregulate the production of reactive oxygen species (ROS) and nitric oxide (NO), which suppress T-cell activation and proliferation.[30]

Apart from these immediate impacts, metabolic reprogramming brought on by hypoxia also affects the synthesis and release of several chemokines and cytokines that inhibit the immune system. HIFs are stabilized by hypoxia and stimulate the transcription of genes related to lactate generation and glycolysis. These metabolic pathways facilitate the release of many substances, including adenosine, TGF-β, and vascular endothelial growth factor (VEGF), all working together to create an immunosuppressive milieu.[11] TGF-β and adenosine further reduce effector immune cell activation and function, strengthening the immunosuppressive environment. The intricate relationship between immunological suppression and metabolic reprogramming emphasizes how difficult it is to stop hypoxia-associated immune evasion in cancer.[31]

ALTERED IMMUNE CELL TRAFFICKING AND FUNCTION

The expression of essential adhesion molecules and chemokines is altered in hypoxic environments, influencing immune cell movement and infiltration. CCL28 is upregulated by HIFs, and this attracts regulatory T cells (Tregs), which inhibit effector immunological responses. The overexpression of CXCR4 in hypoxic tumor and immune cell populations facilitates the recruitment of MDSCs to the hypoxic areas, therefore fostering an immunosuppressive environment.[32] This altered trafficking favors the accumulation of immunosuppressive cells while hindering the infiltration of effector T cells and NK cells that are crucial for anti-tumor immunity.[33]

In addition to altering immune cell trafficking, hypoxia directly impacts the function of infiltrating immune cells. Effector T cells, for instance, experience reduced proliferation and cytokine production under hypoxic conditions. The hypoxia-induced metabolic shift toward glycolysis and the accumulation of lactate create an acidic microenvironment that impairs T cell receptor (TCR) signaling and the cytotoxic function of CD8+ T cells.[34] NK cells exhibit diminished cytotoxic activity and cytokine secretion in hypoxic conditions, weakening their ability to control tumor growth and spread.[35] DCs exposed to hypoxia show impaired antigen presentation and reduced ability to activate T cells.[36]

Hypoxia also fosters the development of an immunosuppressive network within the tissue microenvironment through the induction of various immunomodulatory molecules. HIFs drive the expression of VEGF, adenosine, and TGF-β, which collectively create a hostile environment for effector immune cells.[10] VEGF, for instance, not only promotes angiogenesis but also modulates the endothelial barrier, reducing the extravasation of effector T cells into the tumor tissue. Adenosine, produced in large amounts under hypoxia, binds to its receptors on immune cells, inhibiting their function and promoting the development of Tregs. TGF-β further inhibits effector T cell and NK cell activity while promoting the differentiation and maintenance of Tregs and MDSCs.[37]

REGULATORY IMMUNE CELLS

The regulatory T cells and MDSCs play pivotal roles in immune suppression. Under hypoxic conditions, Tregs are recruited to hypoxic regions to undergo enhanced proliferation and activation. This process is driven by HIFs, particularly HIF-1α, which upregulate the expression of FOXP3, a transcription factor critical for Treg development and function.[38] The increased presence of Tregs in hypoxic areas contributes to an immunosuppressive microenvironment by secreting high levels of immunosuppressive cytokines such as TGF-β and interleukin-10 (IL-10). These cytokines inhibit the activation and proliferation of effector T cells, dampening the overall immune response against tumors.[39]

Another critical factor in the hypoxia-induced regulation of the immune system is MDSCs. Through stabilizing HIF-1α, which triggers the production of several proteins that enhance MDSC survival and function, hypoxia encourages the accumulation and activation of MDSCs.[40] Multiple mechanisms, such as the generation of ROS, NO, and arginase-1, are employed by MDSCs to exert their immunosuppressive effects. These processes collectively impede T-cell function and proliferation. Additionally, MDSCs produce high levels of immunosuppressive cytokines like TGF-β and IL-10, further contributing to the suppression of effector immune responses.[36,41]

The coexistence and function of Tregs and MDSCs in hypoxic environments pose a strong obstacle to efficient anti-tumor immunity. To strengthen their immunosuppressive properties, Tregs and MDSCs interact with one another and other elements of the TME.[42] The immunosuppressive effects in hypoxic areas are amplified by this synergistic interaction, which makes it difficult for the immune system to generate a robust anti-tumor response. A viable therapeutic strategy to combat hypoxia-induced immune suppression and boost the effectiveness of cancer immunotherapies is to target these regulatory immune cells and the manner they interact.[43]

VASCULAR ABNORMALITIES IN HYPOXIC TUMORS

Under low oxygen conditions, HIFs induce the expression of VEGF and other pro-angiogenic factors, prompting the rapid and disorganized growth of new blood vessels.[21] These vessels are structurally and functionally abnormal, characterized by irregular shapes, disorganized architecture, and increased permeability. The resultant leaky vasculature not only fails to provide adequate oxygen and nutrients but also creates regions of persistent hypoxia within the tumor. This abnormal vascular network impedes the efficient delivery of immune cells to the tumor site, thereby limiting the effectiveness of anti-tumor immune responses.[13]

The impaired immune cell infiltration due to vascular abnormalities significantly contributes to the immune suppression observed in hypoxic tumors. The disorganized and dysfunctional blood vessels hinder the extravasation of effector immune cells, CTLs and NK cells, into the TME.[6] Even when immune cells manage to infiltrate, the chaotic blood flow and high interstitial fluid pressure within the tumor stroma can restrict their movement and reduce their ability to locate and eliminate tumor cells.[18] The poor vascularization also hampers the delivery of therapeutic agents, including immunotherapies, reducing their efficacy.[44]

Moreover, the abnormal vasculature fosters a hostile environment for effective immune responses by promoting the secretion of immunosuppressive factors. Hypoxia and the resulting vascular abnormalities increase the production of VEGF, which not only stimulates angiogenesis but also has direct immunosuppressive effects. VEGF can inhibit the maturation and function of DCs, essential for antigen presentation and T-cell activation.[45] VEGF and other hypoxia-induced factors, such as adenosine and TGF-β, create an immunosuppressive milieu by promoting the recruitment and activation of Tregs and MDSCs. These cells secrete additional immunosuppressive cytokines, perpetuating a cycle of immune evasion.[44]

TARGETING HYPOXIA TO ENHANCE IMMUNE RESPONSES

Targeting hypoxia is a strategic approach to enhancing anti-tumor immunity by addressing the factors that limit immune cell effectiveness in the TME. Hypoxia, a common feature in tumors, drives the expression of immunosuppressive factors and creates barriers that hinder immune cell infiltration and function.[40] By targeting hypoxia, such as through inhibiting HIFs or normalizing the abnormal tumor vasculature, we can mitigate these suppressive effects and improve the immune system's ability to combat cancer.

Key strategies include using anti-angiogenic therapies to correct the dysfunctional blood vessels in tumors, which enhances oxygen delivery and allows for better immune cell infiltration.[46] Additionally, combining these approaches with ICIs or other immunotherapies can further amplify the anti-tumor response.[14]

HIF INHIBITORS TO TARGET HYPOXIA

Small molecule inhibitors targeting HIFs, specifically HIF-1α and HIF-2α, are emerging as promising tools to combat hypoxia-induced immunosuppression in tumors[37] (Table 4.2). HIFs are crucial regulators of the cellular response to low oxygen levels, orchestrating a range of adaptive mechanisms that enable tumor survival and growth under hypoxic conditions. By stabilizing HIF-1α and HIF-2α, hypoxia drives the expression of genes involved in angiogenesis, metabolic reprogramming, and immunosuppression.[5]

HIF inhibitors work by interfering with the stabilization and activity of HIF-1α and HIF-2α, thus preventing the transcription of hypoxia-responsive genes that promote tumor progression and immune evasion.[4] For instance, by inhibiting HIF activity, these agents can reduce the expression of VEGF, leading to the normalization of abnormal, leaky blood vessels within the tumor. This vascular normalization not only improves oxygenation but also facilitates the infiltration of effector immune cells, such as CTLs and NK cells, into the tumor.[47] Enhanced immune cell infiltration, in turn, boosts the immune system's ability to target and destroy cancer cells.

TABLE 4.2
Various HIF Inhibitors to Target Hypoxia

HIF Inhibitor	Mechanism of Action	Targeted HIF Subunit	Clinical/Preclinical Status	Reference
Acriflavine	Directly binds to HIF-1α and prevents the dimerization of HIF-1α with HIF-1β, inhibiting HIF transcriptional activity	HIF-1α	Preclinical	48
PT2385	Allosterically inhibits the HIF-2α-ARNT (HIF-2β) interaction, specifically targeting HIF-2α	HIF-2α	Phase 1/2 clinical trials	49
PT2977 (Belzutifan)	Selectively inhibits HIF-2α by disrupting HIF-2α-ARNT dimerization	HIF-2α	FDA-Approved (2021)	50
YC-1	Inhibits HIF-1α by promoting its degradation and suppressing HIF-1 transcriptional activity	HIF-1α	Preclinical	51
PX-478	Inhibits HIF-1α expression and activity, possibly by inhibiting translation and promoting degradation	HIF-1α	Phase 1 clinical trials	52
EZN-2208	A pegylated SN38 (topoisomerase I inhibitor) conjugate that downregulates HIF-1α and shows anti-tumor activity	HIF-1α	Phase 1/2 clinical trials	53
FG-4592 (Roxadustat)	Inhibits prolyl hydroxylase enzymes (PHDs), preventing HIF-α degradation and stabilizing HIF under normoxia	HIF-1α, HIF-2α	FDA-approved (2021, for anemia)	54
BAY 87-2243	Inhibits mitochondrial complex I, indirectly suppressing HIF-1α activity by reducing cellular oxygen consumption	HIF-1α	Preclinical	55

Additionally, HIF inhibitors can directly restore immune function by modulating the metabolic and immunosuppressive environment of tumors.[8] By inhibiting HIF activity, these agents can reverse the metabolic shifts, reducing lactate production and improving the functionality of immune cells.[27] Moreover, HIF inhibitors can decrease the recruitment and activity of immunosuppressive cells, such as regulatory T cells (Tregs) and MDSCs, further enhancing anti-tumor immunity.[39,56]

NORMALIZING TUMOR VASCULATURE AND ANTI-ANGIOGENIC THERAPIES

Normalizing tumor vasculature through anti-angiogenic therapies, such as VEGF inhibitors, is a critical strategy to counteract the immunosuppressive effects of hypoxia within the TME.[21] Tumors often induce the formation of abnormal, leaky, and dysfunctional blood vessels, driven by high levels of pro-angiogenic factors like VEGF.[45] These aberrant vessels fail to provide adequate oxygen, resulting in persistent hypoxia and creating physical barriers that hinder immune cell infiltration. This vascular normalization improves oxygen delivery and also reduces interstitial fluid pressure, thereby enhancing the penetration and distribution of immune cells within the tumor.[30]

Better oxygen delivery alleviates hypoxia, reducing the stabilization of HIFs and their downstream immunosuppressive effects.[8] As the TME becomes less hypoxic, the metabolic reprogramming of immune cells is reversed, leading to enhanced functionality and cytotoxicity of effector T cells and NK cells.[57] Moreover, normalized blood vessels facilitate efficient trafficking and infiltration of these immune cells into the tumor cells.[35] This improved immune cell access is crucial for the effectiveness of immunotherapies, as it ensures that therapeutic agents and immune cells can reach and act on their targets within the tumor (Figure 4.3).

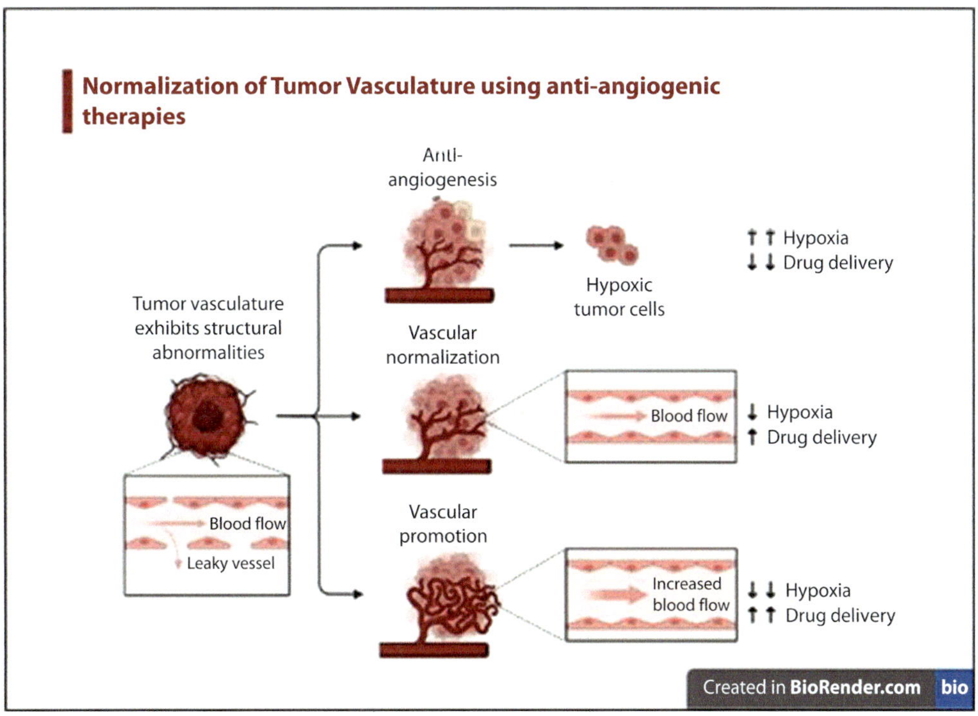

FIGURE 4.3 Normalization of tumor vasculature using anti-angiogenic therapies. By inhibiting excessive angiogenesis, these therapies reduce abnormal vessel formation, improving oxygen and drug delivery. The figure illustrates the transition from disorganized, leaky blood vessels to more normalized and efficient vasculature, enhancing the therapeutic response and reducing tumor hypoxia.

Combining anti-angiogenic therapies with ICIs has shown synergistic effects in preclinical and clinical studies. ICIs, such as anti-PD-1 and anti-CTLA-4 antibodies, work by blocking inhibitory signals that prevent immune cells from attacking tumor cells.[58] When used alongside VEGF inhibitors, the normalization of tumor vasculature enhances the infiltration and activity of immune cells, thereby amplifying the anti-tumor effects of checkpoint blockade.[3]

METABOLIC MODULATION FOR TARGETING HYPOXIA

Hypoxia drives tumor cells to switch from oxidative phosphorylation to glycolysis, a phenomenon known as the Warburg effect, leading to the excessive production of lactate and acidification of the TME.[33] This metabolic reprogramming not only supports tumor growth and survival but also creates an immunosuppressive environment that impairs the function of effector immune cells. By targeting key metabolic pathways, such as glycolysis or lactate production, it is possible to reprogram the TME and reduce immunosuppression.[43]

Glycolysis-inhibiting agents such as 2-deoxy-D-glucose (2-DG) reduce the production of lactate and restore a more favorable metabolic environment for immune cells. By blocking glycolysis, these inhibitors decrease the levels of lactate and alleviate the associated acidification of the TME.[32] This reduction in lactate levels enhances the function and proliferation of effector T cells and NK cells, otherwise impaired by the acidic and hypoxic conditions. Moreover, glycolysis inhibitors potentially disrupt the energy supply of tumor cells.[59] The reprogramming of the TME through metabolic modulation thus creates a less hostile and more supportive environment for immune cell activity.[42]

Additionally, targeting lactate production or transport is another effective approach to modulate tumor metabolism and enhance immune responses. Lactate dehydrogenase (LDH) inhibitors, which block the conversion of pyruvate to lactate, can reduce lactate accumulation in the TME.[23] Similarly, agents that inhibit monocarboxylate transporters (MCTs), responsible for lactate export from tumor cells, can prevent lactate-induced immunosuppression.[60] These strategies not only improve the functionality of effector immune cells but also reduce the recruitment and activity of immunosuppressive cells such as regulatory T cells (Tregs) and MDSCs.[25] This integrated approach holds significant potential for improving the efficacy of cancer treatments by overcoming the challenges posed by metabolic reprogramming in the TME.[20]

ROLE OF IMMUNE CHECKPOINT INHIBITORS IN CANCER THERAPY

Modulating immune checkpoints through the use of ICIs has revolutionized cancer therapy by enabling the immune system to more effectively recognize and attack tumor cells. ICIs, such as anti-PD-1 and anti-CTLA-4 antibodies, work by blocking the inhibitory signals that prevent T cells from attacking cancer cells.[16] However, the hypoxic TME often limits the efficacy of ICIs by promoting immune evasion mechanisms. Hypoxia-induced factors, such as HIFs, enhance the expression of immune checkpoint molecules like PD-L1 on tumor cells and immunosuppressive cells, thereby attenuating the effectiveness of ICIs. Combining ICIs with agents that target hypoxia pathways can potentiate anti-tumor immune responses by reversing hypoxia-induced immune evasion.[61]

Targeting hypoxia pathways can enhance the effectiveness of ICIs by normalizing the TME and mitigating the immunosuppressive effects of hypoxia. For example, inhibiting HIF activity or normalizing tumor vasculature with anti-angiogenic therapies can improve oxygenation and reduce the expression of immune checkpoint molecules induced by hypoxia.[20] This normalization process not only alleviates the hypoxic conditions that favor immune evasion but also enhances the infiltration and function of effector T cells within the tumor.[62] By creating a more favorable environment for immune cell activity, these combined therapies can significantly boost the efficacy of ICIs, leading to more robust and sustained anti-tumor responses.

Clinical and preclinical studies have demonstrated the synergistic effects of combining ICIs with agents targeting hypoxia pathways.[63] The combination of VEGF inhibitors with anti-PD-1 therapy suggests alleviating hypoxia and enhancing immune cell infiltration can enhance the therapeutic benefits of ICIs.[43] Additionally, targeting metabolic pathways influenced by hypoxia, such as glycolysis and lactate production, support the immune response by reducing the metabolic barriers to T-cell function. By integrating ICIs with strategies that target the hypoxic TME, it is possible to overcome the limitations imposed by hypoxia-induced immune suppression.[14]

HYPOXIA-ACTIVATED PRODRUGS

Hypoxia-activated prodrugs (HAPs) represent a novel approach to targeting hypoxic tumor regions (Table 4.3). HAPs are designed to remain inactive under normal oxygen conditions but become activated in the low-oxygen environments characteristic of tumors.[64] Once activated, these prodrugs release cytotoxic agents specifically within hypoxic regions, effectively targeting cancer cells that are typically resistant to conventional therapies.[65,66]

HAPs have the ability to directly modulate the TME by reducing the population of hypoxic, treatment-resistant cancer cells. This reduction in hypoxic cells can alleviate the pressure on immune cells and reduce the levels of VEGF and TGF-β.[67] By decreasing the immunosuppressive milieu, HAPs can enhance the activation and effector functions of T cells and other immune cells within the TME. This can be particularly beneficial when combined with other immunotherapies, such as ICIs, as the reduction in hypoxia-induced immune evasion mechanisms can potentiate the efficacy of ICIs.[68]

Moreover, the use of HAPs can synergize with other therapeutic strategies aimed at normalizing the TME.[76] This multi-pronged approach can disrupt the vicious cycle of hypoxia, immunosuppression, and tumor growth, leading to more effective and durable anti-tumor responses. Clinical trials are underway to evaluate the efficacy of HAPs in various cancers. These prodrugs hold significant promise as a complementary strategy to enhance the outcomes of existing immunotherapies and overcome the challenges posed by hypoxia in the TME.[77]

TABLE 4.3
List of Hypoxia-Activated Prodrugs

Prodrug	Mechanism of Action	Target	Reference
Tirapazamine (TPZ)	Selectively activated under hypoxic conditions, generating DNA-damaging radicals	DNA, topoisomerase II	69
TH-302 (evofosfamide)	Activated under hypoxia to release the alkylating agent bromo-isophosphoramide mustard (Br-IPM)	DNA alkylation	70
PR-104	A nitroaromatic prodrug converted to DNA cross-linking agents in hypoxic cells	DNA cross-linking	71
AQ4N (banoxantrone)	Activated to AQ4, a DNA intercalator, under hypoxic conditions, leading to DNA strand breaks	DNA intercalation	72
TH-4000 (tarloxotinib)	Activated under hypoxia to release a potent EGFR tyrosine kinase inhibitor	EGFR inhibition	73
SN30000	A second-generation TPZ analog that generates DNA-damaging radicals in hypoxic cells	DNA, topoisomerase II	74
Apaziquone	A prodrug converted to an active DNA-damaging agent by reductases in hypoxic tumor cells	DNA damage	75

IMMUNOTHERAPY-BASED APPROACHES TO TARGET HYPOXIA

Immunotherapies specifically designed to target hypoxia within the TME are emerging as a promising strategy to enhance anti-tumor immune responses. Hypoxia, a hallmark of solid tumors, creates a challenging environment for immune cells, promoting immunosuppression and aiding in tumor evasion.[78] To counteract these effects, novel immunotherapies are being developed that can either directly target hypoxic areas or modulate the immune system to better function under low-oxygen conditions. These therapies include the use of engineered T cells, vaccines, and checkpoint inhibitors that are optimized to work more effectively in hypoxic environments.[62]

One approach involves engineering T cells, such as CAR-T cells, to express hypoxia-responsive elements or be resistant to the suppressive effects of hypoxia.[79] These modified T cells are designed to retain their cytotoxic function even in low-oxygen conditions, allowing them to effectively target and destroy tumor cells that reside in hypoxic regions of the tumor. Additionally, vaccines targeting antigens expressed preferentially in hypoxic tumor cells can help to elicit a robust immune response specifically against these difficult-to-reach cells (Figure 4.4). By focusing on the unique metabolic and physiological characteristics of hypoxia, these therapies aim to improve the precision and efficacy of the immune response.[80]

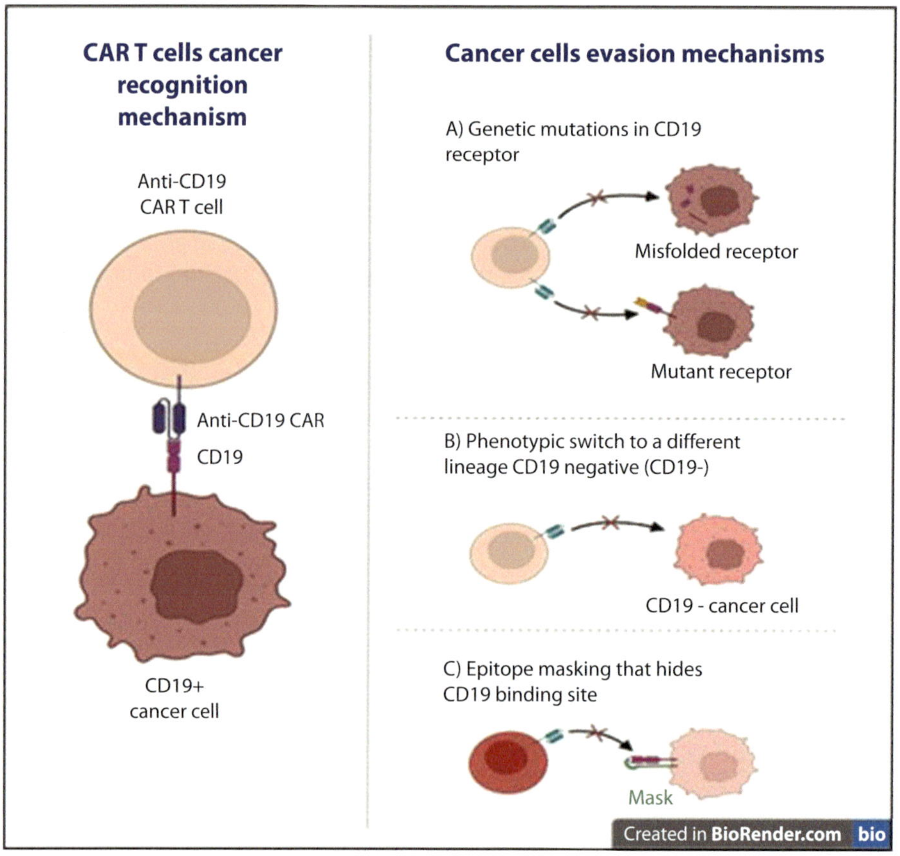

FIGURE 4.4 The CAR-T cell cancer recognition mechanism involves engineered T cells that express chimeric antigen receptors (CARs) on cancer cells. However, hypoxia within the tumor microenvironment can impede CAR-T cell function by promoting immune evasion mechanisms. Hypoxic conditions lead to the upregulation of immune checkpoint molecules and the secretion of immunosuppressive factors by cancer cells, which inhibit CAR-T cell activity. The figure depicts the dual processes of CAR-T cell-mediated cancer cell recognition and the hypoxia-driven evasion tactics employed by the tumor.

Hypoxia-induced factors like HIFs can increase the expression of immune checkpoints such as PD-L1, which helps tumors evade immune detection.[81] By using ICIs in conjunction with treatments that reduce hypoxia, such as anti-angiogenic agents or metabolic modulators, it is possible to lower the expression of these checkpoints and restore immune cell function.[46] This combination approach has shown synergistic effects in preclinical and clinical studies, resulting in improved infiltration and activity of immune cells within the TME.[68] Thus, targeting hypoxia through tailored immunotherapies and combination strategies offers a comprehensive solution to overcome the immunosuppressive barriers presented by hypoxic tumors, enhancing the overall effectiveness of cancer treatment.

NANOPARTICLE-BASED THERAPY TO TARGET HYPOXIA

Perfluorocarbon-based nanoparticles can carry and release oxygen, alleviating hypoxia and enhancing the effectiveness of radiotherapy and chemotherapy. Nanoparticles can deliver hypoxia-activating prodrugs to release their cytotoxic agents upon encountering the low-oxygen environment, sparing normal tissues and targeting hypoxic tumor cells effectively.[82] Nanoparticles deliver genes that encode for anti-hypoxia factors or oxygen-regulating proteins (Table 4.4). By introducing these genes into tumor cells, the hypoxic environment can be altered, making it more conducive to immune cell infiltration and activity.[83]

Zheng et al. (2018) developed calcium peroxide (CaO_2) nanoparticles that generate oxygen upon decomposition.[91] Liu et al. (2017) designed hypoxia-responsive lipid nanoparticles that release their drug cargo specifically in hypoxic conditions.[92,93] These nanoparticles delivered doxorubicin effectively to hypoxic tumor regions, resulting in significant tumor regression. Wang et al. (2019) created nanoparticles encapsulating VEGF inhibitors that normalized tumor vasculature and improved oxygen delivery. This approach reduced hypoxia and enhanced the response to immunotherapy in preclinical models.[94]

By precisely locating the hypoxic microenvironment of pancreatic cancer and irradiating it with multiple wavelength lasers, the nanocomposite PSPP-Au980-D, also known as the "oxygen bomb," can ameliorate hypoxia, produce singlet oxygen, and increase the effectiveness of photodynamic treatment (PDT). MnO_2 and H_2O_2 combine in an acidic environment, producing a significant amount of oxygen to relieve intra-tumoral hypoxia. Cancer-sharing antigens released by fragmented human induced pluripotent stem cells (iPSCs) stimulate robust innate and adaptive immune responses against malignancies, encourage DC maturation, and activate effector T and NK cells.[95]

CLINICAL APPLICATIONS OF STRATEGIES TO TARGET HYPOXIA IMMUNE ESCAPE MECHANISM

Hypoxia-Activated Prodrugs (HAPs)

HAPs are designed to remain inactive under normal oxygen conditions but become activated in the hypoxic regions of tumors. The prodrug TH-302 (evofosfamide) releases a DNA cross-linking agent specifically in low-oxygen conditions.[96] Reduction in hypoxia-induced immune suppression can enhance the efficacy of concurrent immunotherapies such as ICIs. The strategic use of HAPs in combination with ICIs is currently being explored.[97]

Vascular Normalization Strategies

Anti-angiogenic therapies, such as VEGF inhibitors (e.g., bevacizumab), normalize the abnormal tumor vasculature, improving oxygen delivery and reducing hypoxia. Clinical applications of these strategies have shown improved oxygenation into the TME.[98] When combined with ICIs, such as

TABLE 4.4
Overview of Nanoparticle-Based Therapies to Target Hypoxia

Nanoparticle Type	Composition	Mechanism of Action	Therapeutic Application	Clinical/Preclinical Status	Reference
Oxygen-loaded liposomes	Lipid bilayer encapsulating oxygen	Releases oxygen in hypoxic tumor microenvironment, improving radiotherapy efficacy	Radiotherapy enhancement	Preclinical	84
Hypoxia-responsive liposomes	Lipid bilayer with hypoxia-sensitive polymers	Releases encapsulated drugs selectively in hypoxic conditions by degrading in low oxygen environments	Targeted chemotherapy	Preclinical	85
pH sensitive nanogels	Polymers with hypoxia-sensitive linkers	Swell and release drugs in acidic and hypoxic tumor microenvironments	Targeted chemotherapy	Preclinical	85
MnO_2 nanoparticles	Manganese dioxide nanoparticles	Reacts with tumor-generated hydrogen peroxide to produce oxygen, alleviating hypoxia	Combined chemotherapy and PDT	Preclinical	86
$CaCO_3$ nanoparticles	Calcium carbonate nanoparticles	Decomposes in acidic and hypoxic tumor microenvironments to release calcium ions and oxygen	Combined chemotherapy and PDT	Preclinical	87
Poly(lactic-co-glycolic acid) (PLGA) nanoparticles	Biodegradable polymer with encapsulated HAPs	Controlled release of hypoxia-activated prodrugs in hypoxic tumors, increasing local drug concentration	Targeted chemotherapy	Preclinical	88
Upconversion nanoparticles (UCNPs)	Lanthanide-doped nanocrystals	Converts near-infrared light to visible light to activate photodynamic therapy (PDT) in deep hypoxic tissues	Photodynamic therapy	Preclinical	89
Silica-coated gold nanorods	Gold nanorods coated with mesoporous silica	Absorbs near-infrared light and generates heat, improving tumor oxygenation and sensitizing to radiotherapy	Photothermal and radiotherapy	Preclinical	90

anti-PD-1 or anti-CTLA-4 antibodies, this approach has demonstrated enhanced therapeutic efficacy. The vascular normalization not only reduces the immunosuppressive effects of hypoxia but also improves the distribution and penetration of immunotherapeutic agents, making this combination a promising avenue in clinical oncology.[99]

Metabolic Modulation

Agents that inhibit glycolysis, such as 2-DG, and LDH inhibitors, aim to decrease lactate production and normalize the TME.[100,101] Clinical trials are investigating the efficacy of these metabolic modulators in combination with ICIs. By reducing the acidic, immunosuppressive environment, these agents can enhance the function and proliferation of effector immune cells.[46]

Hypoxia-Targeted Immunotherapies

CAR-T cells can be modified to express hypoxia-responsive elements, ensuring that they retain their cytotoxic activity even in low-oxygen environments.[102] Clinical applications of these hypoxia-resistant CAR-T cells are being explored, with the goal of improving their infiltration and persistence in hypoxic tumor regions.[79] Additionally, vaccines targeting antigens specific to hypoxic tumor cells are being developed to elicit a robust immune response against these cells (Figure 4.5).[103]

Challenges and Limitations

Targeting hypoxia-induced immune suppression and immune escape mechanisms offers promising advancements in cancer therapy, but several challenges and limitations must be addressed. These include the complexity and heterogeneity of the TME, limited therapeutic penetration, adaptive resistance mechanisms, systemic toxicity, difficulties in patient selection, and regulatory hurdles.[99]

Complexity of the Tumor Microenvironment

Targeting hypoxia-induced immune suppression presents several obstacles, one of which is the TME's complexity and heterogeneity. It is challenging to create treatments that reliably and

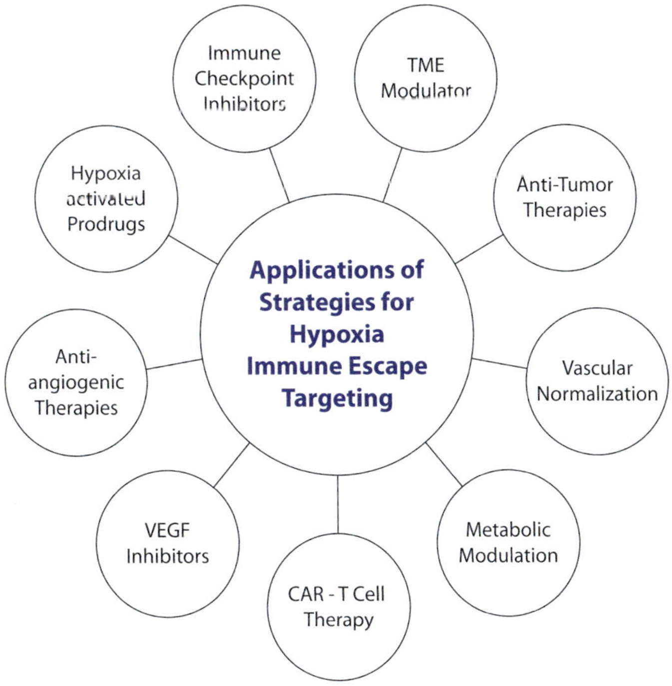

FIGURE 4.5 Illustration depicting various applications of strategies to target hypoxia mediated immune escape mechanism and immune suppression. The applications include hypoxia activated prodrugs, CAR-T therapy, anti-angiogenic therapy, vascular normalization, metabolic modulations, and immune checkpoint inhibitors amongst various others.

successfully target hypoxic areas because of this diversity. In addition, various cell types, including stromal, endothelial, immunological, and cancer cells, are present in the TME and interact intricately with one another. These interactions can contribute to resistance mechanisms that diminish the efficacy of hypoxia-targeting therapies.[28]

LIMITED PENETRATION OF THERAPEUTICS

The hypoxic tumor possesses abnormal and leaky vasculature. Anti-angiogenic therapies aim to normalize these blood vessels, but achieving optimal vascular normalization can be challenging. Over-normalization can lead to reduced blood flow, while under-normalization may not sufficiently improve drug delivery. Additionally, the high interstitial fluid pressure within tumors can further hinder the penetration and distribution of drugs, including HAPs and metabolic modulators.[104]

ADAPTIVE RESISTANCE MECHANISMS

Tumor cells often acquire adaptive resistance to treatment, especially targeting hypoxia and this relaxation of treatment has implications for long-term management of the tumor. Inhibiting HIFs helps in the disruption of the hypoxia signaling pathway but tumor cells can develop alternative mechanisms toward growth and survival. There are also cases where the tumor, with the help of metabolic reprogramming, adapts its energy production capacity and survives the thermodynamic constraints posed by metabolic inhibitors.[105] This plasticity in tumor cells requires combination therapies to pre-emptively address potential resistance mechanisms, but identifying and optimizing such combinations remains a significant challenge.[106]

SYSTEMIC TOXICITY AND SEVERE ADVERSE EFFECTS

Adverse side effects and systemic toxicity may result from targeting hypoxia and associated mechanisms. Anti-angiogenic treatments, such as VEGF inhibitors, may result in thromboembolic events, hypertension, and bleeding. Metabolic inhibitors may have off-target effects on normal cells since they depend on the same metabolic pathways as cancer cells. Balancing the therapeutic benefits with the potential for systemic toxicity requires careful dose optimization and monitoring, complicating the clinical application of these strategies.[107]

PATIENT SELECTION AND BIOMARKER IDENTIFICATION

Identifying the right patient populations who will benefit most from hypoxia-targeting therapies is crucial but challenging. Biomarkers that accurately reflect hypoxia levels and predict response to treatment are still under development.[28] Additionally, the variability in hypoxia levels among different tumor types and even within the same tumor necessitates robust and precise diagnostic tools to guide therapy selection.

REGULATORY AND DEVELOPMENTAL HURDLES

Demonstrating the efficacy and safety of these novel approaches requires extensive preclinical and clinical studies. The complexity of combination therapies, involving multiple agents targeting different aspects of the TME, adds to the regulatory challenges.[63] In addition, strong and accurate diagnostic methods are required for therapy selection to overcome the heterogeneity in hypoxia levels among different tumor types and within the same tumor.

CONCLUSION

There is great promise in optimizing cancer immunotherapy by addressing immune escape mechanisms linked to hypoxia. New age approaches of hypoxia-targeted immunotherapies, vascular normalization, metabolic modulation, and HAPs seek to disrupt the hypoxia-induced mechanisms that promote tumor growth while suppressing deterrence of the immune system. Each of these strategies has its own merits and avenues for promoting better infiltration, function, and efficacy of immune cells in anti-tumor intervention.

HAPs take advantage of the low oxygen levels in the TME to activate prodrugs that release toxic compounds resulting in cytotoxicity toward otherwise non-responsive tumor cells and altering the immunosuppressive milieu. Use of agents like VEGF inhibitors aims to normalize vessels so as to enhance oxygen perfusion and promote the infiltration of immune effector cells into tumors. These strategies have shown some degree of success in clinical trials indicating a likelihood of increased effectiveness in treating cancer with a combination of active immunotherapy with ICIs.

In addition, vaccines and modified T cells that combat hypoxia have been developed to be effective in conditions of low oxygen in the tissue. This effectively counterbalances some of the immune evasion strategies adopted by tumors in this case hypoxia, thereby boosting immunity against tumors.

FUTURE PROSPECTS OF IMMUNOTHERAPY TO TREAT HYPOXIA

Immune cell function can be greatly impacted by hypoxia, especially when it comes to T-cell activation and the growth of regulatory T cells (Tregs), which are immune response suppressors. Preclinical research indicates that immune checkpoint blockade combined with targeting VEGF, a chemical increased in hypoxia, may improve T-cell infiltration into hypoxic tumor areas and bolster the anti-tumor immune response.

Apart from cancer, immunotherapies can also effectively target hypoxia-induced damage in ischemia disorders like heart disease and stroke. Treatments for these illnesses may undergo a revolutionary change if therapies are developed that alter the immune system's reaction to hypoxia by promoting tissue repair processes while reducing inflammation. Hypoxia-driven diseases may be efficiently treated by utilizing bioengineered immune cells that can operate well in low-oxygen situations or by combining immunotherapy with oxygen-modulating drugs.

Tumors undergo metabolic adaptation, become more aggressive, and inhibit anti-tumor immune responses when exposed to hypoxia. HIFs, which control angiogenesis, cell survival, and immunological suppression, are mostly responsible for this. By reversing immune exhaustion and reactivating T-cells, current immunotherapies, which include ICIs (such as anti-PD-1/PD-L1 and anti-CTLA-4 antibodies), are starting to demonstrate efficacy in targeting hypoxic tumors. But T-cell activity is frequently compromised by the hypoxic microenvironment, which reduces the effectiveness of these treatments. In order to improve immune infiltration and response, future initiatives will therefore involve investigating combinations of immunotherapies with medicines that target the HIF pathway or modify the hypoxic habitat. Future therapy approaches for hypoxia-driven disorders could greatly benefit from the integration of immunotherapies with drugs that adjust oxygen levels, such as oxygen carriers or hypoxia-reducing drugs.

REFERENCES

1. Chiang AC, Massagué J. Molecular basis of metastasis. *N Engl J Med*. 2008;359(26):2814–2823. doi: 10.1056/NEJMra0805239.
2. Vaupel P. The role of hypoxia-induced factors in tumor progression. *Oncologist*. 2004;9(S5):10–17. doi: 10.1634/theoncologist.9-90005-10.
3. Niu M, Yi M, Li N, Luo S, Wu K. Predictive biomarkers of anti-PD-1/PD-L1 therapy in NSCLC. *Exp Hematol Oncol*. 2021;10(1):18. doi: 10.1186/s40164-021-00211-8.

4. Abou Khouzam R, Brodaczewska K, Filipiak A, et al. Tumor hypoxia regulates immune escape/invasion: Influence on angiogenesis and potential impact of hypoxic biomarkers on cancer therapies. *Front Immunol*. 2021;11:613114. doi: 10.3389/fimmu.2020.613114.
5. Mangraviti A, Raghavan T, Volpin F, et al. HIF-1α-targeting acriflavine provides long term survival and radiological tumor response in brain cancer therapy. *Sci Rep*. 2017;7(1):14978. doi: 10.1038/s41598-017-14990-w.
6. Chaurasiya S, Warner S. Viroimmunotherapy for colorectal cancer: Clinical studies. *Biomedicines*. 2017;5(1):11. doi: 10.3390/biomedicines5010011.
7. Tirpe AA, Gulei D, Ciortea SM, Crivii C, Berindan-Neagoe I. Hypoxia: Overview on hypoxia-mediated mechanisms with a focus on the role of HIF genes. *Int J Mol Sci*. 2019;20(24):6140. doi: 10.3390/ijms20246140.
8. Poblete JMS, Ballinger MN, Bao S, et al. Macrophage HIF-1α mediates obesity-related adipose tissue dysfunction via interleukin-1 receptor-associated kinase M. *Am J Physiol-Endocrinol Metab*. 2020;318(5):E689–E700. doi: 10.1152/ajpendo.00174.2019.
9. Schito L, Semenza GL. Hypoxia-inducible factors: Master regulators of cancer progression. *Trends Cancer*. 2016;2(12):758–770. doi: 10.1016/j.trecan.2016.10.016.
10. Huang H, Zhong P, Zhu X, et al. Immunotherapy combined with rh-endostatin improved clinical outcomes over immunotherapy plus chemotherapy for second-line treatment of advanced NSCLC. *Front Oncol*. 2023;13:1137224. doi: 10.3389/fonc.2023.1137224.
11. Jain RK. Antiangiogenesis strategies revisited: From starving tumors to alleviating hypoxia. *Cancer Cell*. 2014;26(5):605–622. doi: 10.1016/j.ccell.2014.10.006.
12. Ray SK, Mukherjee S. Interaction among noncoding RNAs, DNA damage reactions, and genomic instability in the hypoxic tumor: Is it therapeutically exploitable practice? *Curr Mol Med*. 2023;23(3):200–215. doi: 10.2174/1566524022666220120123557.
13. Barth S, Edlich F, Berchner-Pfannschmidt U, et al. Hypoxia-inducible factor prolyl-4-hydroxylase PHD2 protein abundance depends on integral membrane anchoring of FKBP38. *J Biol Chem*. 2009;284(34):23046–23058. doi: 10.1074/jbc.M109.032631.
14. Palazon A, Goldrath AW, Nizet V, Johnson RS. HIF transcription factors, inflammation, and immunity. *Immunity*. 2014;41(4):518–528. doi: 10.1016/j.immuni.2014.09.008.
15. Peng S, Wang G, Cheng Z, Guo Z. IRF7 as an immune-related prognostic biomarker and associated with tumor microenvironment in low-grade glioma. *Int J Gen Med*. 2021;14:4381–4393. doi: 10.2147/IJGM.S324307.
16. Abou Khouzam R, Zaarour RF, Brodaczewska K, et al. The effect of hypoxia and hypoxia-associated pathways in the regulation of antitumor response: Friends or foes? *Front Immunol*. 2022;13:828875. doi: 10.3389/fimmu.2022.828875.
17. Ray SK, Mukherjee S. Hyperoxic-hypoxic paradox: Breast cancer microenvironment and an innovative treatment strategy. *Anticancer Agents Med Chem*. 2024;24(10):729–732. doi: 10.2174/0118715206290816240220062545.
18. Ma S, Zhao Y, Lee WC, et al. Hypoxia induces HIF1α-dependent epigenetic vulnerability in triple negative breast cancer to confer immune effector dysfunction and resistance to anti-PD-1 immunotherapy. *Nat Commun*. 2022;13(1):4118. doi: 10.1038/s41467-022-31764-9.
19. Roth S, Cao J, Singh V, et al. Post-injury immunosuppression and secondary infections are caused by an AIM2 inflammasome-driven signaling cascade. *Immunity*. 2021;54(4):648–659.e8. doi: 10.1016/j.immuni.2021.02.004.
20. Leone RD, Emens LA. Targeting adenosine for cancer immunotherapy. *J Immunother Cancer*. 2018;6(1):57. doi: 10.1186/s40425-018-0360-8.
21. Han Z, Dong Y, Lu J, Yang F, Zheng Y, Yang H. Role of hypoxia in inhibiting dendritic cells by VEGF signaling in tumor microenvironments: Mechanism and application. *Am J Cancer Res*. 2021;11(8):3777–3793.
22. Bray MA, Sartain SE, Gollamudi J, Rumbaut RE. Microvascular thrombosis: Experimental and clinical implications. *Transl Res*. 2020;225:105–130. doi: 10.1016/j.trsl.2020.05.006.
23. Mishra D, Banerjee D. Lactate dehydrogenases as metabolic links between tumor and stroma in the tumor microenvironment. *Cancers*. 2019;11(6):750. doi: 10.3390/cancers11060750.
24. Lin YH, Duong HG, Limary AE, et al. Small intestine and colon tissue-resident memory CD8+ T cells exhibit molecular heterogeneity and differential dependence on Eomes. *Immunity*. 2023;56(1):207–223.e8. doi: 10.1016/j.immuni.2022.12.007.
25. Zalfa C, Paust S. Natural killer cell interactions with myeloid derived suppressor cells in the tumor microenvironment and implications for cancer immunotherapy. *Front Immunol*. 2021;12:633205. doi: 10.3389/fimmu.2021.633205.

26. Singleton DC, Macann A, Wilson WR. Therapeutic targeting of the hypoxic tumour microenvironment. *Nat Rev Clin Oncol*. 2021;18(12):751–772. doi: 10.1038/s41571-021-00539-4.
27. Paredes F, Williams HC, San Martin A. Metabolic adaptation in hypoxia and cancer. *Cancer Lett*. 2021;502:133–142. doi: 10.1016/j.canlet.2020.12.020.
28. Chen Z, Han F, Du Y, Shi H, Zhou W. Hypoxic microenvironment in cancer: Molecular mechanisms and therapeutic interventions. *Signal Transduct Target Ther*. 2023;8(1):70. doi: 10.1038/s41392-023-01332-8.
29. Semenza GL. Hypoxia-inducible factors in physiology and medicine. *Cell*. 2012;148(3):399–408. doi: 10.1016/j.cell.2012.01.021.
30. Mezzadra R, Sun C, Jae LT, et al. Identification of CMTM6 and CMTM4 as PD-L1 protein regulators. *Nature*. 2017;549(7670):106–110. doi: 10.1038/nature23669.
31. Brehme M, Voisine C, Rolland T, et al. A chaperome subnetwork safeguards proteostasis in aging and neurodegenerative disease. *Cell Rep*. 2014;9(3):1135–1150. doi: 10.1016/j.celrep.2014.09.042.
32. Boehler C, Kleber C, Martini N, et al. Actively controlled release of Dexamethasone from neural microelectrodes in a chronic in vivo study. *Biomaterials*. 2017;129:176–187. doi: 10.1016/j.biomaterials.2017.03.019.
33. Riera-Domingo C, Audigé A, Granja S, et al. Immunity, hypoxia, and metabolism–the Ménage à trois of cancer: Implications for immunotherapy. *Physiol Rev*. 2020;100(1):1–102. doi: 10.1152/physrev.00018.2019.
34. Ray SK, Mukherjee S. Imitating hypoxia and tumor microenvironment with immune evasion by employing three dimensional *in vitro* cellular models: Impressive tool in drug discovery. *Recent Patents Anticancer Drug Discov*. 2022;17(1):80–91. doi: 10.2174/1574892816666210728115605.
35. Labiano S, Palazón A, Bolaños E, et al. Hypoxia-induced soluble CD137 in malignant cells blocks CD137L-costimulation as an immune escape mechanism. *OncoImmunology*. 2016;5(1):e1062967. doi: 10.1080/2162402X.2015.1062967.
36. Hatfield SM, Kjaergaard J, Lukashev D, et al. Immunological mechanisms of the antitumor effects of supplemental oxygenation. *Sci Transl Med*. 2015;7(277). doi: 10.1126/scitranslmed.aaa1260.
37. Ou ZL, Luo Z, Wei W, Liang S, Gao TL, Lu YB. Hypoxia-induced shedding of MICA and HIF1A-mediated immune escape of pancreatic cancer cells from NK cells: Role of circ_0000977/miR-153 axis. *RNA Biol*. 2019;16(11):1592–1603. doi: 10.1080/15476286.2019.1649585.
38. Duan S, Guo W, Xu Z, et al. Natural killer group 2D receptor and its ligands in cancer immune escape. *Mol Cancer*. 2019;18(1):29. doi: 10.1186/s12943-019-0956-8.
39. Liang B, Deng L, Zhou X. Targeting hypoxia-related metabolism molecules: How to improve tumour immune and clinical treatment? *Biomed Pharmacother*. 2022;156:113917. doi: 10.1016/j.biopha.2022.113917.
40. Luan M, Si H. Novel hypoxia features with appealing implications in discriminating the prognosis, immune escape and drug responses of 947 hepatocellular carcinoma patients. *Transl Cancer Res*. 2022;11(7):2097–2121. doi: 10.21037/tcr-22-253.
41. Wang B, Zhao Q, Zhang Y, et al. Targeting hypoxia in the tumor microenvironment: A potential strategy to improve cancer immunotherapy. *J Exp Clin Cancer Res*. 2021;40(1):24. doi: 10.1186/s13046-020-01820-7.
42. Rankin EB, Giaccia AJ. Hypoxic control of metastasis. *Science*. 2016;352(6282):175–180. doi: 10.1126/science.aaf4405.
43. Musleh Ud Din S, Streit SG, Huynh BT, Hana C, Abraham AN, Hussein A. Therapeutic targeting of hypoxia-inducible factors in cancer. *Int J Mol Sci*. 2024;25(4):2060. doi: 10.3390/ijms25042060.
44. Du S, Xiong H, Xu C, Lu Y, Yao J. Attempts to strengthen and simplify the tumor vascular normalization strategy using tumor vessel normalization promoting nanomedicines. *Biomater Sci*. 2019;7(3):1147–1160. doi: 10.1039/C8BM01350K.
45. LaValley DJ, Zanotelli MR, Bordeleau F, Wang W, Schwager SC, Reinhart-King CA. Matrix stiffness enhances VEGFR-2 internalization, signaling, and proliferation in endothelial cells. *Converg Sci Phys Oncol*. 2017;3(4):044001. doi: 10.1088/2057-1739/aa9263.
46. Wu Q, You L, Nepovimova E, et al. Hypoxia-inducible factors: Master regulators of hypoxic tumor immune escape. *J Hematol OncolJ Hematol Oncol*. 2022;15(1):77. doi: 10.1186/s13045-022-01292-6.
47. Kelly RJ, Rixe O. Axitinib—A selective inhibitor of the vascular endothelial growth factor (VEGF) receptor. *Target Oncol*. 2009;4(4):297–305. doi: 10.1007/s11523-009-0126-9.
48. Martí-Díaz R, Montenegro MF, Cabezas-Herrera J, Goding CR, Rodríguez-López JN, Sánchez-del-Campo L. Acriflavine, a potent inhibitor of HIF-1α, disturbs glucose metabolism and suppresses ATF4-protective pathways in melanoma under non-hypoxic conditions. *Cancers*. 2020;13(1):102. doi: 10.3390/cancers13010102.
49. Xie C, Gao X, Sun D, et al. Metabolic profiling of the novel hypoxia-inducible factor 2α inhibitor PT2385 in vivo and in vitro. *Drug Metab Dispos*. 2018;46(4):336–345. doi: 10.1124/dmd.117.079723.

50. Jonasch E, Donskov F, Iliopoulos O, et al. Belzutifan for renal cell carcinoma in von Hippel–Lindau disease. *N Engl J Med*. 2021;385(22):2036–2046. doi: 10.1056/NEJMoa2103425.
51. Sun HL, Liu YN, Huang YT, et al. YC-1 inhibits HIF-1 expression in prostate cancer cells: Contribution of Akt/NF-κB signaling to HIF-1α accumulation during hypoxia. *Oncogene*. 2007;26(27):3941–3951. doi: 10.1038/sj.onc.1210169.
52. Villa-Roel N, Ryu K, Gu L, et al. Hypoxia inducible factor 1α inhibitor PX-478 reduces atherosclerosis in mice. *Atherosclerosis*. 2022;344:20–30. doi: 10.1016/j.atherosclerosis.2022.01.002.
53. Valsecchi R, Coltella N, Magliulo D, et al. EZN-2208 treatment suppresses chronic lymphocytic leukaemia by interfering with environmental protection and increases response to fludarabine. *Open Biol*. 2020;10(5):190262. doi: 10.1098/rsob.190262.
54. Zhu X, Jiang L, Wei X, Long M, Du Y. Roxadustat: Not just for anemia. *Front Pharmacol*. 2022;13:971795. doi: 10.3389/fphar.2022.971795.
55. Ellinghaus P, Heisler I, Unterschemmann K, et al. BAY 87-2243, a highly potent and selective inhibitor of hypoxia-induced gene activation has antitumor activities by inhibition of mitochondrial complex I. *Cancer Med*. 2013;2(5):611–624. doi: 10.1002/cam4.112.
56. Fan P, Zhang N, Candi E, et al. Alleviating hypoxia to improve cancer immunotherapy. *Oncogene*. 2023;42(49):3591–3604. doi: 10.1038/s41388-023-02869-2.
57. Ou Z, Lu Y, Xu D, Luo Z. Hypoxia mediates immune escape of pancreatic cancer cells by affecting miR-1275/AXIN2 in natural killer cells. *Front Immunol*. 2023;14:1271603. doi: 10.3389/fimmu.2023.1271603.
58. Mukherjee S, Ray SK. Targeting tumor hypoxia and hypoxia-inducible factors (HIFs) for the treatment of cancer – A story of transcription factors with novel approach in molecular medicine. *Curr Mol Med*. 2022;22(4):285–286. doi: 10.2174/1566524022204220325161921.
59. Zhang W, Zhang Q, Yang N, et al. Crosstalk between IL-15Rα+ tumor-associated macrophages and breast cancer cells reduces CD8+ T cell recruitment. *Cancer Commun*. 2022;42(6):536–557. doi: 10.1002/cac2.12311.
60. Valvona CJ, Fillmore HL, Nunn PB, Pilkington GJ. The regulation and function of lactate dehydrogenase a: Therapeutic potential in brain tumor. *Brain Pathol*. 2016;26(1):3–17. doi: 10.1111/bpa.12299.
61. Choonoo G, Blucher AS, Higgins S, et al. Illuminating biological pathways for drug targeting in head and neck squamous cell carcinoma. *PLOS ONE*. 2019;14(10):e0223639. doi: 10.1371/journal.pone.0223639.
62. Iorgulescu JB, Braun D, Oliveira G, Keskin DB, Wu CJ. Acquired mechanisms of immune escape in cancer following immunotherapy. *Genome Med*. 2018;10(1):87. doi: 10.1186/s13073-018-0598-2.
63. Huang M, Yang S, Tai WCS, et al. Bioinformatics identification of regulatory genes and mechanism related to hypoxia-induced PD-L1 inhibitor resistance in hepatocellular carcinoma. *Int J Mol Sci*. 2023;24(10):8720. doi: 10.3390/ijms24108720.
64. Mathur S, Chen S, Rejniak KA. Exploring chronic and transient tumor hypoxia for predicting the efficacy of hypoxia-activated pro-drugs. *npj Syst Biol Appl*. 2024;10(1):1. doi: 10.1038/s41540-023-00327-z.
65. Baran N, Konopleva M. Molecular pathways: Hypoxia-activated prodrugs in cancer therapy. *Clin Cancer Res*. 2017;23(10):2382–2390. doi: 10.1158/1078-0432.CCR-16-0895.
66. Petrova V, Annicchiarico-Petruzzelli M, Melino G, Amelio I. The hypoxic tumour microenvironment. *Oncogenesis*. 2018;7(1):10. doi: 10.1038/s41389-017-0011-9.
67. Phillips RM. Targeting the hypoxic fraction of tumours using hypoxia-activated prodrugs. *Cancer Chemother Pharmacol*. 2016;77(3):441–457. doi: 10.1007/s00280-015-2920-7.
68. Wen Q, Han T, Wang Z, Jiang S. Role and mechanism of programmed death-ligand-1 in hypoxia-induced liver cancer immune escape (review). *Oncol Lett*. Published online February 5, 2020. doi:10.3892/ol.2020.11369.
69. Reddy SB, Williamson SK. Tirapazamine: A novel agent targeting hypoxic tumor cells. *Expert Opin Investig Drugs*. 2009;18(1):77–87. doi: 10.1517/13543780802567250.
70. Brenner AJ, Floyd J, Fichtel L, et al. Phase 2 trial of hypoxia activated evofosfamide (TH302) for treatment of recurrent bevacizumab-refractory glioblastoma. *Sci Rep*. 2021;11(1):2306. doi: 10.1038/s41598-021-81841-0.
71. Konopleva M, Thall PF, Yi CA, et al. Phase I/II study of the hypoxia-activated prodrug PR104 in refractory/relapsed acute myeloid leukemia and acute lymphoblastic leukemia. *Haematologica*. 2015;100(7):927–934. doi: 10.3324/haematol.2014.118455.
72. Mehibel M, Singh S, Cowen RL, Williams KJ, Stratford IJ. Radiation enhances the therapeutic effect of Banoxantrone in hypoxic tumour cells with elevated levels of nitric oxide synthase. *Oncol Rep*. 2016;35(4):1925–1932. doi: 10.3892/or.2016.4555.

73. Estrada-Bernal A, Le AT, Doak AE, et al. Tarloxotinib is a hypoxia-activated pan-her kinase inhibitor active against a broad range of her-family oncogenes. *Clin Cancer Res*. 2021;27(5):1463–1475. doi: 10.1158/1078-0432.CCR-20-3555.
74. Mao X, McManaway S, Jaiswal JK, et al. An agent-based model for drug-radiation interactions in the tumour microenvironment: Hypoxia-activated prodrug SN30000 in multicellular tumour spheroids. *PLOS Comput Biol*. 2018;14(10):e1006469. doi: 10.1371/journal.pcbi.1006469.
75. Phillips RM, Loadman PM, Reddy G. Inactivation of apaziquone by haematuria: Implications for the design of phase III clinical trials against non-muscle invasive bladder cancer. *Cancer Chemother Pharmacol*. 2019;83(6):1183–1189. doi: 10.1007/s00280-019-03812-7.
76. Smith PJ, McKeown SR, Patterson LH. Targeting DNA topoisomerase IIα (TOP2A) in the hypoxic tumour microenvironment using unidirectional hypoxia-activated prodrugs (uHAPs). *IUBMB Life*. 2023;75(1):40–54. doi: 10.1002/iub.2619.
77. Hunter FW, Wouters BG, Wilson WR. Hypoxia-activated prodrugs: Paths forward in the era of personalised medicine. *Br J Cancer*. 2016;114(10):1071–1077. doi: 10.1038/bjc.2016.79.
78. Iyer S, Radwan AE, Hafezi-Moghadam A, Malyala P, Amiji M. Long-acting intraocular delivery strategies for biological therapy of age-related macular degeneration. *J Controlled Release*. 2019;296: 140–149. doi: 10.1016/j.jconrel.2019.01.007.
79. Feldman L, Brown C, Badie B. Chimeric antigen receptor (CAR) T cell therapy for glioblastoma. *NeuroMolecular Med*. 2022;24(1):35–40. doi: 10.1007/s12017-021-08689-5.
80. Sharma A, Arambula JF, Koo S, et al. Hypoxia-targeted drug delivery. *Chem Soc Rev*. 2019;48(3): 771–813. doi: 10.1039/c8cs00304a.
81. Bui BP, Nguyen PL, Lee K, Cho J. Hypoxia-inducible factor-1: A novel therapeutic target for the management of cancer, drug resistance, and cancer-related pain. *Cancers*. 2022;14(24):6054. doi: 10.3390/cancers14246054.
82. Gavas S, Quazi S, Karpiński TM. Nanoparticles for cancer therapy: Current progress and challenges. *Nanoscale Res Lett*. 2021;16(1):173. doi: 10.1186/s11671-021-03628-6.
83. Carvalho A, Fernandes AR, Baptista PV. Nanoparticles as delivery systems in cancer therapy. In: *Applications of Targeted Nano Drugs and Delivery Systems*. Elsevier; 2019:257–295. doi: 10.1016/B978-0-12-814029-1.00010-7.
84. Deng W, Chen W, Clement S, et al. Controlled gene and drug release from a liposomal delivery platform triggered by X-ray radiation. *Nat Commun*. 2018;9(1):2713. doi: 10.1038/s41467-018-05118-3.
85. Xia Y, Duan S, Han C, Jing C, Xiao Z, Li C. Hypoxia-responsive nanomaterials for tumor imaging and therapy. *Front Oncol*. 2022;12:1089446. doi: 10.3389/fonc.2022.1089446.
86. Murphy DA, Cheng H, Yang T, Yan X, Adjei IM. Reversing hypoxia with plga-encapsulated manganese dioxide nanoparticles improves natural killer cell response to tumor spheroids. *Mol Pharm*. 2021;18(8):2935–2946. doi: 10.1021/acs.molpharmaceut.1c00085.
87. Zhang Y, Dong Z, Hao Y, et al. Synthesis of fluorinated $CaCO_3$-based oxygen-supplying nanophotosensitizers to potentiate photodynamic immunotherapy by reversing tumor hypoxia and immunosuppression. *Nano Res*. 2023;16(7):9815–9825. doi: 10.1007/s12274-023-5698-7.
88. Ferreira LAB, Garcia-Fossa F, Radaic A, Durán N, Fávaro WJ, De Jesus MB. Biogenic silver nanoparticles: In vitro and in vivo antitumor activity in bladder cancer. *Eur J Pharm Biopharm*. 2020;151: 162–170. doi: 10.1016/j.ejpb.2020.04.012.
89. Du K, Feng J, Gao X, Zhang H. Nanocomposites based on lanthanide-doped upconversion nanoparticles: Diverse designs and applications. *Light Sci Appl*. 2022;11(1):222. doi: 10.1038/s41377-022-00871-z.
90. Trayford C, Crosbie D, Rademakers T, et al. Mesoporous silica-coated gold nanoparticles for multimodal imaging and reactive oxygen species sensing of stem cells. *ACS Appl Nano Mater*. 2022;5(3):3237–3251. doi: 10.1021/acsanm.1c03640.
91. Zheng D, Li B, Xu L, et al. Normalizing tumor microenvironment based on photosynthetic abiotic/biotic nanoparticles. *ACS Nano*. 2018;12(6):6218–6227. doi: 10.1021/acsnano.8b02977.
92. Liu C, Wu T, Liu C, et al. Self-supplying O_2 through the catalase-like activity of gold nanoclusters for photodynamic therapy against hypoxic cancer cells. *Small*. 2017;13(26):1700278. doi: 10.1002/smll.201700278.
93. Liu J, nan, Bu W, Shi J. Chemical design and synthesis of functionalized probes for imaging and treating tumor hypoxia. *Chem Rev*. 2017;117(9):6160–6224. doi: 10.1021/acs.chemrev.6b00525.
94. Wang W, Cheng Y, Yu P, et al. Perfluorocarbon regulates the intratumoural environment to enhance hypoxia-based agent efficacy. *Nat Commun*. 2019;10(1):1580. doi: 10.1038/s41467-019-09389-2.

95. Yang XY, Lu YF, Xu JX, Du YZ, Yu RS. Recent advances in well-designed therapeutic nanosystems for the pancreatic ductal adenocarcinoma treatment dilemma. *Molecules*. 2023;28(3):1506. doi: 10.3390/molecules28031506.
96. Li Y, Zhao L, Li XF. The hypoxia-activated prodrug TH-302: Exploiting hypoxia in cancer therapy. *Front Pharmacol*. 2021;12:636892. doi: 10.3389/fphar.2021.636892.
97. Kishimoto S, Brender JR, Chandramouli GVR, et al. Hypoxia-activated prodrug evofosfamide treatment in pancreatic ductal adenocarcinoma xenografts alters the tumor redox status to potentiate radiotherapy. *Antioxid Redox Signal*. 2021;35(11):904–915. doi: 10.1089/ars.2020.8131.
98. Fukumura D, Kloepper J, Amoozgar Z, Duda DG, Jain RK. Enhancing cancer immunotherapy using antiangiogenics: Opportunities and challenges. *Nat Rev Clin Oncol*. 2018;15(5):325–340. doi: 10.1038/nrclinonc.2018.29.
99. Li DD, Tang YL, Wang X. Challenges and exploration for immunotherapies targeting cold colorectal cancer. *World J Gastrointest Oncol*. 2023;15(1):55–68. doi: 10.4251/wjgo.v15.i1.55.
100. Li J, Eu JQ, Kong LR, et al. Targeting metabolism in cancer cells and the tumour microenvironment for cancer therapy. *Molecules*. 2020;25(20):4831. doi: 10.3390/molecules25204831.
101. Varghese E, Samuel SM, Líšková A, Samec M, Kubatka P, Büsselberg D. Targeting glucose metabolism to overcome resistance to anticancer chemotherapy in breast cancer. *Cancers*. 2020;12(8):2252. doi: 10.3390/cancers12082252.
102. Laskowski TJ, Biederstädt A, Rezvani K. Natural killer cells in antitumour adoptive cell immunotherapy. *Nat Rev Cancer*. 2022;22(10):557–575. doi: 10.1038/s41568-022-00491-0.
103. Fan T, Zhang M, Yang J, Zhu Z, Cao W, Dong C. Therapeutic cancer vaccines: Advancements, challenges, and prospects. *Signal Transduct Target Ther*. 2023;8(1):450. doi: 10.1038/s41392-023-01674-3.
104. Matuszewska K, Pereira M, Petrik D, Lawler J, Petrik J. Normalizing tumor vasculature to reduce hypoxia, enhance perfusion, and optimize therapy uptake. *Cancers*. 2021;13(17):4444. doi: 10.3390/cancers13174444.
105. Liao C, Liu X, Zhang C, Zhang Q. Tumor hypoxia: From basic knowledge to therapeutic implications. *Semin Cancer Biol*. 2023;88:172–186. doi: 10.1016/j.semcancer.2022.12.011.
106. Codony VL, Tavassoli M. Hypoxia-induced therapy resistance: Available hypoxia-targeting strategies and current advances in head and neck cancer. *Transl Oncol*. 2021;14(3):101017. doi: 10.1016/j.tranon.2021.101017.
107. Santorsola M, Capuozzo M, Nasti G, et al. Exploring the spectrum of VEGF inhibitors' toxicities from systemic to intra-vitreal usage in medical practice. *Cancers*. 2024;16(2):350. doi: 10.3390/cancers16020350.

5 Role of Hypoxia in Cancer Stem Cell Characteristics

Zirha Saleem and Sukhes Mukherjee
Department of Biochemistry, All India Institute of Medical Sciences, Bhopal, Madhya Pradesh, India

INTRODUCTION

Twenty-five per cent of deaths in India are caused by cancer, and the number of incidences increases due to population growth, prolonged life expectancy, and an abundance of risk factors including smoking, a lack of activity, and obesity [1]. A common of most tumours is a low level of oxygen, called hypoxia, the severity of which varies between tumour types. It has been shown that the lack of efficient oxygenation within the tumour centre induces hypoxia and hypoxia-related factors, which correlate with tumour progression [2]. Hypoxia is one of the most common features of solid tumours and is a key link in the tumour microenvironment. During hypoxia, tumour cells tend to be more prone to proliferation, metastasis, drug resistance, and poor prognosis [2, 3].

Although hypoxia is one of the important escape mechanisms within the tumour microenvironment, it should be noted that hypoxia generation is a function of tumour growth and it is a physiological effect of fast growth and not enough circulation [4]. The tumour microenvironment's low oxygen levels activate hypoxia-inducible factors (HIFs), which play crucial roles in tumour progression and metastasis [5].

Hypoxia extensively shapes the tumour microenvironment by modulating the transcription of hundreds of genes, which regulate tumorigenesis, angiogenesis, invasion, metastasis, drug resistance, and immune suppression [6]. Hypoxia is a condition characterized by low oxygen levels and is a critical microenvironmental factor that significantly influences the behaviour and properties of cancer stem cells (CSCs) [7]. These cells, which possess the ability to self-renew and differentiate, are implicated in tumour initiation, progression, metastasis, and recurrence [8, 9].

The hypoxic tumour microenvironment fosters the maintenance and triggers the expression of pluripotency factors like KLF4, NANOG, OCT4, and SOX2 and plasticity of CSCs through the activation of HIFs promoting breast CSC (BCSC) specification [9], which regulate a plethora of genes involved in stemness, survival, angiogenesis, and metabolic adaptation [10]. Hypoxia significantly influences the metastatic potential of CSCs by altering cellular behaviour and promoting aggressive traits [6, 11]. Some studies delve into the molecular mechanisms by which hypoxia contributes to the CSC phenotype, highlighting key pathways such as HIF signalling, Notch, Wnt/β-catenin, and PI3K/Akt and discussed how hypoxia-induced metabolic reprogramming and epigenetic modifications enhance CSC resistance to conventional therapies, contributing to the difficulty in eradicating these cells and achieving lasting treatment success [12]. Hypoxia strongly correlates to poor patient survival, therapeutic resistance, and an aggressive tumour phenotype, but the full contribution of hypoxia and the HIFs to tumour biology is an area of active investigation [13]. Hypoxia plays a critical role in the maintenance and development of CSCs, influencing their behaviour and contributing to tumour aggressiveness [12, 13]. The interplay between hypoxia and CSCs is multifaceted,

DOI: 10.1201/9781003477419-5

involving various molecular pathways and mechanisms that promote stemness and resistance to therapies [14].

MECHANISMS OF HYPOXIA IN CANCER STEM CELLS

- *HIF Activation*: Under hypoxic conditions, HIF-1α and HIF-2α are activated, leading to changes in gene expression that enhance cell survival, proliferation, and invasion. HIF-2α, in particular, has been linked to increased stem cell characteristics and aggressive tumour growth [15, 16].
- *Cell Reprogramming*: Hypoxia can induce dedifferentiation of cancer cells into stem-like cells, which express pluripotency markers, thereby enhancing their metastatic potential [16].
- Therapy Resistance: Hypoxic CSCs exhibit resistance to conventional therapies, contributing to poor patient outcomes and increased mortality [17].

BIOLOGICAL PROPERTIES OF CANCER STEM CELLS

Cancer-initiating cells, also known as tumour stem cells, are small subpopulations of cancer cells that have the capacity for excessive self-renewal and tumour development [18]. The idea behind CSC dates back to Julius Friedrich Cohnheim's discovery in the early 1900s that the tissues of teratocarcinoma and embryonic tissue were comparable [19]. Cohnheim used the similarity to support the hypothesis of "embryonic rests." G. Barry Pierce demonstrated in 1964 that when embryonal carcinoma (EC) cells produced from embryonal teratocarcinoma and carcinomas are transplanted into mice, they can produce various differentiated tissues and induce EC [20]. Following this discovery, he explained his observation in terms of the CSC theory and claimed that EC cells possess multipotency [21]. During the 1980s, oncogenes' effects on genomic stability and proliferation received greater attention than their effects on tumour differentiation [21, 22]. It went on until the 1990s because teratocarcinomas, which offered a model for examining the phenomena of differentiation, were viewed by many researchers as a special case with minimal bearing on the study of other malignancies [23]. Research on acute myelogenous leukaemia has sparked a greater interest in learning more about the theory behind CSCs [24]. Tissues like the breast, brain, lung, liver, ovary, and testis have CSCs, albeit it is still unclear where these cells came from.

Many intracellular signal transduction pathways, including the Wnt/β-catenin signalling, Notch signalling, transforming growth factor-β signalling, and Hedgehog signalling, enable these cells to differentiate and have the ability to self-renew [25]. Because they are immune to established treatment approaches that primarily target the majority of tumour cells, they can also play a significant role in developing various malignancies and are a major cause of tumour recurrence and metastasis [26]. The tumour's microenvironment determines tumorigenesis and cell behaviour, and surface markers determine the potency of the markers' self-renewal and propagation [27]. By controlling essential malignant behaviours including invasion, metastasis, and treatment resistance, which are brought on by genetic and epigenetic mechanisms, CSCs contribute to the heterogeneity of tumours [28].

CSC activity is regulated by a variety of extracellular and intracellular variables that can be targeted by cancer-treating medications. Because CSCs are difficult for chemotherapy and radiation to destroy, some residual CSCs may survive after the majority of the tumour has been effectively destroyed by different therapies [29]. This can lead to invasiveness and therapy resistance, which is why CSCs are essential to the progression of cancer and therapy resistance. A thorough understanding of CSC biology is crucial to the development of potent treatments aimed at preventing this illness [30].

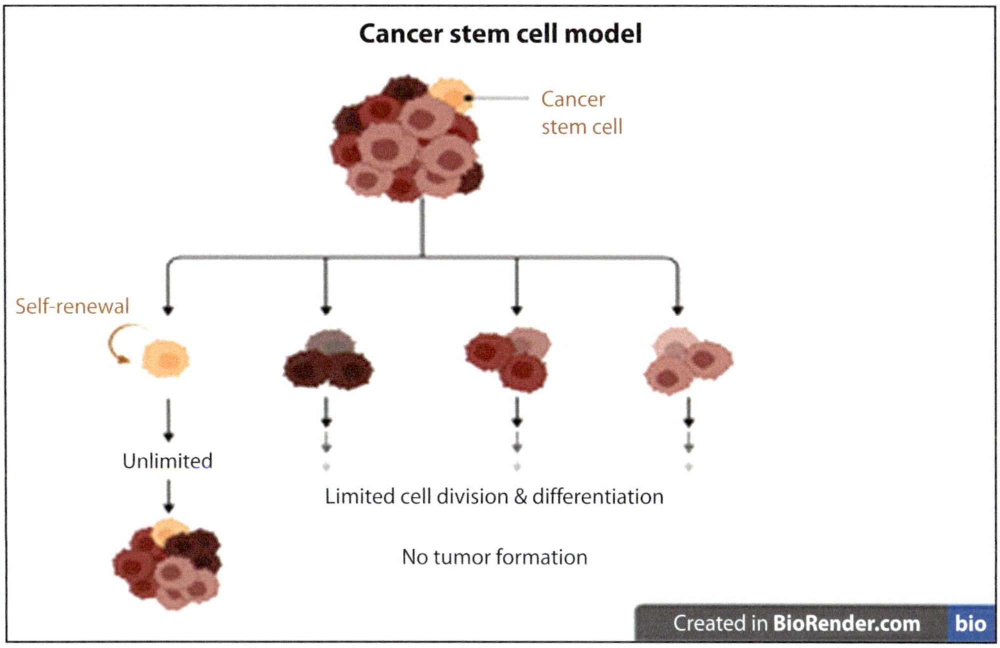

FIGURE 5.1 The self-renewable capacity of cancer stem cells is shown in this image which leads to the unlimited growth of cancer cells promoting tumour growth and diversity.

Around the world, a number of CSC-specific medicines are being developed to increase cancer patients' chances of survival and quality of life, particularly for those with metastatic disease [31]. Their biological features are important targets for novel cancer therapeutics because they greatly contribute to tumour heterogeneity, metastasis, and treatment failure [31, 32] (Figure 5.1).

KEY BIOLOGICAL PROPERTIES OF CANCER STEM CELLS

- *Self-Renewal and Differentiation*: CSCs can self-renew and differentiate into various cell types, promoting tumour growth and diversity [32].
- *Drug Resistance*: CSCs are inherently resistant to chemotherapy and radiation, often leading to tumour recurrence and metastasis [33].
- *Surface Markers*: Common markers like CD44 and CD133 are used to identify and isolate CSCs, aiding in understanding their role in cancer [34].
- *Microenvironment Interactions*: The tumour microenvironment, including stromal and immune cells, supports CSC survival and proliferation, complicating treatment strategies [35].

HYPOXIA AND CANCER STEM CELLS

Cancer incidence, recurrence, metastasis, and resistance to chemotherapy and radiation are all linked to CSCs, a group of cells that resemble stem cells [36]. The presence of CSCs presents a problem for the treatment of tumours, but it can also offer a fresh approach to therapeutic therapy [37]. Though there have been many theories regarding the existence of CSCs, nothing is known for sure. Advanced cancer typically has hypoxia in the tumour microenvironment, which is linked to a poor prognosis and low survival rates [38]. Because of their high plasticity, ability to establish a quiescent state with basal activity, enhanced ability to survive in a stressful tumour environment with reduced oxygen and nutrient levels, and increased resistance to chemotherapy, radiotherapy, and immunotherapy, CSCs can differentiate into a variety of cells that may be found in the tumour. As a result, tumours can escape treatment and recurrence [38, 39].

CSCs play a significant role in managing the hypoxic tumour microenvironment through several mechanisms:

1. *Stemness and Tumorigenicity*: CSCs possess unique properties that allow them to survive and thrive in hypoxic conditions [38, 40]. They can maintain their stemness and tumorigenic capabilities, which contribute to tumour development, metastasis, and recurrence [40]. This resilience makes them less susceptible to conventional therapies that primarily target the bulk tumour population, thereby allowing them to repopulate the tumour after treatment [41].
2. *Adaptation to Hypoxia*: CSCs can adapt to low oxygen levels by altering their metabolic pathways. They often rely on glycolysis for energy production, which is more efficient under hypoxic conditions [42]. This metabolic shift supports their survival and promotes the expression of HIFs, which regulate genes involved in angiogenesis, metabolism, and cell survival [43].
3. *Microenvironmental Interactions*: CSCs can influence their surrounding microenvironment by secreting factors that modify the behaviour of other cells [44]. For instance, they can promote angiogenesis through the release of vascular endothelial growth factor (VEGF), which helps to improve oxygen supply to the tumour [45]. Additionally, CSCs can interact with stromal cells and immune cells, further shaping the tumour microenvironment to their advantage [46].
4. *Therapeutic Resistance*: The presence of CSCs in a hypoxic environment contributes to resistance against chemotherapy, radiotherapy, and immunotherapy [47]. Their ability to survive in low-oxygen conditions allows them to evade the effects of these treatments, leading to tumour recurrence and progression [48].

Hypoxia can prevent embryonic stem cells and progenitor cells from differentiating, according to a number of recent studies [49]. Hypoxic tumour cells exhibit stem cell markers and appear to be poorly differentiated. Tumour cells exhibit greater clonogenic capacity when exposed to hypoxia. Increased tumorigenic potential in vivo is another effect of hypoxia exposure in vitro [50].

Tumour hypoxia may promote the formation of malignant clones by keeping CSCs in their undifferentiated stem cell state, which allows for self-renewal and the continuous accumulation of genetic and epigenetic modifications over an extended period [47]. These intriguing findings support this novel theory. The current understanding of hypoxia and its role in stem cell maintenance is briefly reviewed in this chapter. Research on CSCs is rapidly growing in this area [6].

EFFECT OF CANCER STEM CELLS ON HYPOXIA

CSCs are neoplastic cells that can self-renew, differentiate, and start tumour growth in vivo [25]. They are also referred to as cancer-initiating cells or tumour-propagation cells. It is thought that CSCs are the primary causes of tumour development and treatment resistance [38]. Although several normal stem cell populations have been demonstrated to benefit from hypoxia, its functions

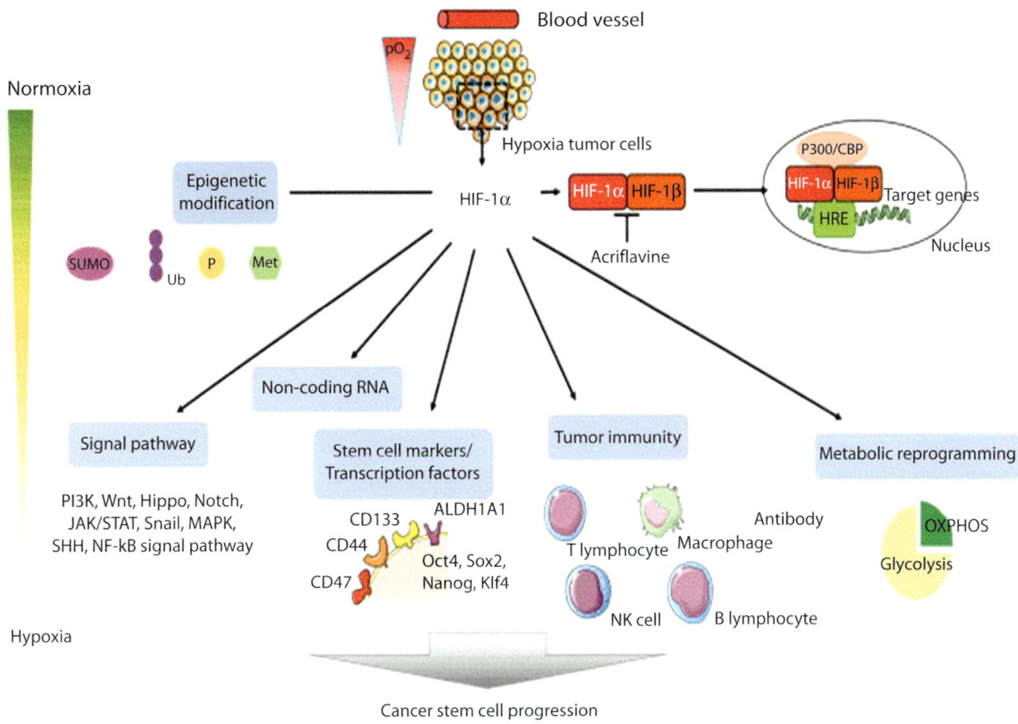

FIGURE 5.2 The induction of various factors such as epigenetic modification, signalling pathways, stem cell markers induction, tumour immunity, and metabolic reprogramming by the activation of hypoxia inducible factor-1 which eventually leads to cancer stem cell progression.

for CSCs are still mainly unclear [51]. There is growing evidence that hypoxia has an impact on CSC upkeep and functions. Within the tumour heterogeneous cell types, CSCs are an undifferentiated stem-like cell fraction that plays a role in cancer start, development, metastasis, treatment resistance, and recurrence [47].

CSCs have characteristics in common with their normal stem cell counterparts in solid tumours and haematological malignancies, such as self-renewal and the ability to differentiate into many cell types [52]. Moreover, CSCs are capable of forming spheres. The definitive universal indicators for CSCs in solid tumours are yet unclear, even though various putative markers for CSCs in haematological malignancies have been proposed [53]. Haematopoietic stem cells, for example, are kept in a hypoxic zone that is separated from the vasculature, which helps to preserve their stem cell characteristics [54]. These characteristics (stem and progenitor qualities referred to as stemness) are lost when oxygen levels rise. Likewise, CSCs tend to localize to hypoxic regions within tumours, which probably favour the preservation the stemness, as well as to generate highly invasive tumours [55] (Figure 5.2).

Through the control of octamer-binding transcription factor 4 (Oct4), sex determining region Y box 2 (SOX2), kruppel-like factor 4 (KLF4), myelocytomatosis oncogene product (Myc), Tir nan Og (NANOG), and polycomb complex protein BMI-1 (BMI1), HIF signalling improves the maintenance of a CSC phenotype [56]. Hypoxia has been shown to trigger EMT and CSC characteristics through HIF signalling. Tumour cells undergo detachment and develop a mesenchymal phenotype during this process. They also exhibit stemness characteristics such as tumorigenesis, lack of differentiation, and enhanced therapeutic resistance [57]. NF-κB, PI3K/Akt, Wnt/β-catenin, Hedgehog, and Notch are comparable signalling pathways that promote hypoxia/HIF-induced EMT and CSC phenotype [58]. Evidence suggests that HIF-1α and HIF-2α play a part in the growth and recurrence of cancer generated by CSC. Thus, it has been shown that Sox2, Nanog, and Oct4 expression are all increased by direct binding of HIF-2α to the HRE found in the promoter regions [59]. CSCs can be identified from other types of cells by expressing certain markers on their surface, like CD133, CD24, and CD44. As a result, HIFs regulate CD133 promoter activity and boost the differentiation of CSCs that express CD133 [60]. A possible tactic to prevent CSC-associated cancer recurrence and chemo-resistance is to target hypoxia-related variables, even if the exact molecular pathways that promote the creation of CSCs by HIFs are not fully understood [61].

HIF ACTIVITY PROMOTES GENERATION OF CANCER STEM CELL

By controlling the transcription of target genes, HIF-1 plays a crucial role in the regulation of CSCs by hypoxia and contributes to tumour development, immunological evasion, metabolic reprogramming, and drug resistance [62]. HIF-1 appears to be crucial, if not essential, for the development and upkeep of CSCs, albeit the precise process is still unknown. The regulation of many signalling pathways, which CSCs use to control stemness in hypoxic and therapeutic environments, is greatly influenced by HIF signalling [63].

Activator of transcription (JAK/STAT), Notch, Hedgehog, Hippo, Wnt (wingless)/β-catenin, Janus-activated kinase/signal transducer, phosphatidylinositol 3-kinase/phosphatase, tensin homolog (PI3K/PTEN), and nuclear factor-kB (NF-kB) pathways are some of these pathways [64]. An increasing amount of research suggests that CSCs depend on HIFs to maintain their phenotypic and function [65] (Figure 5.3).

HIFs induce numerous gene products, including pluripotency-related transcription factors, epithelial-to-mesenchymal transition (EMT) programmers, glycolysis-associated molecules, drug resistance-associated molecules, miRNAs, and VEGF [63, 65].

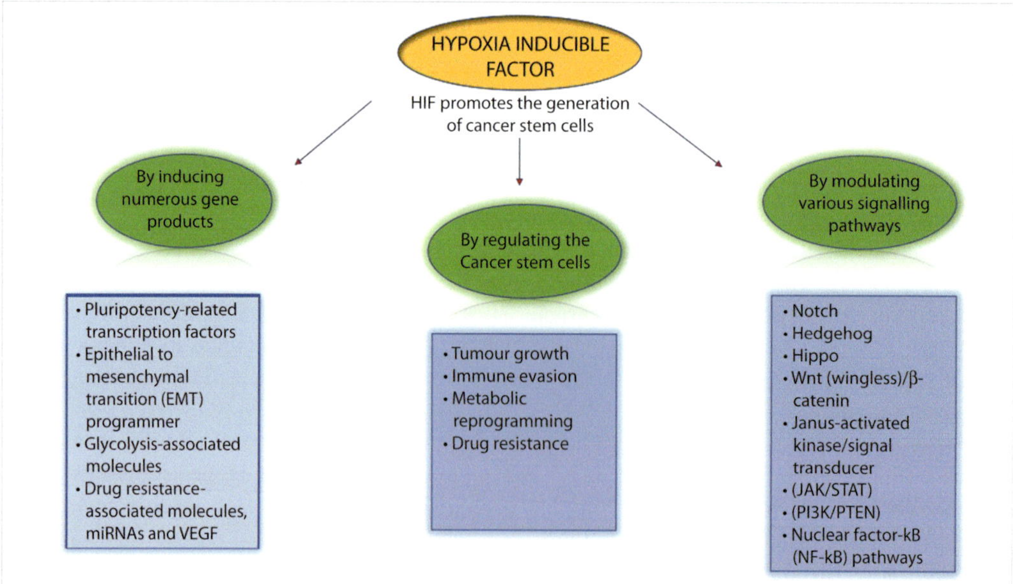

FIGURE 5.3 Role of hypoxia-inducible factor in the generation of cancer stem cell.

ROLE OF HIF IN CANCER STEM CELLS MARKER

Cancer cells are made pluripotent by CSC markers, which are also used to identify subpopulations of CSCs, some of which are linked to metastasis. Research has revealed a connection between HIF-1 and the production of CSC markers [66]. Based on available evidence, HIF-1α has the ability to stimulate the expression of several stem cell markers, including OCT4, SOX2, NANOG, and Krüppel-like factor 4 (KLF4). Furthermore, by preventing the production of markers associated with stem cells, HIF-1α silencing can impede the advancement of cancer [67] (Table 5.1).

TABLE 5.1
Induction of Cancer Stem Cell Markers by the Activation of Hypoxia-Inducible Factor in Different Types of Cancer

S.no.	Type of Cancer	Stem Cell Marker	HIF Subunits	Role of HIF and Markers	References
1.	Breast cancer	CD44/CD24, CD29, CD133, CD200	HIF-1α	A decline in the characteristics of stem cells due to a decrease in the mRNA levels of genes connected to the epithelial-mesenchymal transition.	[68]
2.	Pancreatic cancer	CD44/CD24, CD133, ESA, CXCR4	HIF-2α	Upregulation of these markers under hypoxic conditions is mediated by HIFs, with a longer-lasting effect of HIF-2α.	[69]
3.	Head and neck	CD44, BMI-1	HIF-2α	Hypoxia leads to a selection of genotypes favouring survival and promoting tumour angiogenesis, epithelial-to-mesenchymal transition, invasiveness, and metastasis, as well as suppressing immune reactivity.	[70]
4.	Brain tumour	CD33, CD200	HIF-2α	Hypoxia induces tumour cell invasion, cellular adaptations to hypoxia, and tumour cell radioresistance. In addition, hypoxia limits the efficacy of immunotherapy and hinders antitumour responses.	[71]
5.	Bone cancer	Stro-1, CD105, CD44	HIF-1α	HIF may induce spontaneous metastasis to the bone and promote tumour colonization of bone, in particular in the case of breast cancer dissemination to the bone marrow.	[72]
6.	Colorectal cancer	EpCAM, CD44, CD166, CD133	HIF-1α	HIF-1alpha expression is correlated with tumour invasion, tumour stage, lymphatic invasion, venous invasion, and liver metastasis in colorectal cancer.	[73]
7.	Prostate cancer	CD133, CD44, Integrin 12 b1	HIF-1α	HIF by integrin 12 b1 mediates multiple intracellular processes that drive cellular metabolism and induce proliferation. Dysregulated HIF expression is associated with oncogenic cellular transformation.	[60, 74]
8.	Lung cancer	ALDH	HIF-1α	HIF-1α promotes the expression of ALDH1, identifying the cancer stem cells that exhibit increased tumorigenicity and drug resistance.	[63]
9.	Glioblastoma	CD133	HIF-2α	HIF-2α is overexpressed in CSCs, promoting proliferation and undifferentiated markers like CD133. Production of genes necessary in maintaining the stem-like features. Also stimulates angiogenesis, which contributes to metastasis.	[75]

TABLE 5.2
Cancer Stem Cell Markers and Their Functions

S. No.	Cancer Stem Cell Markers	Functions	Reference
1.	CD44	CD44 is a transmembrane receptor for hyaluronic acid, which is highly expressed in many cancers and regulates cell migration and invasion processes by increasing self-renewal capacity, cell survival, and drug resistance.	[68, 69]
2.	CD133	CD133 is a 5-pass transmembrane glycoprotein, identified as a novel marker for haematopoietic stem/precursor cells and can also be used as a marker for the identification of CSCs in many solid tumours, including hepatocellular carcinoma.	[72, 73]
3.	CD177	CD117, also known as the c-kit receptor, is a transmembrane protein with tyrosine kinase activity that plays a pivotal role in the maintenance and proliferation of haematopoietic stem cells.	[76]
4.	CD24	CD24, a heat-stable antigen, is a surface marker expressed in many tumour types. It has been extensively studied as a cancer stem cell marker in a variety of solid cancers.	[77]
5.	CD33	CD33 is a transmembrane protein that is found on cells of myeloid lineage. It is also intensely expressed on acute myeloid leukaemia progenitor cells but not on normal stem cells.	[78]
6.	CD200	CD200 is a cell surface glycoprotein that has been implicated in a variety of human cancer cells. It has been proposed as a cancer stem cell (CSC) marker in colon cancer and is closely related to tumour immunosuppression.	[78, 79]
7.	EpCAM	Epithelial cell adhesion molecule (EpCAM), also known as CD326 among other names, is a transmembrane glycoprotein mediating Ca^2+-independent homotypic cell-cell adhesion in epithelia. EpCAM is also involved in cell signalling, migration, proliferation, and differentiation.	[80]
8.	Integrin 12 b1	Integrin signalling drives multiple stem cell functions, including tumour initiation, epithelial plasticity, metastatic reactivation, and resistance to oncogene- and immune-targeted therapies.	[81]

Targeting HIF proteins is a compelling approach in the therapy of tumours since they are the master controllers of oxygen homeostasis in hypoxia [63]. Targeting hypoxia and HIF can be accomplished in a number of ways, including by taking advantage of the following: (1) hypoxia-activated prodrugs (HAPs) or drugs; (2) selective targeting of HIFs; and (3) targeting downstream HIF signalling pathways and significant pathways in hypoxic cells (mTOR and UPR) [63] (Table 5.2).

HYPOXIA-MEDIATED RESISTANCE

Radiation, Chemotherapy, and Drug Resistance

Cancer's complexity is matched by the wide range of treatments and strategies available to combat it [82]. These days, treatment management is becoming more individualized and focused, and patients and doctors can discuss immunotherapy, gene therapy, chemotherapy, and radiation [83]. Nevertheless, despite advancements and achievements in cancer treatment, a cure for the disease is still a long way off. Much work has to be done to improve our knowledge of the mechanisms underlying cancer resistance so that patient-specific treatment plans can be developed to maximize cancer eradication. The effectiveness of chimeric antigen receptor (CAR)-T cell immunotherapy is complicated by solid tumour heterogeneity, and only a small percentage of patients respond to immunotherapy [84]. Chemotherapy remains the most widely used anticancer treatment; nonetheless, subpopulations of cancer cells, frequently CSCs, are able to proliferate, survive treatment, and represent a barrier to a disease-free remission. The process of "oxygen fixation," in which free radicals—byproducts of ionizing radiation—react with oxygen molecules inside cells and permanently damage DNA, accounts for the effectiveness of radiation therapy [85, 86]. Nonetheless, this mechanism is less significant in hypoxic cellular settings, where cells are still able to survive [87, 88]. The cytotoxic effects of X- and γ-irradiation are inhibited by low oxygen tension and the death of oxygen radicals, according to early studies made in the 1930s. In hypoxia cells, up to three times the radiation dose is required to have the same cytotoxic effects as in normoxic cells [89].

In addition to cell state (i.e., cell cycle phase), oxygen levels in the target tissue region, and radiation type all affect radiosensitivity. Studies conducted both in vivo and in vitro have demonstrated that greater radiation resistance is a result of both short- and long-term hypoxia [89]. The rise in VEGF brought on by hypoxia aids in angiogenesis, which encourages the recurrence of the illness following radiation therapy [90].

Hypoxia induces drug resistance in cancer cells through multiple mechanisms, the main ones being HIFs and metabolic adaptations. Hypoxia plays a crucial role in these pathways. Patients with cancer have poor treatment outcomes as a result of hypoxia's varied impact [85].

Mechanisms of Drug Resistance

- *HIF Activation*: Hypoxia activates HIF-1, which alters drug target expression and metabolic pathways, enhancing cancer cell survival and resistance to therapies like chemotherapy and radiotherapy [91].
- *Mitochondrial Adaptations*: In colorectal cancer, hypoxia induces the expression of mitochondrial glutathione transporters, which are crucial for maintaining redox balance and contribute to resistance against drugs like oxaliplatin and 5-fluorouracil [92].
- *DNA Damage Prevention*: Hypoxia can prevent drug-induced DNA damage, as seen with etoposide, by downregulating topoisomerase IIα, thereby enhancing cell survival [6].

Although hypoxia plays a significant role in the development of drug resistance, focusing on hypoxic areas inside tumours may present novel therapeutic approaches to address this issue and enhance patient outcomes, and cells that cause tumours. According to Jogi et al., hypoxic cells in neuroblastoma (NB) take on an immature character, which is consistent with this [93, 94]. Within the TME, hypoxic areas appear to harbour cells with phenotypes similar to stem cells, which are less developed and more invasive than oxygenated parts [94].

Mechanisms of CSC Resistance Induced by Hypoxia

Hypoxia induces resistance in CSCs through a number of mechanisms, the main ones being changes in cellular pathways and HIFs. Developing tailored medicines requires an understanding of these pathways [62].

HIF-Dependent Mechanisms

- *HIF Activation*: Hypoxia activates HIF-1, which enhances the expression of genes that promote survival and resistance to chemotherapy, such as those involved in DNA repair and metabolism. HIF-1, participates in tumour growth, immune evasion, metabolic reprogramming, and drug resistance by regulating the transcription of target genes [95]. HIF-1 seems to play an important, or even core, role in the generation and maintenance of CSCs [96]. HIF-1α is a hypoxia-inducible transcription factor that contains two

transactivation domains (C-TAD and N-TAD). C-TAD can interact with co-activators such as CREB binding protein (CBP)/p300 to regulate the transcription of HIF-1α target genes [97]. N-TAD participates in stabilizing HIF-1α. The core complex formed by HIF-1α and CBP/p300 mainly depends on the recognition of the two short-helical domains of C-TAD by CBP/p300. Under normoxic conditions, factor inhibiting HIF-1 (FIH), an asparaginyl hydroxylase, hydroxylates asparagine (N)803 residue within C-TAD in an oxygen-dependent manner to block the cooperative binding of CBP/p300 and C-TAD, thereby eliminating HIF-1α-mediated target gene transcription [98]. However, the oxygen-dependent hydroxylation of N803 is inhibited in hypoxic conditions to promote this binding, leading to the transcriptional activation of target genes. Oxygen-dependent degradation domain, another special structure of HIF-1α, participates in mediating the degradation of HIF-1 [99]. It is worth noting that HIF-1α must form a heterodimer with HIF-1β before exerting its biological function. HIF-1β is stably expressed in cells and maintains the stability of HIF-1 [36]. The structures included in HIF-1α and HIF-1β are basic-helix-loop-helix and PER-ARNT-SIM domain, which promote DNA binding and dimerization. Increasing evidence has indicated that HIF-1α, as the active subunit of HIF-1, is involved in inducing and maintaining the phenotype of various CSCs [100].
- *DNA Damage Prevention*: Hypoxia has been shown to prevent drug-induced DNA damage, particularly in response to agents like etoposide, by downregulating topoisomerase IIα, thereby enhancing cell survival [101].

HIF-Independent Mechanisms

- *Epigenetic Changes*: Hypoxia can induce epigenetic modifications, such as the degradation of ATAD2, which contributes to chemo-resistance [102].
- *Wnt/β-Catenin Pathway*: In lung cancer, hypoxia alters the proportion of ALDHhi CSCs through the Wnt/β-catenin signalling pathway, affecting cell plasticity and resistance [103].

Tumour Microenvironment Interactions

- *Inflammatory Responses*: CSCs in hypoxic niches exhibit heightened inflammatory responses, which can further enhance their aggressive phenotype and resistance to therapies [104].

Although hypoxia plays a significant role in CSC resistance, it is important to remember that not all hypoxic responses result in resistance; some may actually make cells more sensitive to specific treatments, suggesting a complicated interplay that needs more research [105].

Hypoxia Mediates CSC Resistance through Drug Transporters

Additionally, through drug transporters, the hypoxic microenvironment can affect CSCs' resistance to medicines. The majority of CSCs express ATP-binding cassette (ABC) family membrane transporters, ABCG2/breast cancer resistance protein (BCRP), ABCC1/multidrug resistance-related protein (MRP1), and ABCB1 (P-gp)/multidrug resistance gene 1 (MDR1) [106]. Since the majority of these proteins are capable of transporting metabolites, medications, and other materials, CSCs can develop greater resistance to many chemotherapeutic medications [97]. Tumour resistance has been found to be strongly mediated by HIF-1 and drug transporters. It has also been established that HIF-1α and ABCB1 (P-gp) are related [107]. A study has discovered the HIF-1 binding site in the MDR1 gene and found out that there was a positive correlation between the expression of HIF-1 and MDR1 [108]. Furthermore, studies have shown that MDR1/P-gp and HIF-1α are overexpressed in colon cancer that is generated by hypoxia, and that the production of

HIF-1α may contribute to the development of tumour multidrug resistance [109]. The multidrug resistance of CSCs is tightly associated with ABCG2, often referred to as BCRP. HIF-1 binds to the HRE site at base pair -115 in acute myeloid leukaemia, activating the transcription of BCRP [110]. This implies that LSCs with high BCRP levels under hypoxia may be resistant to numerous chemotherapy drugs, including mitoxantrone, and survive chemotherapy [111]. Moreover, HIF-1α can influence ABCG2 α expression in Ovarian Cancer Stem Cells (OCSCs). Furthermore, HIF-2 has been shown to facilitate e resistance to Adriamycin and encourage the development of BCRP in OCSCs.

POTENTIAL TARGETS FOR CSC THERAPY BASED ON HIF

Tumorigenesis, development, treatment resistance, recurrence, invasion, and metastasis are all significantly influenced by CSCs. While there exist numerous methods to influence the stemness of CSCs, it is important to take into account hypoxia and its related elements. The hypoxic microenvironment preserves the stemness of CSCs by means of pathways, microRNA regulation, drug transporter expression, and enhanced mobile transition to evade the impacts of radiation and chemotherapy. This chapter primarily focuses on the potential mechanisms of hypoxia-mediated CSC resistance and strategies for tumour treatment. Nevertheless, hypoxia is a vital component that triggers HIF signalling in tumours; HIF inhibitors can combat hypoxic crises in tumours in a variety of ways. We hope that as HIF inhibitors are developed further, cancers' resistance to chemotherapy and radiation will be lessened.

The development of HIF-1α and HIF-2α inhibitors has made it possible to employ combination therapies or better, more effective, and less toxic medicines in the clinic.

In many studies, the use of HIFs as new targets for tumour therapy and reversing or reducing tumour resistance has been stated. It is noteworthy that distinct cancer types have distinct HIF-1 regulation effects. Since HIF-1/HIF-1α plays a crucial role in controlling CSCs, adjuvant therapy may employ its inhibitor. HIF-1 inhibitor acriflavine stops HIF-1α and HIF-1β from dimerizing, which inhibits hypoxia-induced gene expression and results in the destruction of undimerized HIF-1α. Chronic myeloid leukaemia cells' stemness and proliferation can be efficiently inhibited by acriflavine (Table 5.3).

By lowering the expression of receptors for advanced glycation end products, a membrane receptor that detects the necrotic stimulation of cells that die from hypoxia, digoxin, another HIF-1 inhibitor, or acriflavine can stop glioblastoma stem cells from reacting to hypoxia. The radiation sensitivity of malignant gliomas can be increased by the targeted suppression of HIF-1 by siRNA; however, the restricted delivery efficiency of siRNA still has to be addressed. It is suggested that the HIF-1α vaccination can prevent the spread of breast cancer by impeding tumour immunity. Furthermore, HIF-1α and co-activators together may one day be used as a therapeutic target (Figure 5.4).

3-(5-Hydroxymethyl-2-furyl)-1-benzyl indazole may, in a way that is N803 hydroxylation-independent, promote FIH to bind to C-TAD and decrease the recruitment of p300 to inhibit

TABLE 5.3
HIF-1α and HIF-2α Inhibitors

S. No.	HIF-1α inhibitors	HIF-2α inhibitor
1.	EZN-2968	PT2385
2.	EZN-2208	PT2977
3.	PX-478	–
4.	RAD001	–

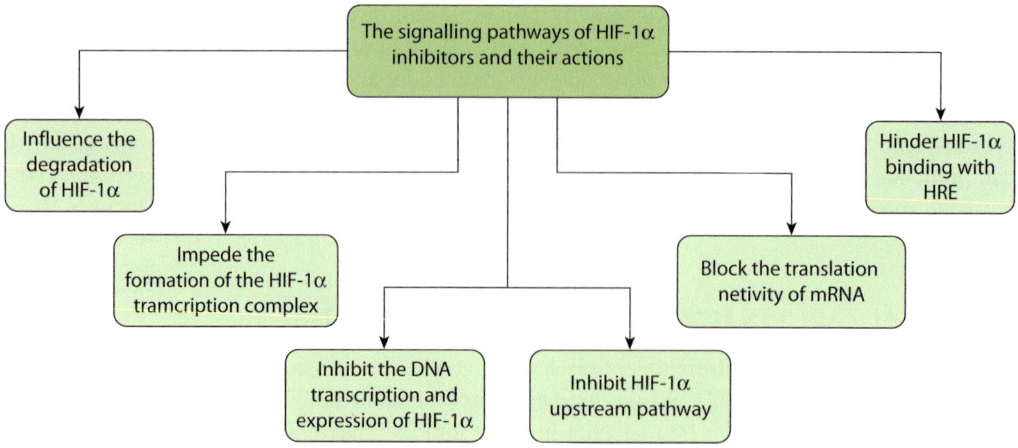

FIGURE 5.4 HIF-1α inhibitors mainly inhibit HIF-1α activity through the above-given actions.

HIF-1α, even in hypoxic environments. Bortezomib exhibits comparable FIH-mediated anticancer effects and is utilized in clinical trials for several tumour types. To directly disrupt the link between HIF-1α and p300, osmium metal complex 1 can be employed as an inhibitor to halt HIF-1α expression and prevent cell division. Melatonin, discorhabdin L, and chelomin all have comparable functions [107].

The proliferation of castration-resistant prostate cancer cells is efficiently inhibited by the combination of chetomin and the androgen receptor antagonist enzalutamide [97, 106]. TEL03, a perylene derivative, functions as a dual-targeted inhibitor of HIF-1α and STAT3; it prevents STAT3 from being phosphorylated and inhibits its transcription; additionally, it prevents HIF-1α and CBP/p300 from working together to cause HIF-1α breakdown, which causes apoptosis and suppresses the growth of tumours [108]. By inhibiting the proliferation of prostate cancer cells through targeting both the HIF-1α and STAT3 pathways, LB-1 also hinders the formation of the HIF-1α/p300/p-STAT3 complex [109].

A phase I trial of advanced gastrointestinal cancers has demonstrated the clinical potential of methylide, a prodrug of triptolide, and a phase II trial is now being planned. Furthermore, CSC-related immunological and metabolic control, critical gene deletion, and the suppression of important enzymes and signalling cascades are also possible targets for CSC therapy [97].

CONCLUSION AND FUTURE PERSPECTIVE

The ability of hypoxia to support tumour survival, dissemination, and invasiveness has been demonstrated, and while there are numerous ways to influence CSC stemness, hypoxia and its related aspects should be taken into account. Through pathways, the control of microRNAs, the production of drug transporters, and EMT to evade the effects of radiation and chemotherapy, the hypoxic microenvironment preserves the stemness of CSCs [110]. The importance of HIFs in CSC formation, stem cell marker production, and HIF-mediated therapy resistance are mostly summarized in this chapter. HIF inhibitors have several strategies for combating hypoxic emergencies in tumours, although hypoxia is a crucial element in the activation of HIF signalling within tumours [111]. We hope that as HIF inhibitors are developed further, cancers' resistance to chemotherapy and radiation will be lessened. The development of HIF-1α and HIF-2α inhibitors has made it possible to employ combination therapies or better, less toxic, more effective medicines in the clinic. The earlier studies suggest that the effects of tumour hypoxia extend beyond its critically important role in driving angiogenesis and modulating cancer cell metabolism and survival. Reducing HIF activity in CSCs may promote their differentiation, thereby reducing their ability to repopulate tumours after chemo and radiation therapies [107, 108]. To test this theory, it will be necessary to ablate the function of HIF-1α, HIF-2α, Notch, Oct4, c-Myc, and other pathway components in carefully defined tumour models.

REFERENCES

1. Rankin, Erinn B., and Amato J. Giaccia. "Hypoxic control of metastasis." *Science* vol. 352, 6282 (2016): 175–180. https://doi.org/10.1126/science.aaf4405
2. Semenza, Gregg Leonard. "Hypoxia-inducible factors in physiology and medicine." *Cell* vol. 148, 3 (2012): 399–408. https://doi.org/10.1016/j.cell.2012.01.021
3. Triner, Daniel., and Yatrik M. Shah. "Hypoxia-inducible factors: A central link between inflammation and cancer." *Journal of Clinical Investigation* vol. 126, 10 (2016): 3689–3698. https://doi.org/10.1172/JCI84430
4. Park, Chung-Ho., Daniel E. Bergsagel, and Ernest A. McCulloch. "Mouse myeloma tumour stem cells: A primary cell culture assay." *Journal of the National Cancer Institute* vol. 46, 2 (1971): 411–422.
5. Bonnet, Dominique., and Jeffrey E. Dick. "Human acute myeloid leukaemia is organized as a hierarchy that originates from a primitive hematopoietic cell." *Nature Medicine* vol. 3, 7 (1997): 730–737.
6. Zhang, Qi et al. "Role of hypoxia-inducible factor-1 in cancer stem cells (review)." *Molecular Medicine Reports* vol. 23, 1 (2021): 17. https://doi.org/10.3892/mmr.2020.11655
7. Zhang, Kun-Dong. et al. "MiR-301a transcriptionally activated by HIF-2alpha promotes hypoxia-induced epithelial-mesenchymal transition by targeting TP63 in pancreatic cancer." *World Journal of Gastroenterology* vol. 26, 19 (2020): 2349–2373.
8. Almiron Bonnin, Damian A. et al. "Secretion-mediated STAT3 activation promotes self-renewal of glioma stem- like cells during hypoxia." *Oncogene* vol. 37, 8 (2018): 1107–1118.
9. Wang, Wen-Jing. et al. "Ursolic acid inhibits proliferation and reverses drug resistance of ovarian cancer stem cells by downregulating ABCG2 through suppressing the expression of hypoxia-inducible factor-1alpha in vitro." *Oncology Reports* vol. 36, 1 (2016): 428–440.
10. Zhang, Zhengle. et al. "Hypoxia potentiates gemcitabine-induced stemness in pancreatic cancer cells through AKT/Notch1 signaling." *Journal of Experimental & Clinical Cancer Research* vol. 37, 1 (2018): 291.
11. Vilchez, Valery., Lilia Turcios, Francesc Marti, and Roberto Gedaly. "Targeting Wnt/beta-catenin pathway in hepatocellular carcinoma treatment." *World Journal of Gastroenterology* vol. 22, 2 (2016): 823–832.
12. Farago, Marganit., Isabel Dominguez, Esther Landesman-Bollag, Xin Xu, Andrea Rosner, Robert D. Cardiff, and David C. Seldin. "Kinase-inactive glycogen synthase kinase 3β promotes Wnt signaling and mammary tumorigenesis." *Cancer Research* vol. 65, 13 (2005): 5792–5801. https://doi.org/10.1158/0008-5472.CAN-05-1021
13. Mazumdar, Jolly., W.Timothy O'Brien, Randall S. Johnson, Joseph C. LaManna, Juan C. Chavez, Peter S. Klein, and M.Celeste Simon. "O2 regulates stem cells through Wnt/beta-catenin signalling." *Nature Cell Biology* vol. 12, 10 (2010): 1007–1013. https://doi.org/10.1038/ncb2102
14. Santoyo-Ramos, Paula., María Likhatcheva, Eduardo A. Garcia-Zepeda, M.Cristina Castaneda-Patlan, and Martha Robles-Flores. "Hypoxia-inducible factors modulate the stemness and malignancy of colon cancer cells by playing opposite roles in canonical Wnt signaling." *PLoS One* vol. 9, 11 (2014): e112580. https://doi.org/10.1371/journal.pone.0112580
15. Giambra, Vincenzo et al. "Leukemia stem cells in T-ALL require active Hif1alpha and Wnt signaling." *Blood* vol. 125, 25 (2015): 3917–3927. https://doi.org/10.1182/blood-2014-10-609370
16. Yan, Guang-Ning et al. "Endothelial cells promote stem-like phenotype of glioma cells through activating the hedgehog pathway." *The Journal of Pathology* vol. 234, 1 (2014): 11–22. https://doi.org/10.1002/path.4349
17. He, Miao et al. "The Hedgehog signalling pathway mediates drug response of MCF-7 mammosphere cells in breast cancer patients." *Clinical Science (London)* vol. 129, 9 (2015): 809–822.
18. Roscigno, Giuseppina et al. "MiR-24 induces chemotherapy resistance and hypoxic advantage in breast cancer." *Oncotarget* vol. 8, 12 (2017): 19507–19521. https://doi.org/10.18632/oncotarget.14470

19. Chen, Ke, Ying-Hui Huang, and Ji-Long Chen. "Understanding and targeting cancer stem cells: Therapeutic implications and challenges." *Acta Pharmacologica Sinica* vol. 34, 6 (2013): 732–740. https://doi.org/10.1038/aps.2013.27
20. Clarke, Michael F. et al. "Cancer stem cells–perspectives on current status and future directions: AACR workshop on cancer stem cells." *Cancer Research* vol. 66, 19 (2006): 9339–9344. https://doi.org/10.1158/0008-5472.CAN-06-3126
21. Comerford, Katrina M., Timothy J. Wallace, Jörn Karhausen, Nancy A. Louis, Michael C. Montalto, and Sean P. Colgan. "Hypoxia-inducible factor-1-dependent regulation of the multidrug resistance (MDR1) gene." *Cancer Research* vol. 62, 12 (2002): 3387–3394.
22. Ding, Zhenyu et al. "Expression and significance of hypoxia-inducible factor-1 alpha and MDR1/P-glycoprotein in human colon carcinoma tissue and cells." *Journal of Cancer Research and Clinical Oncology* vol. 136, 11 (2010): 1697–1707.
23. Sell, S., and G.B. Pierce. "Maturation arrest of stem cell differentiation is a common pathway for the cellular origin of teratocarcinomas and epithelial cancers." *Laboratory Investigation; a Journal of Technical Methods and Pathology* vol. 70, 1 (1994): 6–22.
24. Kantarjian, Hagop M. et al. "Acute myeloid leukemia management and research in 2025." *CA: a Cancer Journal for Clinicians* vol. 75, 1 (2025): 46–67. https://doi.org/10.3322/caac.21873
25. Bisht, Shweta et al. "Cancer stem cells: From an insight into the basics to recent advances and therapeutic targeting." *Stem Cells International* vol. 2022 (2022): 9653244. https://doi.org/10.1155/2022/9653244
26. Barros, Luciana et al. "Immunological-based approaches for cancer therapy." *Clinics (Sao Paulo, Brazil)* vol. 73, 1 (2018): e429s. https://doi.org/10.6061/clinics/2018/e429s
27. Wang, Maonan et al. "Role of tumor microenvironment in tumorigenesis." *Journal of Cancer* vol. 8, 5 (2017): 761–773. https://doi.org/10.7150/jca.17648
28. Chen, Jocelyn F., and Qin Yan. "The roles of epigenetics in cancer progression and metastasis." *The Biochemical Journal* vol. 478, 17 (2021): 3373–3393. https://doi.org/10.1042/BCJ20210084
29. Phi, Lan Thi Hanh et al. "Cancer stem cells (CSCs) in drug resistance and their therapeutic implications in cancer treatment." *Stem Cells International* vol. 2018 (2018): 5416923. https://doi.org/10.1155/2018/5416923
30. Huang, Tianzhi et al. "Stem cell programs in cancer initiation, progression, and therapy resistance." *Theranostics* vol. 10, 19 (2020): 8721–8743. https://doi.org/10.7150/thno.41648
31. Kharkar, Prashant S. "Cancer stem cell (CSC) inhibitors in oncology-a promise for a better therapeutic outcome: State of the art and future perspectives." *Journal of Medicinal Chemistry* vol. 63, 24 (2020): 15279–15307. https://doi.org/10.1021/acs.jmedchem.0c01336
32. Yoo, Young Dong, and Yong Tae Kwon. "Molecular mechanisms controlling asymmetric and symmetric self-renewal of cancer stem cells." *Journal of Analytical Science and Technology* vol. 6, 1 (2015): 28. https://doi.org/10.1186/s40543-015-0071-4
33. Malik, Babar, and Daotai Nie. "Cancer stem cells and resistance to chemo and radio therapy." *Frontiers in Bioscience (Elite Edition)* vol. 4, 6 (2012): 2142–2149. https://doi.org/10.2741/531
34. Wang, Chunxia et al. "Evaluation of CD44 and CD133 as cancer stem cell markers for colorectal cancer." *Oncology Reports* vol. 28, 4 (2012): 1301–1308. https://doi.org/10.3892/or.2012.1951
35. Desai, Sharav A. et al. "The tumor microenvironment: Shaping cancer progression and treatment response." *Journal of Chemotherapy (Florence, Italy)* vol. 37, 1 (2025): 15–44. https://doi.org/10.1080/1120009X.2023.2300224
36. Chang, Jenny C. "Cancer stem cells: Role in tumor growth, recurrence, metastasis, and treatment resistance." *Medicine* vol. 95, Suppl 1 (2016): S20–S25. https://doi.org/10.1097/MD.0000000000004766
37. Liao, Wenhao et al. "Natural products-based nanoformulations: A new approach targeting CSCs to cancer therapy." *International Journal of Nanomedicine* vol. 17 (2022): 4163–4193. https://doi.org/10.2147/IJN.S380697
38. Atashzar, Mohammad Reza et al. "Cancer stem cells: A review from origin to therapeutic implications." *Journal of Cellular Physiology* vol. 235, 2 (2020): 790–803. https://doi.org/10.1002/jcp.29044
39. Chen, Wanyin et al. "Cancer stem cell quiescence and plasticity as major challenges in cancer therapy." *Stem Cells International* vol. 2016 (2016): 1740936. https://doi.org/10.1155/2016/1740936
40. Aponte, Pedro M., and Andrés Caicedo. "Stemness in cancer: Stem cells, cancer stem cells, and their microenvironment." *Stem Cells International* vol. 2017 (2017): 5619472. https://doi.org/10.1155/2017/5619472
41. Lei, Zi-Ning et al. "Understanding and targeting resistance mechanisms in cancer." *MedComm* vol. 4, 3 (2023): e265. https://doi.org/10.1002/mco2.265

42. Lee, Pearl et al. "Cellular adaptation to hypoxia through hypoxia inducible factors and beyond." *Nature Reviews. Molecular Cell Biology* vol. 21, 5 (2020): 268–283. https://doi.org/10.1038/s41580-020-0227-y
43. Mylonis, Ilias et al. "Hypoxia-inducible factors and the regulation of lipid metabolism." *Cells* vol. 8, 3 (2019): 214. https://doi.org/10.3390/cells8030214
44. Ravindran, Shilpa et al. "The cross talk between cancer stem cells/cancer initiating cells and tumor microenvironment: The missing piece of the puzzle for the efficient targeting of these cells with immunotherapy." *Cancer Microenvironment: Official Journal of the International Cancer Microenvironment Society* vol. 12, 2–3 (2019): 133–148. https://doi.org/10.1007/s12307-019-00233-1
45. Melincovici, Carmen Stanca et al. "Vascular endothelial growth factor (VEGF) – Key factor in normal and pathological angiogenesis." *Romanian Journal of Morphology and Embryology = Revue roumaine de morphologie et embryologie* vol. 59, 2 (2018): 455–467.
46. Wu, Bo et al. "Cross-talk between cancer stem cells and immune cells: Potential therapeutic targets in the tumor immune microenvironment." *Molecular Cancer* vol. 22, 1 (2023): 38. https://doi.org/10.1186/s12943-023-01748-4
47. Najafi, Masoud et al. "Hypoxia in solid tumors: A key promoter of cancer stem cell (CSC) resistance." *Journal of Cancer Research and Clinical Oncology* vol. 146, 1 (2020): 19–31. https://doi.org/10.1007/s00432-019-03080-1
48. Boothby, Thomas C. "Mechanisms and evolution of resistance to environmental extremes in animals." *EvoDevo* vol. 10 (2019): 30. https://doi.org/10.1186/s13227-019-0143-4
49. Podkalicka, Paulina et al. "Hypoxia as a driving force of pluripotent stem cell reprogramming and differentiation to endothelial cells." *Biomolecules* vol. 10, 12 (2020): 1614. https://doi.org/10.3390/biom10121614
50. Kim, Yuri et al. "Hypoxic tumor microenvironment and cancer cell differentiation." *Current Molecular Medicine* vol. 9, 4 (2009): 425–434. https://doi.org/10.2174/156652409788167113
51. Yun, Zhong, and Qun Lin. "Hypoxia and regulation of cancer cell stemness." *Advances in Experimental Medicine and Biology* vol. 772 (2014): 41–53. https://doi.org/10.1007/978-1-4614-5915-6_2
52. Ju, Feng et al. "Characteristics of the cancer stem cell niche and therapeutic strategies." *Stem Cell Research & Therapy* vol. 13, 1 (2022): 233. https://doi.org/10.1186/s13287-022-02904-1
53. Mehta, Pooja et al. "Self-renewal and CSCs in vitro enrichment: Growth as floating spheres." *Methods in Molecular Biology (Clifton, N.J.)* vol. 1692 (2018): 61–75. https://doi.org/10.1007/978-1-4939-7401-6_6
54. Ganuza, Miguel, and Shannon McKinney-Freeman. "Hematopoietic stem cells under pressure." *Current Opinion in Hematology* vol. 24, 4 (2017): 314–321. https://doi.org/10.1097/MOH.0000000000000347
55. Chagastelles, Pedro C., and Nance B. Nardi. "Biology of stem cells: An overview." *Kidney International Supplements* vol. 1, 3 (2011): 63–67. https://doi.org/10.1038/kisup.2011.15
56. Zhang, Shuchen, and Wei Cui. "Sox2, a key factor in the regulation of pluripotency and neural differentiation." *World Journal of Stem Cells* vol. 6, 3 (2014): 305–311. https://doi.org/10.4252/wjsc.v6.i3.305
57. Bao, Bin et al. "The biological kinship of hypoxia with CSC and EMT and their relationship with deregulated expression of miRNAs and tumor aggressiveness." *Biochimica et biophysica acta* vol. 1826, 2 (2012): 272–296. https://doi.org/10.1016/j.bbcan.2012.04.008
58. Zhao, Xiaopeng et al. "PI3K/Akt and Wnt/β-catenin signaling cross-regulate NF-κB signaling in TNF-α-induced human Lgr5+ intestinal stem cells." *Anticancer Research* vol. 42, 7 (2022): 3325–3340. https://doi.org/10.21873/anticanres.15820
59. Befani, Christina, and Panagiotis Liakos. "The role of hypoxia-inducible factor-2 alpha in angiogenesis." *Journal of Cellular Physiology* vol. 233, 12 (2018): 9087–9098. https://doi.org/10.1002/jcp.26805
60. Sahlberg, Sara Häggblad et al. "Evaluation of cancer stem cell markers CD133, CD44, CD24: Association with AKT isoforms and radiation resistance in colon cancer cells." *PloS One* vol. 9, 4 (2014): e94621. https://doi.org/10.1371/journal.pone.0094621
61. Raghav, Pawan Kumar, and Zoya Mann. "Cancer stem cells targets and combined therapies to prevent cancer recurrence." *Life Sciences* vol. 277 (2021): 119465. https://doi.org/10.1016/j.lfs.2021.119465
62. Bui, Bich Phuong et al. "Hypoxia-inducible factor-1: A novel therapeutic target for the management of cancer, drug resistance, and cancer-related pain." *Cancers* vol. 14, 24 (2022): 6054. https://doi.org/10.3390/cancers14246054
63. Qannita, Reem A. et al. "Targeting hypoxia-inducible factor-1 (HIF-1) in cancer: Emerging therapeutic strategies and pathway regulation." *Pharmaceuticals (Basel, Switzerland)* vol. 17, 2 (2024): 195. https://doi.org/10.3390/ph17020195

64. Raychaudhuri, Smriti K., and Siba P. Raychaudhuri. "Janus kinase/signal transducer and activator of transcription pathways in spondyloarthritis." *Current Opinion in Rheumatology* vol. 29, 4 (2017): 311–316. https://doi.org/10.1097/BOR.0000000000000399
65. Schöning, Jennifer Petra et al. "Drug resistance and cancer stem cells: The shared but distinct roles of hypoxia-inducible factors HIF1α and HIF2α." *Clinical and Experimental Pharmacology & Physiology* vol. 44, 2 (2017): 153–161. https://doi.org/10.1111/1440-1681.12693
66. Lim, Jacqueline R. et al. "Cancer stem cell characteristics and their potential as therapeutic targets." *Medical Oncology (Northwood, London, England)* vol. 38, 7 (2021): 76–29. https://doi.org/10.1007/s12032-021-01524-8
67. Cui, Peng et al. "HIF-1α affects the neural stem cell differentiation of human induced pluripotent stem cells via MFN2-mediated Wnt/β-catenin signaling." *Frontiers in Cell and Developmental Biology* vol. 9 (2021): 671704. https://doi.org/10.3389/fcell.2021.671704
68. Lee, Jin Woo, and Hwa-Yong Lee. "Targeting cancer stem cell markers or pathways: A potential therapeutic strategy for oral cancer treatment." *International Journal of Stem Cells* vol. 14, 4 (2021): 386–399. https://doi.org/10.15283/ijsc21084
69. Wang, Chongwu et al. "A low MW inhibitor of CD44 dimerization for the treatment of glioblastoma." *British Journal of Pharmacology* vol. 177, 13 (2020): 3009–3023. https://doi.org/10.1111/bph.15030
70. Gong, Liang et al. "Prognostic value of HIFs expression in head and neck cancer: A systematic review." *PloS One* vol. 8, 9 (2013): e75094. https://doi.org/10.1371/journal.pone.0075094
71. Park, Jang Hyun et al. "Tumor hypoxia represses γδ T cell-mediated antitumor immunity against brain tumors." *Nature Immunology* vol. 22, 3 (2021): 336–346. https://doi.org/10.1038/s41590-020-00860-7
72. Johnson, Rachelle W. et al. "Hypoxia and bone metastatic disease." *Current Osteoporosis Reports* vol. 15, 4 (2017): 231–238. https://doi.org/10.1007/s11914-017-0378-8
73. Kuwai, Toshio et al. "Expression of hypoxia-inducible factor-1alpha is associated with tumor vascularization in human colorectal carcinoma." *International Journal of Cancer* vol. 105, 2 (2003): 176–181. https://doi.org/10.1002/ijc.11068
74. Seguin, Laetitia et al. "Integrins and cancer: Regulators of cancer stemness, metastasis, and drug resistance." *Trends in Cell Biology* vol. 25, 4 (2015): 234–240. https://doi.org/10.1016/j.tcb.2014.12.006
75. Wigerup, Caroline et al. "Therapeutic targeting of hypoxia and hypoxia-inducible factors in cancer." *Pharmacology & Therapeutics* vol. 164 (2016): 152–169. https://doi.org/10.1016/j.pharmthera.2016.04.009
76. Yoshii, Tatsuyuki et al. "Biochemical and biomechanical drivers of cancer cell metastasis, drug response and nanomedicine." *Drug Discovery Today* vol. 21, 9 (2016): 1489–1494. https://doi.org/10.1016/j.drudis.2016.05.011
77. Fong, Emma J. et al. "A perspective on expanding our understanding of cancer treatments by integrating approaches from the biological and physical sciences." *SLAS Discovery: advancing life sciences R & D* vol. 25, 7 (2020): 672–683. https://doi.org/10.1177/2472555220915830
78. Zafar, Aasma et al. "Revolutionizing cancer care strategies: Immunotherapy, gene therapy, and molecular targeted therapy." *Molecular Biology Reports* vol. 51, 1 (2024): 219. https://doi.org/10.1007/s11033-023-09096-8
79. Sadelain, Michel, Isabelle Riviere, and Stanley Riddell. "Therapeutic T cell engineering." *Nature* vol. 545, 7655 (2017): 423–431.
80. Ewing, David. "The oxygen fixation hypothesis: A reevaluation." *American Journal of Clinical Oncology* vol. 21, 4 (1998): 355–361. https://doi.org/10.1097/00000421-199808000-00008
81. Grimes, David Robert, and Mike Partridge. "A mechanistic investigation of the oxygen fixation hypothesis and oxygen enhancement ratio." *Biomedical Physics & Engineering Express* vol. 1, 4 (2015): 045209. https://doi.org/10.1088/2057-1976/1/4/045209
82. Horan, Annamarie D. et al. "Effect of oxygen on radiation-induced DNA damage in isolated nuclei." *Radiation Research* vol. 152, 2 (1999): 144–153.
83. Abdullah, Lissa Nurrul, and Edward Kai-Hua Chow. "Mechanisms of chemoresistance in cancer stem cells." *Clinical and Translational Medicine* vol. 2, 1 (2013): 3. https://doi.org/10.1186/2001-1326-2-3
84. Shi, Rachel et al. "Hypoxia-driven effects in cancer: Characterization, mechanisms, and therapeutic implications." *Cells* vol. 10, 3 (2021): 678. https://doi.org/10.3390/cells10030678
85. Ortmann, Brian et al. "Cell cycle progression in response to oxygen levels." *Cellular and Molecular Life Sciences: CMLS* vol. 71, 18 (2014): 3569–3582. https://doi.org/10.1007/s00018-014-1645-9

86. Ramakrishnan, S. et al. "Vascular endothelial growth factor signaling in hypoxia and inflammation." *Journal of Neuroimmune Pharmacology: The Official Journal of the Society on NeuroImmune Pharmacology* vol. 9, 2 (2014): 142–160. https://doi.org/10.1007/s11481-014-9531-7
87. Minassian, Lori M. et al. "Hypoxia-induced resistance to chemotherapy in cancer." *Advances in Experimental Medicine and Biology* vol. 1136 (2019): 123–139. https://doi.org/10.1007/978-3-030-12734-3_9
88. Infantino, Vittoria et al. "Cancer cell metabolism in hypoxia: Role of HIF-1 as key regulator and therapeutic target." *International Journal of Molecular Sciences* vol. 22, 11 (2021): 5703. https://doi.org/10.3390/ijms22115703
89. Jin, Ping et al. "Mitochondrial adaptation in cancer drug resistance: prevalence, mechanisms, and management." *Journal of Hematology & Oncology* vol. 15, 1 (2022): 97. https://doi.org/10.1186/s13045-022-01313-4
90. Codony, Victoria L., and Mahvash Tavassoli. "Hypoxia-induced therapy resistance: Available hypoxia-targeting strategies and current advances in head and neck cancer." *Translational Oncology* vol. 14, 3 (2021): 101017. https://doi.org/10.1016/j.tranon.2021.101017
91. Li, Xin et al. "Hypoxia-induced metabolic and functional changes in oral CSCs: Implications for stemness and viability modulation through BNIP3-driven mitophagy." *Journal of Cellular and Molecular Medicine* vol. 29, 3 (2025): e70400. https://doi.org/10.1111/jcmm.70400
92. Basheeruddin, Mohd, and Sana Qausain. "Hypoxia-inducible factor 1-alpha (HIF-1α): An essential regulator in cellular metabolic control." *Cureus* vol. 16, 7 (2024): e63852. https://doi.org/10.7759/cureus.63852
93. Shi, Yong-Hong, and Wei-Gang Fang. "Hypoxia-inducible factor-1 in tumour angiogenesis." *World Journal of Gastroenterology* vol. 10, 8 (2004): 1082–1087. https://doi.org/10.3748/wjg.v10.i8.1082
94. Rani, Soniya et al. "Regulation of transactivation at C-TAD domain of HIF-1α by factor-inhibiting HIF-1α (FIH-1): A potential target for therapeutic intervention in cancer." *Oxidative Medicine and Cellular Longevity* vol. 2022 (2022): 2407223. https://doi.org/10.1155/2022/2407223
95. Comerford, Katrina M. et al. "Hypoxia-inducible factor-1-dependent regulation of the multidrug resistance (MDR1) gene." *Cancer Research* vol. 62, 12 (2002): 3387–3394.
96. Chen, Jianfang et al. "HIF-1α inhibition reverses multidrug resistance in colon cancer cells via downregulation of MDR1/P-glycoprotein." *PloS One* vol. 9, 6 (2014): e98882. https://doi.org/10.1371/journal.pone.0098882
97. Dei, Silvia et al. "Recent advances in the search of BCRP- and dual P-gp/BCRP-based multidrug resistance modulators." *Cancer Drug Resistance (Alhambra, Calif.)* vol. 2, 3 (2019): 710743. https://doi.org/10.20517/cdr.2019.31
98. Natarajan, Karthika et al. "Role of breast cancer resistance protein (BCRP/ABCG2) in cancer drug resistance." *Biochemical Pharmacology* vol. 83, 8 (2012): 1084–1103. https://doi.org/10.1016/j.bcp.2012.01.002
99. He, Xiaodan et al. "Hypoxia regulates ABCG2 activity through the activation of ERK1/2/HIF-1α and contributes to chemoresistance in pancreatic cancer cells." *Cancer Biology & Therapy* vol. 17, 2 (2016): 188–198. https://doi.org/10.1080/15384047.2016.1139228
100. Lin, Qun, and Zhong Yun. "Impact of the hypoxic tumor microenvironment on the regulation of cancer stem cell characteristics." *Cancer Biology & Therapy* vol. 9, 12 (2010): 949–956. https://doi.org/10.4161/cbt.9.12.12347
101. Onnis, Barbara et al. "Development of HIF-1 inhibitors for cancer therapy." *Journal of Cellular and Molecular Medicine* vol. 13, 9A (2009): 2780–2786. https://doi.org/10.1111/j.1582-4934.2009.00876.x
102. Masoud, Georgina N., and Wei Li. "HIF-1α pathway: Role, regulation and intervention for cancer therapy." *Acta Pharmaceutica Sinica. B* vol. 5, 5 (2015): 378–389. https://doi.org/10.1016/j.apsb.2015.05.007
103. Magar, Anuja Gajanan et al. "A molecular perspective on HIF-1α and angiogenic stimulator networks and their role in solid tumors: An update." *International Journal of Molecular Sciences* vol. 25, 6 (2024): 3313. https://doi.org/10.3390/ijms25063313
104. Xu, Renfeng et al. "Action sites and clinical application of HIF-1α inhibitors." *Molecules (Basel, Switzerland)* vol. 27, 11 (2022): 3426. https://doi.org/10.3390/molecules27113426
105. Li, Wen et al. "Roles of the receptor for advanced glycation end products and its ligands in the pathogenesis of Alzheimer's disease." *International Journal of Molecular Sciences* vol. 26, 1 (2025): 403. https://doi.org/10.3390/ijms26010403
106. Shin, Dong Hoon et al. "Bortezomib inhibits tumor adaptation to hypoxia by stimulating the FIH-mediated repression of hypoxia-inducible factor-1." *Blood* vol. 111, 6 (2008): 3131–3136. https://doi.org/10.1182/blood-2007-11-120576

107. Huynh, Jasmine C. et al. "Recent advances in targeted therapies for advanced gastrointestinal malignancies." *Cancers* vol. 12, 5 (2020): 1168. https://doi.org/10.3390/cancers12051168
108. Emami Nejad, Asieh et al. "The role of hypoxia in the tumor microenvironment and development of cancer stem cell: a novel approach to developing treatment." *Cancer Cell International* vol. 21, 1 (2021): 62. https://doi.org/10.1186/s12935-020-01719-5
109. Jun, Jonathan C. et al. "Hypoxia-inducible factors and cancer." *Current Sleep Medicine Reports* vol. 3, 1 (2017): 1–10. https://doi.org/10.1007/s40675-017-0062-7
110. Muz, Barbara et al. "The role of hypoxia in cancer progression, angiogenesis, metastasis, and resistance to therapy." *Hypoxia (Auckland, N.Z.)* vol. 3 (2015): 83–92. https://doi.org/10.2147/HP.S93413
111. Keith, Brian, and M. Celeste Simon. "Hypoxia-inducible factors, stem cells, and cancer." *Cell* vol. 129, 3 (2007): 465–472. https://doi.org/10.1016/j.cell.2007.04.019

6 Stemness Maintenance at Hypoxic Niches and Therapeutic Opportunities in Targeting Hypoxic Cancer Stem Cells

Suman Kumar Ray and Sukhes Mukherjee
Department of Biochemistry, All India Institute of Medical Sciences, Bhopal, Madhya Pradesh, India

INTRODUCTION

Animals can't exist without molecular oxygen (O_2), which is critical for several biological activities that ensure the continued existence of both prokaryotic and eukaryotic cell types. Different cell types and functions use oxygen at different rates. The mitochondria in eukaryotic cells use up 90% of the oxygen that is taken in during respiration and oxidative phosphorylation, and this uptake happens via direct transport across the cell membrane [1]. In addition, the synthesis of adenosine triphosphate (ATP) is closely linked to the citric acid cycle and the β-oxidation of fatty acids. So, O_2 availability is crucial for cellular processes, and a reduction in O_2 concentration is a big stressor for cells. Cells need an oxygen level between 2 and 9% (14.4–64.8 mmHg) when they are in a homeostatic condition, and lower levels of oxygen, 0.5–2% (<10 mmHg) when they are in a hypoxic state [2]. In reaction to oxygen levels, cells alter gene expression, which in turn impacts cellular metabolism, immunity, and reorganization of tissues [3]. The transcription factor hypoxia-inducible factor-1 (HIF-1) is the primary molecule responsible for mediating cellular adaptive responses to hypoxia. It activates a number of genes that aid in angiogenesis, cell proliferation, and survival under hypoxic conditions. In order to adapt to oxygen supply, cells do several things: (1) slow down oxidative phosphorylation, (2) stop the cell cycle, (3) release the major angiogenic factors (such as vascular endothelial growth factor (VEGF), angiopoietin-1 (Ang-1), transforming growth factor β1 (TGF-β1), and fibroblast growth factor (FGF-2) to encourage the formation of new blood vessels, and (4) transition to anaerobic glycolysis [4]. Hypoxia also causes morphological alterations in the cytoskeleton of cells, which include changes in protein aggregation and polarization, which in turn increase membrane permeability [5]. Because it is used up in the process of creating reactive oxygen species (ROS), O_2 dyshomeostasis, like high O_2 levels, can also cause cytotoxicity. Peroxides, singlet O_2, hydroxy radicals, and superoxide are all ROS that cause cellular dysfunction by oxidizing lipids, proteins, and nucleic acids. Antioxidants and redox enzyme levels vary between cells, which contrasts with the formation of ROS. Disappointingly, there is a wide range of ROS tolerance because these defense mechanisms aren't always sufficient to compare ROS output.

DOI: 10.1201/9781003477419-6

Two models have been proposed to explain tumor progression: the clonal evolution hypothesis, which suggests that aggressive cancer cells drive tumor progression through genetic and epigenetic alterations, and the cancer stem cell (CSC) paradigm, which suggests that CSCs are responsible for tumor initiation, development, and recurrence, and that these cells are the direct cause of tumor metastasis and treatment resistance [6, 7].

The possibility that cancers might originate from stem cells that persist after embryonic development was proposed by Julius Cohnheim in 1875 [8]. On the other hand, CSCs were initially introduced in 1971 [9]. It was thought that tumors were caused by a group of self-renewing CSCs that could produce the various differentiated cell types that make up the tumor mass [10]. Isolation of CD34+ CD38 cells from acute myeloid leukemia (AML) patients was the initial step in proving the idea in 1994 [11], and further work in 1997 [12] confirmed that these cells were the sole ones capable of instigating hematological malignancies in immunodeficient animals. In subsequent years, CSCs were also extracted from solid tumors caused by breast cancer [13].

Stem cells in cancer can self-renew and develop much like any other kind of stem cell. A tiny subset of a tumor's cell population consists of CSCs. The terms "tumorigenic cells" and "tumor-initiating cells" are interchangeable. Cell surface indicators are shared between regular stem cells and CSCs [14], and both types of cells can self-renew, differentiate into various offspring, and use the same signaling pathways [15]. The following can be derived from CSCs: (1) every single tumor cell in a cancer; (2) cells that develop resistance to the chemotherapy drug, leading to recurrence; and (3) cells that cause the cancer to spread to other parts of the body. Tumors of the same origin and type can vary in the percentage of CSCs (Figure 6.1). There is high diversity among CSCs, with isolated CSCs from main tumors and metastatic growths being distinct. Recent studies suggest CSCs are more accurately described as a cell status than a static category, with potential for interconversion.

The embryonic rest theory, introduced by Virchow 50 years ago, links cancer cells to healthy cells. CSCs, also known as tumor-initiating or propagating cells, use survival strategies to continue tumor

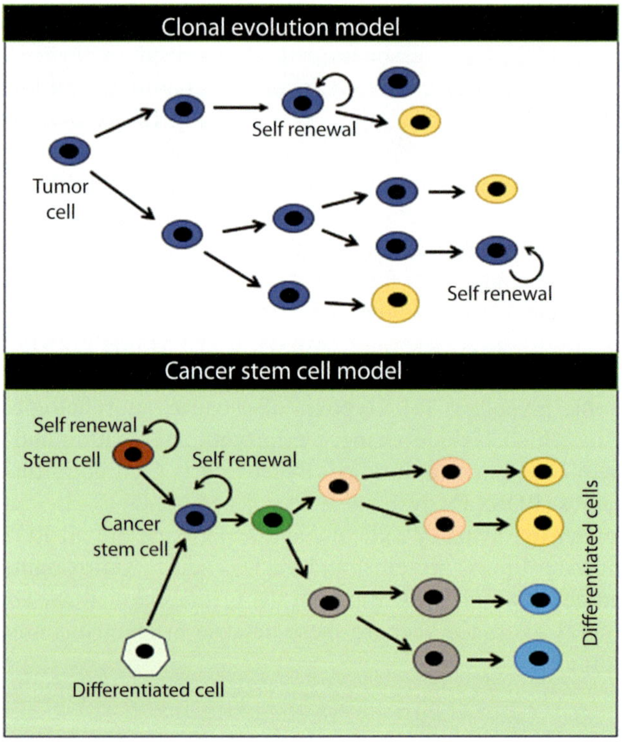

FIGURE 6.1 Archetypal outline of cancer stem cell model vs clonal evolution model of tumorigenesis.

growth. They contribute to tumor growth, maintenance, and recurrence by lowering ROS and increasing DNA checkpoint kinase activity. Recent experimental data show that CSCs play a significant role in tumor angiogenesis regulation through VEGF signaling [16, 17]. Angiogenesis is crucial in cancer treatment [18], as the neoplastic compartment grows larger than the oxygen diffusion distance in tissue, leading to hypoxic conditions. The generation of VEGF by CSC subpopulation controls tumor angiogenesis, causing a steady oxygen flux in solid tumors and decreased patient survival rates [19].

THE DIFFERENT THEORIES OF HOW CANCER STEM CELLS ARISE

Two main ideas in the stem cell theory of cancer are: (1) cancer develops from stem cells found in both adult and pediatric tissues; (2) cancer cells start out as stem cells, proliferating cells, or terminally differentiated cells in healthy tissues [20]. Multiple cancer origin theories point to stem cells as the primary culprit, including field theory, chemical carcinogenesis, infection, mutation, and genetic change.

The stem cell theory postulates that cancer develops when stem cells are unable to complete their maturation process. In addition to stem cells, transit amplifying cells, and terminally differentiated cells, CSCs and cancer cells can also originate from and contain cells present in healthy tissues. Another theory postulated that tumors develop as a result of stem cell maturation arrest, based on observations of teratocarcinomas and hepatocellular carcinomas [21]. Studies on tumor transplantation that were conducted in the same decade provided evidence that cancer might be sustained by a small number of cells with stem-like properties [22, 23].

The somatic stem cell concept, which is more up-to-date [24], proposes that CSC development could be triggered by mutations or chromosomal rearrangements in dormant stem cells. There are three constants about somatic stem cells: (1) they can self-renew indefinitely and produce new cells of the same kind; (2) their offspring can develop into diverse types of cells that are both functional and specialized; and (3) they faithfully react to environmental homeostatic controls [24]. On the other hand, CSCs self-renew while undergoing abnormal differentiation and are unresponsive to homeostatic regulation [25].

The Cell Reversal Theory suggests that cells undergo carcinogenic events, changing their epigenetic state, leading to aberrant proliferation. Some cells choose an evolutionary advantage, such as stem cells or pluripotents, rather than waiting for correct environmental inputs [26]. The stem cell misplacement theory suggests that in situ carcinomas develop when epithelial stem cells get mixed up and end up in the wrong connective tissue stroma [27]. Evidence suggests that HER2 gene amplification/overexpression is more common in ductal carcinoma in situ than in invasive breast cancer. Most theories agree that CSCs arise from accumulated epigenetic and genetic changes originating from normal stem cells or cancer cells.

CANCER STEM CELL ORIGIN

A cancer cell or a CSC—which came first? Tumor cells can develop from transformed resident stem cells or transformed differentiated cells, which helps to shed light on this subject [28, 29]. Environmental variables such as tissue regeneration, infections, poisons, and both intrinsic and extrinsic factors that cause DNA mutations, are likely to cause transformation [30]. Cells undergo de-differentiation, unchecked proliferation, and stem-like traits as a result of oncogene overexpression and tumor suppressor gene deactivation throughout the transformation process in differentiated cells [26]. It is believed that tumors originating from CSCs adhere to a unidirectional hierarchy, which implies that the CSC population starts the tumor growth process [29]. So, CSCs divide asymmetrically to keep some CSCs around and produce some transitory cells that divide symmetrically and are very proliferative [31]. Three non-exclusive models for CSCs have been proposed based on recent evidence on solid and hematological cancers: first, there is the hierarchical model, which states that any cell in the stem/progenitor hierarchy has the potential to transform. Second, there is the CSC model, which states that a small subset of cells encourages tumor initiation and growth. Lastly, there is the clonal evolution model, which states that genetic instability due to genetic alterations becomes worse with time, resulting in stronger tumors with more resistance and heterogeneity.

Cellular plasticity in CSCs is supported by various hypotheses, including cell reversal, stem cell misplacement, somatic stem cell, and stem cell theory of cancer [30, 32]. However, leukemias have distinct environments where CSCs might originate or develop. Leukemic cells that express the same markers as adult human hematopoietic stem cells (CD34+CD38–) have been found to develop hematopoietic malignancy [33]. CSCs in leukemias cause unchecked growth of cancer cells and disease recurrence. They are often identified by specific cell surface markers. Genetic abnormalities and mutations in blood-forming stem cells cause leukemia. Theories include progenitor cells with somatic mutations in genes controlling cell proliferation and differentiation, or clonal evolution. Genetic diversity in leukemia may result from clonal evolution, increasing treatment resistance and relapse risk [34, 35].

MICROENVIRONMENTAL CONTRIBUTIONS TO CSC PHENOTYPE

The original tumorigenic potential of the cells can be altered by the host microenvironment in which the CSCs or progenitor cells are positioned. A big tumor mass can be formed when the most robust clone is selected by the precise microenvironment conditions and then allowed to evolve hierarchically. On the flip side, CSCs or progenitors found in an unfriendly environment might not be able to aid in tumor development.

Cocultivation of normal fibroblast with tumor cells improves the tumorigenicity of the tumor cells, according to a lot of evidence in the literature [36, 37]. An obvious and reasonable explanation for this impact can be found in the fact that senescent fibroblasts secrete a multitude of molecules called senescence-associated secretory phenotype (SASP), which can alter the growth properties of cells [38–40]. Newer research, however, reveals that CSCs can alter the microenvironment by converting nearby fibroblasts into cancer-associated fibroblasts (CAFs), which differ from regular fibroblasts in their secretory factors and proliferative rates [41, 42].

But the pluripotent stromal stem cells known as mesenchymal stem cells release a number of cytokines that help restore the CSC pool by triggering self-renewal. By secreting CXCL12 and IL6/8, these substances help promote stemness through the nuclear factor-κB (NF-κB) pathway [43]. In addition to promoting tumor growth and an undifferentiated state, mesenchymal stem cells limit bone morphogenetic protein (BMP) protein synthesis by releasing Gremlin1 [44].

Proliferation and metastasis of tumor cells are facilitated by inflammation, another feature of many cancers' microenvironments [45]. One manner in which inflammation might aid carcinogenesis is by preventing cyclin-dependent kinase (CDK) inhibitor production during senescence, which promotes immortalization and tumor formation. Another way inflammation can contribute is by reducing the immunosurveillance of natural killer (NK) and CD8+ T cells [46]. The immunosuppression is a result of the recruitment of many cell types by the substances generated by tumor cells. As an example, tumor-associated macrophages can promote cancer growth and metastasis by penetrating other cell types with exosomes that contain messenger RNAs and microRNAs [47, 48].

Normal stem cell niches can be "hijacked" by CSCs, which can then alter their own microenvironment. Factors like TGF-β are part of the typical stem cell milieu and help keep resident stem cells; however, CSCs can use these factors to their advantage and survive. In order to facilitate metastasis, CSCs can also control distant niches within the same or other organs. The pre-metastatic niche is formed when factors such as VEGF-A, TGF-β, TNF-α, and lysyl oxidase (LOX) are secreted by the main tumor [49]. These factors promote the expression of the chemotactic protein S100A and alter the microenvironment in distant tissues. Activation of mesenchymal-derived stem cells (MDSCs) to promote metastasis occurs in the distant niche, where integrins help CSCs migrate and arrive [50]. Malignant progression and clonal evolution using hypoxia-activated pathways are shown in Figure 6.2.

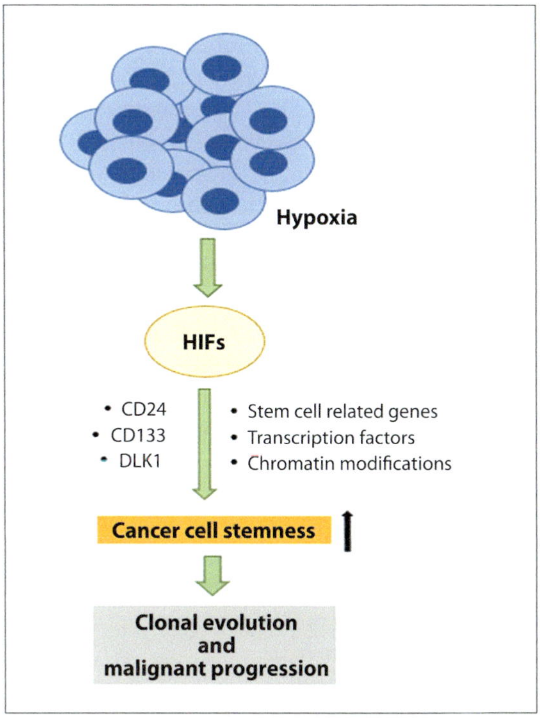

FIGURE 6.2 Clonal evolution and malignant progression using hypoxia-activated pathways.

THE HYPOXIC NICHE

Hypoxia, a feature of locally progressed solid tumors, can enhance tumor initiation, development, and resistance to therapy [51]. It is linked to various characteristics of tumors, including inflammation, metabolic changes, longer life spans, neovascularization, and altered stem cell proliferative dysregulation. Hypoxia may cause cancer through various interrelated routes. von Hippel-Lindau (VHL) tumor suppressor protein interacts with HIF-1α and HIF-2α, which are hydroxylated in proline when oxygen is present [51]. Hypoxia inhibits hydroxylation, leading to the rapid accumulation of HIF-α proteins, which dimerize with HIF-1γ and bind to the promoter of target genes, controlling their transcription [52]. Over a thousand genes are directly regulated by HIF in response to low oxygen levels. HIFs regulate the expression of over a hundred genes involved in various biological processes, including angiogenesis, epithelial-mesenchymal transition (EMT), survival, invasion, metastasis, and cellular energy metabolism. The prognosis is not good when tumor hypoxia is present, and patients' deaths have been linked to tumor hypoxia, HIF-1α and HIF-2α expression, aggressive tumor behavior, bad prognosis, and resistance to therapy. Hypoxia triggers EMT by increasing levels of transcription factors or repressors linked to EMT, which in turn activate the signaling pathways involved with EMT [53, 54]. Hypoxia-regulated EMT impacts cancer resistance to apoptosis, medications, and the immune response. HIFs mediate some of the hypoxia-induced effects on tumor cell differentiation, such as the reduction of survival rates and tumorigenic and angiogenic capabilities of CD133+ glioma stem cells when targeted [55]. Telomerase, an enzyme complex essential for telomere maintenance [56], plays a significant role in maintaining stem cell characteristics in 90% of malignancies. CSCs make up a disproportionate share of the circulating tumor cells (CTC) population in circulation, as they play a role in metastasis. CTCs display characteristics more commonly seen in CSCs, such as CD133 stem cell-like marker expression [57] in castration-resistant prostate cancer (PCa) and CD45 ICAM-1+ phenotype in hepatocarcinoma patients. They also activate HIF genes, which drive angiogenesis through VEGF induction.

HIF is the primary regulator of O_2 homeostasis, consisting of two subunits, HIF-α and HIF-β, and three subunits, HIF-1α, HIF-2α, and HIF-3α. These subunits share a high degree of structural conservation within their respective protein domains and regulate hypoxia-dependent pathways. Vertebrates possess three distinct variants of HIF, which differ in the presence of the oxygen-sensitive α subunit. HIF is usually expressed at the basal level of cells but is ubiquitinated and destroyed in the presence of high and abnormal levels of O_2 [58]. The HIF-1α subunit is destroyed by the proteasome when prolyl hydroxylase domain enzymes (PHDs) hydroxylate its conserved proline residues, forming a binding site for the VHL protein [59]. When hypoxia occurs and there is a low oxygen concentration, PHDs become inactive, and HIF-1α is not increased transcriptionally, but the protein is stabilized. HIF can activate over 70 genes involved in oxygen homeostasis regulation, angiogenesis, mitochondrial metabolism, and adaptive processes such as epigenetic DNA modification, messenger RNA, microRNA, and protein synthesis. The capacity of HIF-1α and HIF-2α to transactivate genes induced by hypoxia varies, with some genes being transactivated solely by HIF-1α, while others are transactivated by both molecules [60]. HIF is engaged in numerous pathways that impact various processes, including cell cycle progression, metabolism, angiogenesis, stem cell plasticity, immunomodulation, and proliferation. It also plays a significant role in inflammatory states by enhancing the activity of NF-κB. The presence or absence of hypoxia response element (HRE) in gene promoters, the structure of variable sequences in HRE elements of genes that affect the selective co-operation of other transcription factors, co-activators, or co-inhibitors with HIF, and the cell type that exhibits specific expression, compartmentalization, and degradation location of HIF-α isomers are some of the factors that impact the final outcome of HIF activity [61, 62] (Figure 6.3).

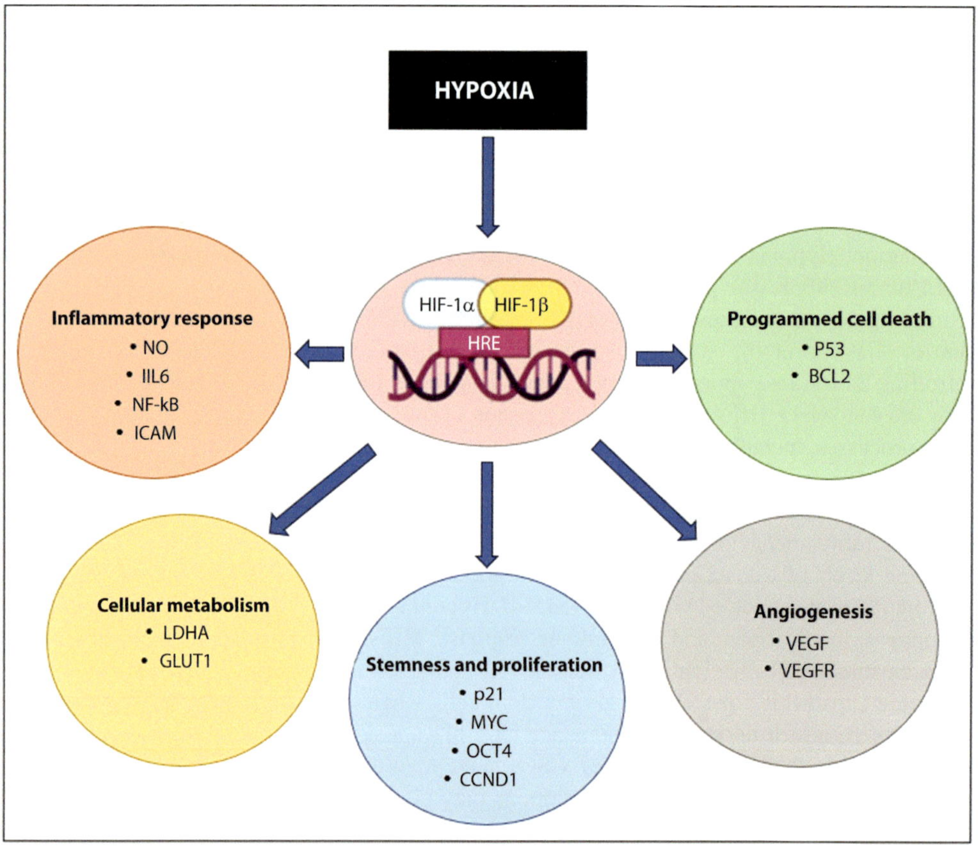

FIGURE 6.3 Activation of HIFs during hypoxia and involvement in different biological responses.

Recent research has shown that hypoxia plays a role in tumor progression, with HIF expression in CSCs associated with increased cell proliferation and survival. Initially, researchers focused on HIF-1α, which stabilized tumor cells in hypoxia, while HIF-2α was not detected or altered between normoxia and hypoxia. However, new data reveal that CSCs and non-stem cells produce HIF-1α and HIF-2α proteins and messenger RNAs (mRNAs) differently, with HIF-2α found exclusively in CSCs. HIFs are essential for the survival of CSCs and tumor development, and recent research suggests that HIF proteins are more important for preserving an undifferentiated phenotype.

HYPOXIA AND STEMNESS

Oxygen concentration is linked to stem cell maintenance in living organisms, with stem cells located in tissue niches that control their involvement in tissue formation, maintenance, and repair. These niches have low oxygen levels, with human studies suggesting an average of 3–13% O_2. Researchers face challenges in simulating native microenvironments' oxygen tension to study stem cells and their potential therapeutic applications in regenerative medicine [63]. In vitro and in vivo methods have been used to recreate the naive hypoxic cellular microenvironment, but results can be variable due to biological factors. Recently, there has been interest in cultivating stem cells in artificially low-oxygen environments to imitate the niche microenvironment in a controlled laboratory setting. Stem cell metabolism, which promotes proliferation, stemness, and commitment, has become an important regulator of cellular activities [64, 65].

EXPLOITATION OF HYPOXIA FOR REGENERATIVE MEDICINE PURPOSES

Stem cell culture conditions are crucial for maintaining stem cell characteristics, but in vitro factors can affect their properties and contribute to aging. Stem cells can thrive in low oxygen environments, and hypoxic conditions are being explored to improve stemness. HIF stabilization, a key regulator of stemness genes and metabolic variables, may indirectly influence O_2's regulation of self-renewal characteristics. Hypoxia induction is relevant to stemness preservation in various cell types, including pluripotent cells (Table 6.1).

HYPOXIA AND STEM CELL TRANSPLANTATION

Mitotic cells in regenerable tissues can stop replicating when damage accumulates, leading to senescence and cell cycle halting, as well as cell death mechanisms like apoptosis [73]. Oxygen gradients within tissues help stem cells avoid senescence, which reduces their ability to regenerate damaged tissue due to their resistance to oxidative stress. As multicellular organisms age, their tissues experience decreased organ function, leading to DNA damage, mutations, epigenetic changes, and significant changes in stem cell functions. Hypoxia has the ability to prolong cell longevity by decreasing the senescent response and increasing telomerase activity.

Tissue origin affects the characteristics of stem cells, and monitoring biological concerns associated with mesenchymal stem cell (MSC) use is crucial for improving efficacy, safety, and quality. Excessive oxidative stress can hasten and even trigger the onset of senescence, and hypoxia preconditioning prior to transplant can reduce ROS generation and improve therapeutic efficacy. Injured or non-vascularized tissues are more vulnerable to cell death caused by a hypoxic microenvironment, impacting patient survival rates through primary graft dysfunctions. The question of whether replicative senescence restricts the therapeutic potential of stem cells warrants further investigation. External stimuli become less supportive as we age, making it difficult to transplant young or rejuvenated stem cells into elderly patients. Hypoxia preconditioned bone marrow-derived mesenchymal stem cells (BMSCs) that up-regulate HIF-1α have shown promising new approaches for regenerative cell therapy in the treatment of bone deformities in the elderly [74, 75].

TABLE 6.1
Role of Hypoxia in Cancer Regenerative Medicine

Role of Hypoxia	Role in Cancer Regenerative Medicine
Pluripotency-Related Markers of Stem Cells	• The expression of transcription factors like Oct-4, Sox-2, and Nanog is crucial for pluripotency in stem cells [66]. • These proteins coordinate a highly interdependent transcriptional network, regulating cell identity, cell cycle progression, self-renewal, and maintaining cell healthiness. • Nanog regulates pluripotency and cell differentiation through interactions with transcription factor complexes. • Rex-1, when combined with Sox-2, Oct-4, and Nanog, promotes cell cycle progression and stemness maintenance [67]. • The diversity of stem cells is influenced by genetic and epigenetic factors, requiring synergistic regulation of these factors and cellular localization.
Metabolic State of Stem Cells	• Stem cells undergo a phenotypic change toward a more differentiated state, resulting in a shift in mitochondrial morphology toward mitochondrial oxidative phosphorylation (OxPhos). • Embryonic stem cells (ESCs) and induced pluripotent stem cells (iPSCs) both rely on glycolysis as their main energy source [68]. • New methods for generating iPSCs rely on compounds that promote glycolytic metabolism, such as transcription factors like Oct-4, which target numerous metabolic genes. • Multipotent stem cells also provide evidence of the association between cellular metabolism and self-renewal capabilities. • Reactive oxygen species (ROS) play an important role in cell fate signaling, influencing signaling pathways and controlling metabolic pathways. • Cells generated from human induced pluripotent stem cells (iPSCs) exhibit antioxidant defenses and ROS levels comparable to those in embryonic stem cells [69].
O_2 for Stemness Preservation	• Hypoxia, is strongly linked to stem cell self-renewal and potency. • Hypoxia slows cell proliferation by lowering respiratory enzyme levels and increasing glycolytic enzyme and lactate synthesis, which improves glycolysis. • The mitochondrial electron transport chain is inhibited in hypoxic environments, facilitating the transition to glycolysis. • HIFs activity downregulates mitochondrial enzyme expression and upregulates glucose transporters and glycolytic enzymes, facilitating the transition to glycolysis. • High oxygen levels can lead to electron leakage from the respiratory chain, leading to high ROS levels. • Stem cells grown in hypoxia can improve self-renewal capacity while maintaining pluripotent potential. • Hypoxia, metabolism, and HIFs are all linked, and simulating the environment can enhance proliferation and the expression of genes relevant to pluripotency.
HIF Role in Stemness	• Hypoxia can control stem cell plasticity by acting on HIFs, which can survive in physiologically low O_2 conditions by relying on glycolysis rather than oxidative phosphorylation for metabolism. • HIF-1α stabilization is linked to keeping anaerobic metabolism going by transcriptionally activating genes that regulate glycolysis and inactivating genes that encode important enzymes in the mitochondrial electron transport chain. • The homeobox transcription factor myeloid ectotrophic viral integration site 1 (Meis1) activates HIF-1α, controlling the metabolism of HSCs and activating HIF-2α [70]. • HIF's participation in their metabolic condition can influence the immunoregulatory features of stem cells, reducing inflammation and inhibiting the production of pro-inflammatory T cells. • HIF can sustain stemness and prevent apoptosis by downregulating p53, an important protein in cell survival. • ALDHs play a role in regulating genes, osmosis, cell signaling, neurotransmission, embryogenesis, development, cell signaling, redox balance, drug metabolism, and protection from ultraviolet radiation [71]. • Research has shown that HIF-1α is part of a mechanism that affects the migration and proliferation of MSCs, such as the HIF-1α/SCAP/SREBP1 pathway [61], which regulates the production of lipogenic enzymes, phosphorylation of mTOR, cyclin D1, cyclin E, F-actin expression, c-Myc, p-cofilin, profilin, and Rho GTPase. • HIF-2α can affect stemness by directing its effects toward Oct-4, which works in tandem with Nanog and Sox-2 to preserve stem cell characteristics and prevent differentiation [72].

CANCER STEM CELLS AND RESISTANCE

Normal stem cells and chronic stem cells share many traits, including defense mechanisms, protective mechanisms against hypoxic microenvironments, drug transporter efflux mechanisms, and DNA damage repair. CSCs are resistant to radiation and chemotherapy due to these defensive mechanisms. Studies have shown that the number of breast cancer stem cells (BCSCs) increases after chemotherapy, and CSCs can impart radioresistance to gliomas by enhancing DNA repair capacity [76, 77]. Hypoxia, a microenvironment that can offer CSCs protection, is a common feature of tumor cells during cancer occurrence and progression. Hypoxia-induced enrichment of prostate CSCs enhances resistance to androgen deprivation therapy (ADT), a major technique for prolonging survival of advanced PCa [78]. Hypoxia may also facilitate the relapse of glioma stem cells, and colorectal cancer patients acquire radioresistance and chemotherapy resistance through hypoxia mediated by HIF-1α [79, 80].

TARGETING HYPOXIA

Recent research has shown that various compounds can suppress HIF-1α function through various pathways, leading to lower amounts of HIF-1α mRNA or protein, DNA binding, and transactivation activity. Many cancers are driven by oncogenes that activate mechanistic target of rapamycin (mTOR) and induce HIF-1 activity, such as HER2, BCR-ABL, EGFR, Ras, and the PI3K/PTEN pathway [81]. Inhibitors of these pathways significantly lower HIF-1 activity and its physiologic effects. However, the effect of mTOR inhibition on other processes beyond HIF-1α protein production cannot be solely attributed to the downregulation of HIF [82]. Camptothecins and other HIF-1α inhibitors work to prevent HIF-1 from triggering transcription of target genes. Researchers are now searching for small compounds that can specifically alter HIF-1α at the protein level, as none of the known regulators of HIF-1α seem to disrupt the HIF pathway selectively. EZN-2968, a third-generation oligonucleotide, has been shown to have significant downregulation of HIF-1α and reduced tumor volume [83].

TARGETED THERAPY BASED ON HYPOXIA-INDUCIBLE FACTORS

Hypoxia is a significant factor in CSCs' radio- and chemoresistance. HIFs have been discussed as potential therapeutic targets for tumors. Research on head and neck squamous cell carcinoma (HNSCC) shows that stem cells in hypoxic conditions become responsive to carbon ions or UV radiation after HIF-1α inhibition [84]. HIFs have shown promise in treating various malignancies, including ovarian, breast, and non-small cell carcinoma. Over 40 HIF inhibitors are currently being studied in clinical studies. Table 6.2 summarizes and analyzes a few clinical studies for HIF inhibitors [85].

CONCLUSIONS AND FUTURE DIRECTIONS

This book chapter highlights the connection between hypoxia and stemness, focusing on cell culture models as a valuable resource for studying physiological hypoxia-induced mechanisms and developing new ways to enhance stem cell-based treatment approaches. To maintain cell phenotypic during expansion for stem cell populations with limited supplies, it has been suggested to lower the O_2 tension to simulate the niche microenvironment. Hypoxia is an effective in vitro stimulation for promoting cell commitment into various tissue lineages, but most protocols for stem cell expansion involve exposing cells to cultural conditions that increase oxidative stress and alter cell metabolism, leading to unpredictable and harmful effects on stem cell phenotype and fate. Precise control of O_2 levels is necessary for improving reproducibility and comparing results across laboratories. Oxygen sensors are seen as a valuable tool for real-time oxygen monitoring in in vitro cultures. Chemical

TABLE 6.2
Different Studies of HIF Inhibitors and Their Key Facts

Inhibitors	Key Roles
HIF-1α inhibitors	• The four functional domains that make up HIF-1α are the basic-helix-loop-helix (bHLH) domain, PER-ARNT-SIM (PAS) domain, oxygen-dependent degradation (ODD) domain, and two transactivation domains (TAD), namely NH2-terminal (N-TAD) and COOH-terminal (C-TAD). • Dimerization of HIF-1α and HIF-1β into HIF-1 complexes allows them to take part in regulation when oxygen levels are low. • Numerous anticancer medications suppress HIF-1α. • The expression of HIF-1α mRNA, levels of HIF-1α protein, formation of dimers of HIF-1α and HIF-1β, binding of HIF-1α to DNA (HIF-1α/HRE), and transcriptional activity of HIF-1α are all impacted by different variations. • EZN-2968 is an antisense oligonucleotide that limits the expression of HIF-1α protein by specifically inhibiting HIF-1α mRNA
EZN-2208	• Irinotecan's (CPT-11) active component is SN38, a prodrug. • An innovative topoisomerase I inhibitor called EZN-2208 is a water-soluble SN38 combination with poly (ethylene) glycol. • In allogeneic implant models, EZN-2208 considerably inhibits tumor growth compared to CPT-11 • Topoisomerase inhibitors can restrict the amounts of HIF-1α translation and accumulation of HIF-1α protein. • EZN-2208 blocks translation of HIF-1α mRNA but has no effect on its transcription. • A phase I dosage-escalation trial found that EZN-2208 is safe for patients with advanced cancers who had already undergone treatment. • In breast tumors of BRCA1-deficient mice, EZN-2208 is effective in overcoming topotecan resistance mediated by ABCG2. • A preclinical study model of arsenic-resistant acute promyelocytic leukemia (APL) indicates that a combination of EZN-2208 and retinoic acid may be an effective choice.
PX-478	• HIF-1α expression can be lower at various levels, including transcription, translation, ubiquitination, and degradation, with PX-478 (S-2-amino-3-[4′-N, N,-bis (chloroethyl) amino] phenyl propanoic acid N-oxide dihydrochloride). • PX-478 plays a role in controlling the ubiquitination of HIF-1α independently of the von Hippel-Lindau protein (pVHL) and P53. • PX-478 significantly enhances the radiosensitivity of cancer cells in various types of cancer, including prostate cancer, glioma, pancreatic cancer, and human pancreatic cancer models. • This effect might be linked to the reduction of HIF-1α-mediated angiogenesis. • An effective combination for the treatment of pancreatic ductal adenocarcinoma is arsenic trioxide and PX-478.
RAD001	• Everolimus, or RAD001, is a drug that has recently hit the market. • It is an mTOR inhibitor that blocks the translation of HIF-1α mRNA, which is dependent on mTOR. • By blocking the mTOR signaling pathway, it can indirectly influence HIF-1α and decrease HIF-1α synthesis. • Preclinical experiments have demonstrated that RAD001 effectively decreases tumor resistance. • According to research, RAD001 can reduce the growth of human ovarian cancer cells and enhance their sensitivity to cisplatin. • The partial chemical resistance of prostate cancer to docetaxel is caused by the accumulation of HIF-1α. • The proof for treating prostate cancer with a clinical RAD001/docetaxel combination was provided by the fact that RAD001 can enhance docetaxel sensitivity in prostate cancer cells by decreasing HIF-1α. • RAD001 works in tandem with cyclophosphamide to make gastric cancer more sensitive to the drug.

PT2977	• An inhibitor of HIF-2α of the second generation is PT2977. • First generation of PT2385, prior clinical trials have demonstrated the efficacy of PT2977 in treating advanced renal cell carcinoma. • Clinical phase II trials for advanced RCC are currently underway, and PT2977 is proving to be a safe and effective treatment option. • Compared to PT2385, PT2977 exhibits better pharmacodynamics and pharmacokinetics. • Clinical trials on advanced renal cell carcinoma (NCT03634540, NCT03401788) are ongoing. • Clinical trials on glioblastoma (NCT02974738) are now underway. • It is important to take hypoxia into account when employing HIF inhibitors as cancer treatments since different findings imply that hypoxia may impact cancer survival in two ways.
SOX2	• One of the transcription factors expressed both throughout embryonic development and adulthood is SOX2. • It regulates a wide range of cellular processes, including metabolism, inflammation, and development, and it also keeps cells pluripotent and able to self-renew. • To keep pluripotency-associated gene expression and differentiation-associated genes inhibited, SOX2 binds directly to DNA sites within the cell. • Several malignancies, including pancreatic cancer, breast cancer, and prostate cancer, have also been linked to increased SOX2 expression. • SOX2 has a role in the progression of breast cancer by facilitating the formation of breast cancer stem cells. • SOX2 expression rises time-dependently in hypoxic circumstances, which helps breast cancer cells migrate in response to hypoxia by increasing NEDD9 expression, which in turn induces Rac1 and HIF-1a expression. • Hypoxia seems to have many roles for SOX2, which promotes tumor invasion and progression. • SOX2 helps with HIF-1a expression and its downstream pathways.
NANOG	• Several human malignancies, such as breast cancer, lung cancer, adenocarcinoma, and gastric cancer, have been found to have abnormal expression of NANOG, a differentiated HOX domain protein. • Expression of NANOG has been linked to the establishment and preservation of CSCs' pluripotent state. • Molecular pathways by which NANOG functions are still largely unknown. • In pancreatic cancer, researchers found that high levels of NANOG expression were associated with a worse prognosis. • NANOG and OCT4 decrease the stemness of pancreatic cancer cells. • NANOG plays an active role in the hypoxic tumor microenvironment • NANOG activates tumor autophagy in non-small cell lung carcinoma cells • HIF-1 and NANOG work together to keep BCSC stem cells alive when oxygen levels are low. • The function of NANOG in stem-cell maintenance requires HIF-1a. • HIF-1a activates transcription of the ALKBH5 gene, which stabilizes NANOG mRNA through demethylation. • NANOG acts as an HIF-1 coactivator to promote its transcription. • Hypoxia-induced NANOG may play a role in melanoma tumor immunosuppression by increasing TGF-β1 expression.

(Continued)

TABLE 6.2 *(Continued)*
Different Studies of HIF Inhibitors and Their Key Facts

Inhibitors	Key Roles
OCT4	• In various cancer types, OCT4, a member of the Pit-Oct-Unc (POU) transcription factor family, is essential for CSC maintenance, self-renewal, and pluripotency. • OCT4A is the most common version of the OCT4 protein, although there are three isoforms in total: OCT4B, OCT4A1, and OCT4A. • Lung, breast, bladder, liver, and pancreatic tumors have all been found to have elevated expression levels of OCT4A. • In germ-line cancers, in particular, it was shown that reducing OCT4 levels directly decreased cell proliferation and stemness. • A recent study discovered that HIF-1α and HIF-2α upregulate SOX2 and OCT4 expression in non-small cell lung cancer cells. • These genes together control CSC development by upregulating CD133 and CD44 stem cell markers. • OCT4 expression, particularly OCT4B, in lung cancer cells is dependent on HIF-2α and not HIF-1α. • Similar to SOX2, it was found that OCT4B expression promotes cancer invasion by increasing SLUG expression. • In liver cancer, OCT4A and OCT4B both help CSCs transform into tumor endothelial-like cells, which is associated with angiogenesis.
KLF4	• The zinc-finger transcriptional factor KLF4 is expressed in a broad variety of tissues. • Cell differentiation, inflammation, apoptosis, inflammation, and angiogenesis are some of the physiological processes in which KLF4 is involved. • KLF4 acts differently in different CSCs because it is oncogenic or anti-oncogenic in cancer. • KLF4 expression stimulates cell proliferation in melanoma despite its role as a strong tumor suppressor in colon cancer. • Hypoxia regulates the cell response to hypoxia, and studies have demonstrated that HIF-1 directly increases KLF4 gene expression in this environment. • KLF4 inhibits the production of HIF-1α, the regulatory subunit of HIF-1, in normoxic circumstances. • KLF4 controls angiogenesis and hypoxia-induced apoptosis. • KLF4 promotes hypoxia-induced apoptosis in some cancer cells by increasing the expression of pro-apoptotic genes • KLF4 inhibits hypoxia-induced angiogenesis by decreasing the expression of pro-angiogenic factors like vascular endothelial growth factor (VEGF). • It would appear that there is a complicated relationship between hypoxia and KLF4, as hypoxia induces KLF4 expression and KLF4 regulates the cellular response to hypoxia.
c-MYC	• Basic helix-loop-helix (bHLH) DNA-binding proteins, of which c-MYC is a crucial component, regulate many cellular activities, including cell division, metabolism, differentiation, cell death, and stem cell traits maintenance. • c-MYC is closely controlled by developmental and mitogenic signals due to its multitude of roles. • Overexpression of c-MYC leads to oncogenic and epigenetic reprogramming via downregulation of lineage-specific transcription factors. • To facilitate CSC development, de-differentiation induces a more progenitor-like state, which in turn enables the acquisition of stem cell features through the activation of de novo oncogenic enhancers by c-MYC. • Hypoxia seems to trigger a complicated interaction between HIF and c-MYC, according to studies. • HIF-1α inhibits c-MYC activity, whereas HIF-2α stabilizes c-MYC's transcriptional activation and repression functions, hence activating c-MYC activity. • To increase HIF levels and activity, overexpression of c-MYC directly enhances HIF-2α expression. • With high c-MYC levels in cancer, HIF and c-MYC work together to alter cellular processes, such as angiogenesis and metastasis, to enhance the disease's oncogenic potential.

methods are ideal for inducing hypoxia and are flexible and reproducible. For interpreting and comparing hypoxia-mediated HIF activation and stem cell response, more standardized in vitro conditions should be used. Hypoxia is a prominent component of the tumor microenvironment that may have a role in CSC phenotype and increased tumorigenicity. Metastasis is caused by a mix of factors, including an acidic environment surrounding hypoxic cells and the activation of certain proteases. Chemotherapy combined with targeting the hypoxic CSC niche might be an effective method for CSC eradication. Genetic and epigenetic alterations, cellular microenvironmental modifications, and other factors contribute to the complicated and multifactorial formation of CSCs. Hypoxia is essential for CSCs to form and stay alive, as it promotes tumor growth and therapy resistance by activating multiple signaling pathways that help CSCs survive and self-renew. Hypoxia may also affect cancer cell Yamanaka factor expression and function, suggesting that this environment may induce a stem-like state. Hypoxia may modulate Yamanaka variables, leading to the acquisition or maintenance of CSC features. Cancer initiation, development, and treatment resistance can be better understood if researchers focus on and analyze these signs. Therapy targeting CSCs and preventing cancer recurrence requires understanding the processes by which hypoxia affects these cells. CSCs are crucial in tumor development, metastasis, and treatment resistance. Understanding the hypoxic tumor microenvironment and CSC interactions could lead to novel therapeutic techniques. Yamanaka factors, which promote pluripotency in somatic cells, can reprogram cancer cells into a stem-like state, potentially halting tumor growth and making traditional treatments more effective. Combinatorial techniques targeting CSCs at the molecular level and within the hypoxic tumor microenvironment could improve therapy efficacy and reduce disease recurrence.

CONSENT FOR PUBLICATION

Not applicable.

FUNDING

None.

CONFLICT OF INTEREST

The authors declare no conflict of interest, financial or otherwise.

ACKNOWLEDGMENTS

Declared none.

REFERENCES

1. Bartz RR, Piantadosi CA. Clinical review: oxygen as a signaling molecule. Crit Care. 2010;14:234.
2. Simon MC, Keith B. The role of oxygen availability in embryonic development and stem cell function. Nat Rev Mol Cell Biol. 2008;9:285–296.
3. Taylor CT, Scholz CC. The effect of HIF on metabolism and immunity. Nat Rev Nephrol. 2022;18(9):573–587.
4. Prabhakar NR, Semenza GL. Oxygen sensing and homeostasis. Physiology. 2015;30:340–348.
5. Glass JJ, Phillips PA, Gunning PW, Stehn JR. Hypoxia alters the recruitment of tropomyosins into the actin stress fibres of neuroblastoma cells. BMC Cancer. 2015;15:712.
6. Greaves M, Maley CC. Clonal evolution in cancer. Nature. 2012;481(7381):306–313. https://doi.org/10.1038/nature10762
7. Ebben JD, Treisman DM, Zorniak M, Kutty RG, Clark PA, Kuo JS. The cancer stem cell paradigm: a new understanding of tumor development and treatment. Expert Opin Ther Targets. 2010;14(6):621–632.

8. Cohnheim J. (1839–1884) experimental pathologist. JAMA. 1968;206:1561–1562.
9. Park CH, Bergsagel DE, McCulloch EA. Mouse myeloma tumor stem cells: a primary cell culture assay. J Natl Cancer Inst. 1971;46:411–422.
10. Gupta PB, Chaffer CL, Weinberg RA. Cancer stem cells: mirage or reality? Nat Med. 2009;15:1010–1012.
11. Lapidot T, Sirard C, Vormoor J, Murdoch B, et al. A cell initiating human acute myeloid leukaemia after transplantation into SCID mice. Nature. 1994;367:645–648.
12. Bonnet D, Dick JE. Human acute myeloid leukemia is organized as a hierarchy that originates from a primitive hematopoietic cell. Nat Med. 1997;3:730–737.
13. Al-Hajj M, Wicha MS, Benito-Hernandez A, Morrison SJ, et al. Prospective identification of tumorigenic breast cancer cells. Proc Natl Acad Sci U S A. 2003;100:3983–3988.
14. Dawood S, Austin L, Cristofanilli M. Cancer stem cells: implications for cancer therapy. Oncology (Williston Park). 2014;28:1101–1107, 1110.
15. Reya T, Morrison SJ, Clarke MF, Weissman IL. Stem cells, cancer, and cancer stem cells. Nature. 2001;414:105–111.
16. Liu ZL, Chen HH, Zheng LL, et al. Angiogenic signaling pathways and anti-angiogenic therapy for cancer. Sig Transduct Target Ther. 2023;8:198.
17. Ghalehbandi S, Yuzugulen J, Pranjol MZI, Pourgholami MH. The role of VEGF in cancer-induced angiogenesis and research progress of drugs targeting VEGF. Eur J Pharmacol. 2023;949:175586.
18. Golhani V, Ray SK, Mukherjee S. Role of MicroRNAs and long non-coding RNAs in regulating angiogenesis in human breast cancer: a molecular medicine perspective. Curr Mol Med. 2022;22(10):882–893.
19. Lugano R, Ramachandran M, Dimberg A. Tumor angiogenesis: causes, consequences, challenges and opportunities. Cell Mol Life Sci. 2020;77(9):1745–1770.
20. Sell S. On the stem cell origin of cancer. Am J Pathol. 2010;176(6):2584. https://doi.org/10.2353/ajpath.2010.091064
21. Sell S. Maturation arrest of stem cell differentiation is a common pathway for the cellular origin of teratocarcinomas and epithelial cancers. Lab Invest. 2022;70(1):6–22.
22. Lapidot T, Sirard C, Vormoor J, Murdoch B, Nature TH. A cell initiating human acute myeloid leukaemia after transplantation into SCID mice. Nature. 2022;367:645–648.
23. Sutherland H, Blair A, Zapf R. Characterization of a hierarchy in human acute myeloid leukemia progenitor cells. Blood. 1996;11:4754–4761.
24. López J, Valdez-Morales FJ, Benıtez-Bribiesca L, Cerbón M, Carrancá AG. Normal and cancer stem cells of the human female reproductive system. Reprod Biol Endocrinol. 2013;11(1):53.
25. Ayob AZ, Ramasamy TS. Cancer stem cells as key drivers of tumour progression. J Biomed Sci. 2018;25(1):20.
26. Carvalho J. Cell reversal from a differentiated to a stem-like state at cancer initiation. Front Oncol. 2020;10:541. https://doi.org/10.3389/fonc.2020.00541
27. Wang RA, Li ZS, Zhang HZ, Zheng PJ, Li QL, Shi JG, Yan QG, Ye J, Wang JB, Guo Y, Huang XF, Yu YH. Invasive cancers are not necessarily from preformed in situ tumours – an alternative way of carcinogenesis from misplaced stem cells. J Cell Mol Med. 2013;17(7):921–926.
28. Walcher L, Kistenmacher AK, Suo H, Kitte R, Dluczek S, Strauß A, et al. Cancer stem cells—Origins and biomarkers: perspectives for targeted personalized therapies. Front Immunol. 2020;11:1280.
29. Afify SM, Seno M. Conversion of stem cells to cancer stem cells: undercurrent of cancer initiation. Cancers (Basel). 2019;11(3):345.
30. Abd GM, Laird MC, Ku JC, Li Y. Hypoxia-induced cancer cell reprogramming: a review on how cancer stem cells arise. Front Oncol. 2023;13:1227884.
31. Li Z, Zhang YY, Zhang H, Yang J, Chen Y, Lu H. Asymmetric cell division and tumor heterogeneity. Front Cell Dev Biol. 2022;10:1374.
32. Paul R, Dorsey JF, Fan Y. Cell plasticity, senescence, and quiescence in cancer stem cells: biological and therapeutic implications. Pharmacol Ther. 2022;231:107985.
33. Brown G. Hematopoietic and chronic myeloid leukemia stem cells: multi-stability versus lineage restriction. Int J Mol Sci. 2022;23(21):13570.
34. Vosberg S, Greif PA. Clonal evolution of acute myeloid leukemia from diagnosis to relapse. Genes Chromosomes Cancer. 2019;58(12):839–849.
35. Onecha E, Rapado I, Luz Morales M, Carreño-Tarragona G, Martinez-Sanchez P, Gutierrez X, Sáchez Pina JM, Linares M, Gallardo M, Martinez-López J, Ayala R. Monitoring of clonal evolution of acute myeloid leukemia identifies the leukemia subtype, clinical outcome and potential new drug targets for post-remission strategies or relapse. Haematologica. 2021;106(9):2325–2333.

36. Wieder R. Fibroblasts as turned agents in cancer progression. Cancers (Basel). 2023;15(7):2014. https://doi.org/10.3390/cancers15072014
37. Gascard P, Tlsty TD. Carcinoma-associated fibroblasts: orchestrating the composition of malignancy. Genes Dev. 2016;30(9):1002–1019.
38. Tchkonia T, Zhu Y, van Deursen J, Campisi J. Cellular senescence and the senescent secretory phenotype: therapeutic opportunities. J Clin Invest. 2013;123:966–972.
39. Acosta JC, Gil J. Senescence: a new weapon for cancer therapy. Trends Cell Biol. 2012;22:211–219.
40. Coppe JP, Desprez PY, Krtolica A, Campisi J. The senescence-associated secretory phenotype: the dark side of tumor suppression. Annu Rev Pathol. 2010;5:99–118.
41. Kalluri R, Zeisberg M. Fibroblasts in cancer. Nat Rev Cancer. 2006;6:392–401.
42. Junttila MR, de Sauvage FJ. Influence of tumour microenvironment heterogeneity on therapeutic response. Nature. 2013;501:346–354.
43. Cabarcas SM, Mathews LA, Farrar WL. The cancer stem cell niche – there goes the neighborhood? Int J Cancer. 2011;129:2315–2327.
44. Davis H, Irshad S, Bansal M, Rafferty H, et al. Aberrant epithelial GREM1 expression initiates colonic tumorigenesis from cells outside the stem cell niche. Nat Med. 2015;21:62–70.
45. Carnero A, Blanco-Aparicio C, Kondoh H, Lleonart ME, MartinezLeal JF, et al. Disruptive chemicals, senescence and immortality. Carcinogenesis. 2015;36(Suppl 1):S19–S37.
46. Casbon AJ, Reynaud D, Park C, Khuc E, et al. Invasive breast cancer reprograms early myeloid differentiation in the bone marrow to generate immunosuppressive neutrophils. Proc Natl Acad Sci U S A. 2015;112:E566–E575.
47. Fabbri M. TLRs as miRNA receptors. Cancer Res. 2012;72:6333–6337.
48. Zhou X, Chen B, Zhang Z, Huang Y, Li J, Wei Q, Cao D, Ai J. Crosstalk between tumor-associated macrophages and microRNAs: a key role in tumor microenvironment. Int J Mol Sci. 2022;23(21):13258.
49. Patras L, Shaashua L, Matei I, Lyden D. Immune determinants of the pre-metastatic niche. Cancer Cell. 2023;41(3):546–572.
50. Plaks V, Kong N, Werb Z. The cancer stem cell niche: how essential is the niche in regulating stemness of tumor cells? Cell Stem Cell. 2015;16:225–238.
51. Mukherjee S, Ray SK. Targeting tumor hypoxia and hypoxia-inducible factors (HIFs) for the treatment of cancer –a story of transcription factors with novel approach in molecular medicine. Curr Mol Med. 2022;22(4):285–286.
52. Ziello JE, Jovin IS, Huang Y. Hypoxia-inducible factor (HIF)-1 regulatory pathway and its potential for therapeutic intervention in malignancy and ischemia. Yale J Biol Med. 2007;80(2):51–60.
53. Gonzalez DM, Medici D. Signaling mechanisms of the epithelial-mesenchymal transition. Sci Signal. 2014;7(344):re8.
54. Tam SY, Wu VWC, Law HKW. Hypoxia-induced epithelial-mesenchymal transition in cancers: HIF-1α and beyond. Front Oncol. 2020;10:486.
55. Li Z, Bao S, Wu Q, Wang H, Eyler C, Sathornsumetee S, Shi Q, Cao Y, Lathia J, McLendon RE, Hjelmeland AB, Rich JN. Hypoxia-inducible factors regulate tumorigenic capacity of glioma stem cells. Cancer Cell. 2009;15(6):501–513.
56. Ray SK, Mukherjee S. Hypoxic regulation of telomerase gene expression in cancer. In: Mukherjee, S., Kanwar, J.R. (eds). Hypoxia in Cancer: Significance and Impact on Cancer Therapy (pp. 251–273). Springer, Singapore.
57. Zhang Q, Rong Y, Yi K, Huang L, Chen M, Wang F. Circulating tumor cells in hepatocellular carcinoma: single-cell based analysis, preclinical models, and clinical applications. Theranostics. 2020;10(26):12060–12071.
58. Smith TG, Robbins PA, Ratcliffe PJ. The human side of hypoxia-inducible factor. Br J Haematol. 2008;141(3):325–334.
59. Fan L, Li J, Yu Z, Dang X, Wang K. The hypoxia-inducible factor pathway, prolyl hydroxylase domain protein inhibitors, and their roles in bone repair and regeneration. Biomed Res Int. 2014;2014:239356.
60. Hu CJ, Wang LY, Chodosh LA, Keith B, Simon MC. Differential roles of hypoxia-inducible factor 1alpha (HIF-1alpha) and HIF-2alpha in hypoxic gene regulation. Mol Cell Biol. 2003;23(24):9361–9374.
61. Di Mattia M, Mauro A, Citeroni MR, Dufrusine B, Peserico A, Russo V, Berardinelli P, Dainese E, Cimini A, Barboni B. Insight into hypoxia stemness control. Cells. 2021;10(8):2161.
62. Yfantis A, Mylonis I, Chachami G, Nikolaidis M, Amoutzias GD, Paraskeva E, Simos G. Transcriptional response to hypoxia: the role of HIF-1-associated co-regulators. Cells. 2023;12(5):798.
63. Mahla RS. Stem cells applications in regenerative medicine and disease therapeutics. Int J Cell Biol. 2016;2016:6940283.

64. Rigaud VOC, Hoy R, Mohsin S, Khan M. Stem cell metabolism: powering cell-based therapeutics. Cells. 2020;9(11):2490.
65. Ito K, Suda T. Metabolic requirements for the maintenance of self-renewing stem cells. Nat Rev Mol Cell Biol. 2014;15(4):243–256.
66. Rodda DJ, Chew JL, Lim LH, Loh YH, Wang B, Ng HH, Robson P. Transcriptional regulation of nanog by OCT4 and SOX2. J Biol Chem. 2005;280(26):24731–24737.
67. Shariati F, Favaedi R, Ramazanali F, Ghoraeian P, Afsharian P, Aflatoonian B, Aflatoonian R, Shahhoseini M. Increased expression of stemness genes REX-1, OCT-4, NANOG, and SOX-2 in women with ovarian endometriosis versus normal endometrium: a case-control study. Int J Reprod Biomed. 2019;16(12):ijrm.v16i12.3684.
68. Varum S, Rodrigues AS, Moura MB, Momcilovic O, Easley CA 4th, Ramalho-Santos J, Van Houten B, Schatten G. Energy metabolism in human pluripotent stem cells and their differentiated counterparts. PLoS One. 2011;6(6):e20914.
69. Chaudhari P, Ye Z, Jang YY. Roles of reactive oxygen species in the fate of stem cells. Antioxid Redox Signal. 2014;20(12):1881–1890.
70. Zhang CC, Sadek HA. Hypoxia and metabolic properties of hematopoietic stem cells. Antioxid Redox Signal. 2014;20(12):1891–1901.
71. Singh S, Brocker C, Koppaka V, Chen Y, Jackson BC, Matsumoto A, Thompson DC, Vasiliou V. Aldehyde dehydrogenases in cellular responses to oxidative/electrophilic stress. Free Radic Biol Med. 2013;56:89–101.
72. Covello KL, Kehler J, Yu H, Gordan JD, Arsham AM, Hu CJ, Labosky PA, Simon MC, Keith B. HIF-2alpha regulates Oct-4: effects of hypoxia on stem cell function, embryonic development, and tumor growth. Genes Dev. 2006;20(5):557–570.
73. Roger L, Tomas F, Gire V. Mechanisms and regulation of cellular senescence. Int J Mol Sci. 2021;22(23):13173.
74. Wei ZZ, Zhu YB, Zhang JY, McCrary MR, Wang S, Zhang YB, Yu SP, Wei L. Priming of the cells: hypoxic preconditioning for stem cell therapy. Chin Med J (Engl). 2017;130(19):2361–2374.
75. Luo Z, Wu F, Xue E, Huang L, Yan P, Pan X, Zhou Y. Hypoxia preconditioning promotes bone marrow mesenchymal stem cells survival by inducing HIF-1α in injured neuronal cells derived exosomes culture system. Cell Death Dis. 2019;10(2):134.
76. Rycaj K, Tang DG. Cancer stem cells and radioresistance. Int J Radiat Biol. 2014;90(8):615–621.
77. Zheng Q, Zhang M, Zhou F, Zhang L, Meng X. The breast cancer stem cells traits and drug resistance. Front Pharmacol. 2021;11:599965.
78. O'Reilly D, Johnson P, Buchanan PJ. Hypoxia induced cancer stem cell enrichment promotes resistance to androgen deprivation therapy in prostate cancer. Steroids. 2019;152:108497.
79. Chédeville AL, Madureira PA. The Role of Hypoxia in Glioblastoma Radiotherapy Resistance. Cancers (Basel). 2021;13(3):542.
80. Xu K, Zhan Y, Yuan Z, Qiu Y, Wang H, Fan G, Wang J, Li W, Cao Y, Shen X, Zhang J, Liang X, Yin P. Hypoxia induces drug resistance in colorectal cancer through the HIF-1α/miR-338-5p/IL-6 feedback loop. Mol Ther. 2019;27(10):1810–1824.
81. Steelman LS, Chappell WH, Abrams SL, Kempf RC, Long J, Laidler P, Mijatovic S, Maksimovic-Ivanic D, Stivala F, Mazzarino MC, Donia M, Fagone P, Malaponte G, Nicoletti F, Libra M, Milella M, Tafuri A, Bonati A, Bäsecke J, Cocco L, Evangelisti C, Martelli AM, Montalto G, Cervello M, McCubrey JA. Roles of the Raf/MEK/ERK and PI3K/PTEN/Akt/mTOR pathways in controlling growth and sensitivity to therapy-implications for cancer and aging. Aging (Albany NY). 2011;3(3):192–222.
82. Dodd KM, Yang J, Shen MH, Sampson JR, Tee AR. mTORC1 drives HIF-1α and VEGF–a signalling via multiple mechanisms involving 4E-BP1, S6K1 and STAT3. Oncogene. 2015;34(17):2239–2250.
83. Jeong W, Rapisarda A, Park SR, Kinders RJ, Chen A, Melillo G, Turkbey B, Steinberg SM, Choyke P, Doroshow JH, Kummar S. Pilot trial of EZN-2968, an antisense oligonucleotide inhibitor of hypoxia-inducible factor-1 alpha (HIF-1α), in patients with refractory solid tumors. Cancer Chemother Pharmacol. 2014;73(2):343–348.
84. Wozny AS, Lauret A, Battiston-Montagne P, Guy JB, Beuve M, Cunha M, Saintigny Y, Blond E, Magne N, Lalle P, Ardail D, Alphonse G, Rodriguez-Lafrasse C. Differential pattern of HIF-1α expression in HNSCC cancer stem cells after carbon ion or photon irradiation: one molecular explanation of the oxygen effect. Br J Cancer. 2017;116(10):1340–1349.
85. Sun X, Lv X, Yan Y, Zhao Y, Ma R, He M, Wei M. Hypoxia-mediated cancer stem cell resistance and targeted therapy. Biomed Pharmacother. 2020;130:110623.

7 Innovative Techniques for Visualization of Cancer Hypoxia

M V Pattarkine and Era Chouhan
Biotechnology, Harrisburg University of Science and Technology, Harrisburg, PA, USA

Pramedha Kamplikar
Department of Biochemistry, All Indian Institute of Medical Sciences, Bhopal, India

INTRODUCTION

Hypoxia, a condition characterized by low concentration of oxygen, is a common feature of various diseases such as tumours, cardiovascular diseases, and stroke.[1,2] In case of tumours/cancers, due to faster proliferation of cancer cells than angiogenesis, the tumour tissues experience an imbalance between supply and consumption of oxygen, leading to an overall reduced oxygen pressure. The hypoxic cancer cells adapt by up regulating the synthesis of proteins that promote cell selection and survival, leading to poor patient outcomes for treatments. Investigating these dynamics between hypoxia, cancer progression, and altered outcomes to therapeutic responses would help design better strategies for treating these cancers.

This hypoxic tumour microenvironment (TME) imposes several changes, such as increased concentration of reactive oxygen species (ROS), modulation of expression of genes regulating metabolic pathways, and interference with other cellular processes, eventually leading to malignancy. Cell migration, proliferation, invasion, and angiogenesis – all these critical cellular processes are impacted due to hypoxia. Hypoxic TME can impact cell cycle regulatory processes, resist therapeutic treatments, and cause cancer recurrence.

The radiosensitivity of any tissue is a function of oxygen tension in tissues, and due to reduced oxygen pressure, hypoxic tissues have been less responsive to radiation.[3] Elimination of the hypoxic TME is therefore a necessary step for successful treatment as well as imaging of these tumours. Several approaches have been attempted to eliminate tumour hypoxia, such as erythropoietin injections, blood transfusion, and vasodilator application,[4–6] but none has been effective.

Innovative and sensitive imaging/visualization of hypoxic tumours has applications in diagnostic, therapeutic, and prognostic fields. While structural imaging provides information about the physical anatomy of a tumour, functional imaging, particularly using techniques like positron emission tomography (PET) scans with hypoxia-specific tracers, allows for direct visualization and quantification of hypoxic regions within a cancer by assessing its physiological activity related to oxygen levels, offering a more detailed understanding of the TME beyond just its structure; essentially, structural imaging shows "where" the tumour is, while functional imaging reveals "how" the tumour is functioning in terms of oxygen deprivation.

This review explores innovative approaches in visualization of hypoxic tissues using conventional scanning techniques such as magnetic resonance imaging (MRI) and PET, with innovations such

DOI: 10.1201/9781003477419-7

as the use of hypoxic-specific reagents, applications of smart nanoparticles that respond uniquely to hypoxic environments, and applications of multi-omics and artificial intelligence (AI).

IMAGING HYPOXIC TUMOURS

Sensitive imaging of hypoxic cancers can provide critical knowledge for cancer care. These non-invasive imaging techniques offer several advantages:

a. Providing information about imaging data and its relationship with specific hypoxic tumours can generate information about cancer proliferation and prognosis.
b. Enable visualizing the entirety of the tissue in a non-invasive manner.
c. Can be optimized for identifying molecular (i.e., PET) and functional (i.e., MRI details.[7,8]

PET SCANNING

PET is a nuclear imaging technology (for molecular imaging) that enables visualization of metabolic processes in the body. The basics of PET imaging are that the technique detects pairs of gamma rays emitted indirectly by a positron-emitting radionuclide (a radiotracer). The tracer is injected into a vein on a biologically active molecule, usually a sugar that is used for cellular energy. PET systems are equipped with sensitive detector panels that can capture gamma ray emissions from inside the body. The PET systems software can plot the signal and pinpoint the source of the emissions to create 3D computed tomography (CT) images of the tracer concentrations within the body (Figure 7.1).[9]

Although this method has considerable potential to be developed as a tumour oximeter, particularly to monitor changes after tumour oxygenation,[10] development of a suitable paramagnetic marker that has low toxicity for humans is currently unavailable. The lack of appropriate enhanced

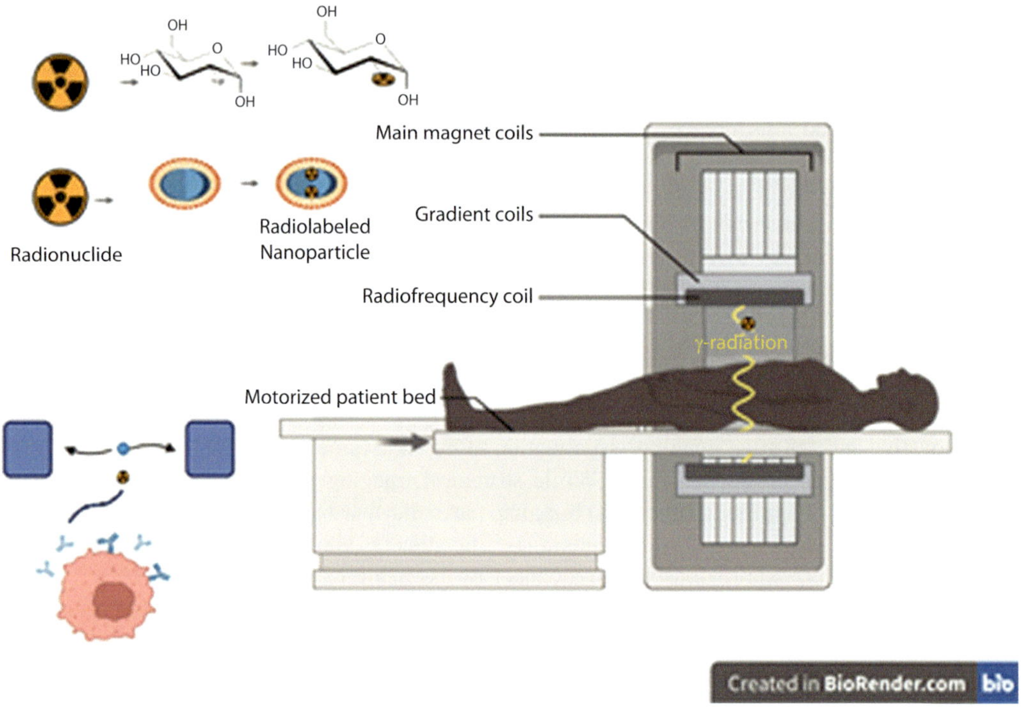

FIGURE 7.1 Schematic for PET scanning using radiolabelled nanoparticles.[43]

permeability and retention (EPR) instrumentation in the clinic also prevents widespread implementation of this otherwise promising technique.[11] Based on the differential optical contrast between oxygenated and deoxygenated Hb, photoacoustic tomography (PAT) can also be used to image blood oxygenation. Though there is no clinical evidence, Wang et al. implemented a PAT scan to image cerebral blood oxygenation of rats *in vivo* and were able to show that the PAT scans could track/image the alternation from hyperoxia to hypoxia.[12]

MRI Scanning

MRI is a non-invasive imaging technique that offers structural images of the anatomical details of tissues. These scans depend on a magnetic field and a radiofrequency pulse to generate images. The contrast between tissue types is determined by the magnetic properties of the tissue matter (Figure 7.2).[13]

Dynamic contrast-enhanced (DCE) MRI employs several contrast agents, the most common of which are gadolinium (Gd) based.[14] DCE-MRI has demonstrated use in the detection of hypoxia in xenograft models of cervical carcinoma, melanoma, and pancreatic ductal adenocarcinoma (PDAC).[15] However, DCE-MRI is limited in the fact that it provides information on perfusion and permeability. Since perfusion is not the only factor influencing tumour oxygenation, the estimates may not be entirely indicative of tumour hypoxia.[16]

Blood-Oxygen-Level-Dependent MRI (BOLD-MRI) scans enable visualization of the increase in concentration of oxygenated haemoglobin.[17] These scans indicated a direct relationship between the concentration of oxygenated blood in the capillaries and the T2_ relaxation time of the protons and vice versa. The relationship between BOLD-MRI signal and vascular oxygenation allowed direct estimation of pO_2.

Another variation of standard MRI, 19F MRI is getting a lot of traction. It uses two types of markers – perfluorocarbons (PFCs) and fluorinated nitroimidazoles – as contrast agents. PFCs are highly hydrophobic but offer exceptional oxygen solubility.[18] The 19F spin lattice relaxation rate of PFCs varies linearly with the dissolved oxygen concentration. Thus, the 19F-based oximetry allows measurements of vascular oxygenation in vivo.[19] The disadvantages of 19F

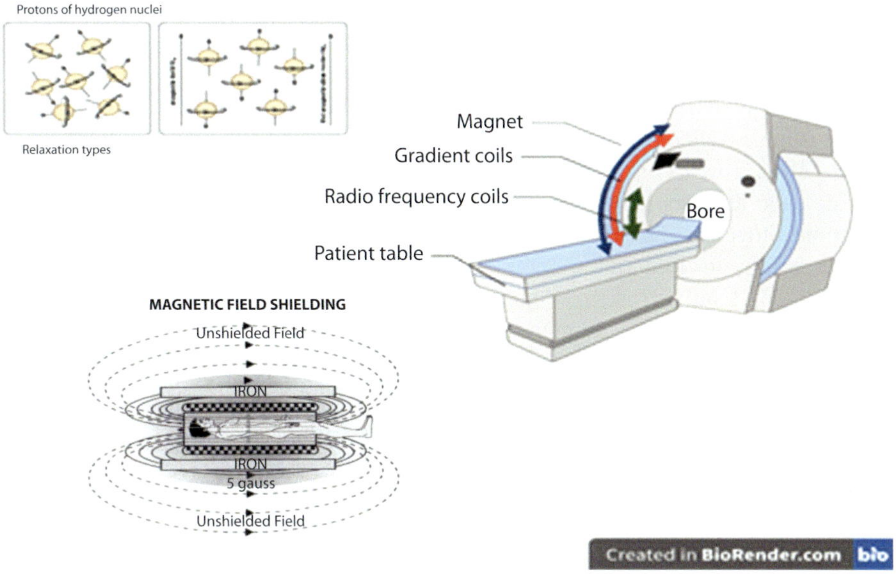

FIGURE 7.2 Schematics for traditional MRI scanning.[43]

MRI are that the measurements are subject to flow artefacts, and the oxygen sensitivity of some 19F MR imaging compounds is easily affected by temperature, dilution, pH, common proteins, and blood.[20]

Optical Imaging Using Fluorescent Probes

PET and MRI techniques have apparent disadvantages such as harmful radiation, lack of precise diagnosis due to a low ratio of signal-to-noise ratio, and inability for real-time monitoring of hypoxic tissues due to the need for significant time to generate the scans.

Fluorescence imaging techniques address the above drawbacks while offering high sensitivity, simplicity and non-invasiveness.[21–23] Especially with the rapid development in materials science and nanotechnology sectors, the design and construction of numerous fluorescent nanomaterial-based probes (nanoprobes) have helped alternative approaches for visualization of intracellular molecular and metabolic process.[24–26] Currently, many fluorescent nanoprobes for imaging of living cells under hypoxic conditions have been developed. Unique properties possessed by nanoparticles, such as ease of cell internalization, higher retention in the circulatory system, targeted and highly specific binding with intracellular biomacromolecules, and the ability to serve as cargo to carry a large amount of imaging agents.[27–29]

Application of Hypoxia-Specific Reagents

In a study, Zhou et al.[30] demonstrated a creative outlook towards the discernment of cancer cells and tumours under hypoxic conditions. The researchers developed a novel method for imaging hypoxic tumours that had improved visualization ability by utilizing hypoxic-specific agents. Use of hypoxic-specific agents increases sensitivity for the detection of hypoxic regions. This provides the ability to detect even the smallest hypoxic cancer cells as the targeted tracers lower the limits of detection.

Certain enzymes such as nitro reductases are not affected by low oxygen pressures and are fully active even under hypoxic conditions, which enables them to be clearly visible with great contrast. These enzymes respond differentially to normoxic and hypoxic tissues by targeting molecules/pathways that are altered due to hypoxia, such as those including HIF-1α (hypoxia-inducible factor 1-alpha). Such agents not only improve visibility in imaging but also provide insights into the TME.[31]

MRI is a significant technique for imaging hypoxic tumours. It can differentiate between variation in levels of hypoxia that influence tumour behaviour and analyse the treatments that are required. By using advanced MRI techniques like BOLD imaging and dynamic contrast-enhanced MRI (DCE-MRI), it assists in identifying the vascularity and oxygenation of the tumour. This type of systematic analysis is necessary for customization of therapies as per the patient and a better outcome altogether. These techniques can also enhance our understanding of how to make strategies, especially for radiation therapy and treatment targeted at oxygen-sensitive cancerous cells. The DCE-MRI and diffusion-weighted imaging (DWI). This kind of approach analyses the perfusion and cellular ability of tumours by assessing the hypoxic images. DCE-MRI also displays the significant effect of a hypoxic tumour by analysing distinguished flow of blood and its permeability.

HYBRID IMAGING APPROACHES

As an innovative combination, Gouel et al.[32] suggested integration of PET and MRI to utilize the strengths of both imaging techniques effectively for diagnosing hypoxia. This hybrid approach may help in better understanding tumour biology as it combines structural and functional results from

MRI with the metabolic knowledge from PET. As these outcomes combine the structural and metabolic aspects of the hypoxic tissue, they have the potential to help design highly efficient treatment strategies

By combining these progressive imaging technologies with clinical practice, it will have a pivotal role in enhancing the tumour response to therapy, especially as the monitoring becomes easier. By proper examination, it helps to improve diagnosis and better personalized treatment for patients.

Emerging Technologies

Nanoparticle-based contrast agents can enhance the detection of hypoxic regions by displaying greater sensitivity and specificity than traditional contrast agents. The evolution of such agents shows a substantial step forward in improving imaging technology.

The researchers also advocate for involving hypoxia imaging in regular check-ups to better make personalized medicine (PM). By accurate assessment of individual tumour hypoxia profiles, health care practitioners can make certain decisions and design improved treatment strategies, therefore leading to better treatment results and reducing the adverse effects.

The integration of hypoxia imaging into the clinical workspace shows a better and customizable cancer treatment. By being informed regarding the treatment choices according to an individual-specific characteristic of each patient's tumour, healthcare providers can improve therapeutic outcomes and thus overall patient survival rates.

IMAGING – MOLECULAR LEVEL – CELL/TISSUE LABELLING – IN-VIVO OR IN-VITRO

The non-invasive observation, description, and measurement of biological processes occurring at the cellular and molecular levels in living things are referred to as molecular imaging. Researchers can observe cellular behaviours, signalling pathways, and molecular interactions by utilizing certain probes and labels.[33] The following are the primary methods for molecular imaging:

a. *Fluorescence imaging*: The use of fluorescent dyes or proteins to label and visualize cellular structures.
b. *Bioluminescence imaging*: Emission of light from biological systems, often used in animal models.
c. *Magnetic resonance imaging (MRI)*: Functional imaging using contrast agents to highlight specific tissues.
d. *Positron emission tomography (PET)*: A nuclear medicine technique using radiolabelled molecules for real-time tracking of metabolic processes.[33,34]

Labelling cells and tissues with high specificity is fundamental to molecular imaging. The labelling procedure involves attaching a marker that can be seen by imaging technology to a biomolecule, cell, or tissue.[35] Biomarkers are biological molecules found in blood, tissue or other body fluids; they are indicative of an alteration in a process that may lead to a condition or disease. Reduced oxygen supply in tumours or cancer hypoxia plays a major role in tumour development, treatment resistance, and metastasis. Its detection and visualization in TMEs is essential for comprehending the biology of tumour development, early detection, and accurate, and targeted therapy.[36]

Hypoxia-responsive reporter gene experiments use genetically modified cells to generate fluorescent or luminous proteins in low-oxygen environments. These reporter assays, controlled by hypoxia-inducible elements, provide dynamic imaging of hypoxic regions in live cells or animal models. This technique is particularly useful for preclinical studies, as it allows for real-time observation of tumour hypoxia and its progression.[37]

Biomarkers-Based Imaging for Hypoxia

Due to their impact on angiogenesis, tumour growth, and treatment resistance, hypoxia biomarkers are essential to our understanding of cancer biology. The most well-known biomarkers for hypoxia are HIFs, especially HIF-1α, which controls the expression of genes involved in the adaptation of cells to hypoxia. Pimonidazole, a synthetic nitroimidazole molecule that binds covalently to thiol groups in hypoxic cells, and carbonic anhydrase IX (CAIX), a cell-surface protein overexpressed in hypoxic circumstances, are two more biomarkers that have proven essential for imaging. These indicators give a comprehensive picture of hypoxic areas by molecular imaging methods such as PET and immunohistochemistry (IHC), which improves our comprehension of TMEs and treatment response.[38]

One of the most popular techniques for identifying hypoxia indicators in tumour tissues is IHC. Using this method, tissue slices are stained with antibodies that specifically target proteins related to hypoxia, like CAIX or HIF-1α. IHC makes it possible to localize hypoxic areas in biopsied tissues with great resolution, which is vital for understanding the distribution of hypoxia in tumours. IHC imaging provides a picture of hypoxia at the time of biopsy, helpful for assessing tumour aggressiveness, forecasting treatment outcomes, and determining diagnoses. Researchers can measure the expression levels of these biomarkers and obtain a precise, localized understanding of hypoxic burden in cancer patients by combining IHC with digital pathology.[39]

Assessing hypoxia *in vivo* with PET imaging using radiolabelled hypoxia indicators is a more dynamic and non-invasive method. Radiotracers, like fluoromisonidazole and fluoroazomycin arabinoside, attach to hypoxic cells and release signals that can be detected by PET scanners, giving a real-time and whole-body picture of the distribution of hypoxia. In clinical settings, PET imaging with these biomarkers is beneficial for assessing the degree of hypoxia in tumours, optimizing radiation therapy, and tracking treatment responses over time. PET imaging, as opposed to tissue-based methods such as IHC, enables longitudinal investigations of hypoxia and allows observation of hypoxia changes throughout the disease.[40]

Another popular method is PET with hypoxia-specific radiotracers such as [18F]-Fluoromisonidazole. These radiotracers provide non-invasive, whole-body hypoxia imaging in clinical settings as they selectively accumulate in hypoxic areas of tumours and are identified by PET scans. For determining the aggressiveness of a tumour and directing hypoxia-targeted therapies, such as radiotherapy, which is less effective in hypoxic environments, PET imaging offers quantitative and geographical information on hypoxia.[41] Clinical and research settings also regularly use fluorescent hypoxia probes, like pimonidazole. Using the covalent binding of these probes to intracellular proteins without oxygen, hypoxic areas in tissue biopsies can be precisely identified using fluorescence microscopy visualization of the resulting adducts[42] (Table 7.1).

Nanoparticles-Based Imaging for Hypoxia

Nanoparticles (gold nanoparticles, magnetic nanoparticles) conjugated to targeting ligands can be used to label specific cell types or tissues. These particles enhance contrast in imaging techniques like MRI or optical imaging.[51] *In vivo* imaging allows for dynamic tracking of biological processes over time, but the challenge lies in delivering the labels specifically to the target cells or tissues

TABLE 7.1
Hypoxia-Specific Probes and Their Intracellular Targets43

	Hypoxia-Specific Probes	Intracellular Target	Mechanism of Action	Ref.
1.	Pimonidazole	Protein thiols	Forms adducts with thiol groups in hypoxic cells, detectable with antibodies for imaging and staining.	44
2.	EF-5 (2-nitroimidazole)	Cellular macromolecules	Binds to hypoxic cell macromolecules, creating adducts that are identifiable with fluorescent or radioactive tags.	45
3.	[18F] FMISO (Fluoromisonidazole)	Intracellular protein macromolecules	Accumulates in hypoxic cells and can be visualized with PET scans due to radioactive fluorine.	46
4.	[64 Cu] Cu-ATSM	Cellular proteins, particularly in mitochondria	Selectively retained in hypoxic cells, emitting positrons for imaging in PET scans.	47
5.	Prodrug reporters	Enzymes such as nitroreductase	Activated by enzymes upregulated in hypoxia, yielding fluorescent or bioluminescent signals.	48
6.	Nitroimidazole-based dyes (for example, SR4554)	Cellular macromolecules	Penetrates hypoxic tissues and binds to cellular macromolecules, then visualized through fluorescence or PET imaging.	49
7.	Carbonic anhydrase IX (CAIX) – targeted probes	CAIX enzyme on cell surface	Binds to CAIX, overexpressed in hypoxic tumours, often used for fluorescence or radiolabelling.	50

without affecting the normal physiological functions. Advancements in molecular imaging will likely focus on improving the specificity, sensitivity, and non-invasiveness of labelling techniques. Developing more biocompatible probes, such as biodegradable nanoparticles, will reduce toxicity concerns *in vivo*.[52] Integrating molecular imaging with other technologies, such as AI and machine learning (ML), may also enhance the interpretation of complex datasets, leading to more precise insights into biological processes[53] (Figure 7.3).

The unique attributes of nanomaterials, such as surface modification capabilities, tunable optical properties, and EPR effects, have made nanomaterials-based imaging for hypoxia has become a potent and adaptable method for observing oxygen-deprived areas in tumours. By functionalizing the nanomaterials with hypoxia-specific ligands, nanoparticles can target hypoxic tissues actively or passively and can accumulate in specific tissues. These nanomaterials are frequently combined with imaging agents, such as radionuclides, fluorescent dyes, or magnetic contrast agents, to allow for the visualization of hypoxia through a variety of imaging modalities, such as PET, fluorescence, and MRI. Several imaging modalities combined into one nanoplatform improve the accuracy of hypoxia detection and offer a more thorough knowledge of the oxygenation status of tumours.[54]

Smart nanoparticles, using oxygen-sensitive nanoparticles, are a noteworthy approach in nanoparticle-based imaging. Real-time imaging of hypoxic zones is made possible by these nanoparticles, which are made to change their chemical or physical characteristics in reaction to oxygen levels (Figure 7.4).

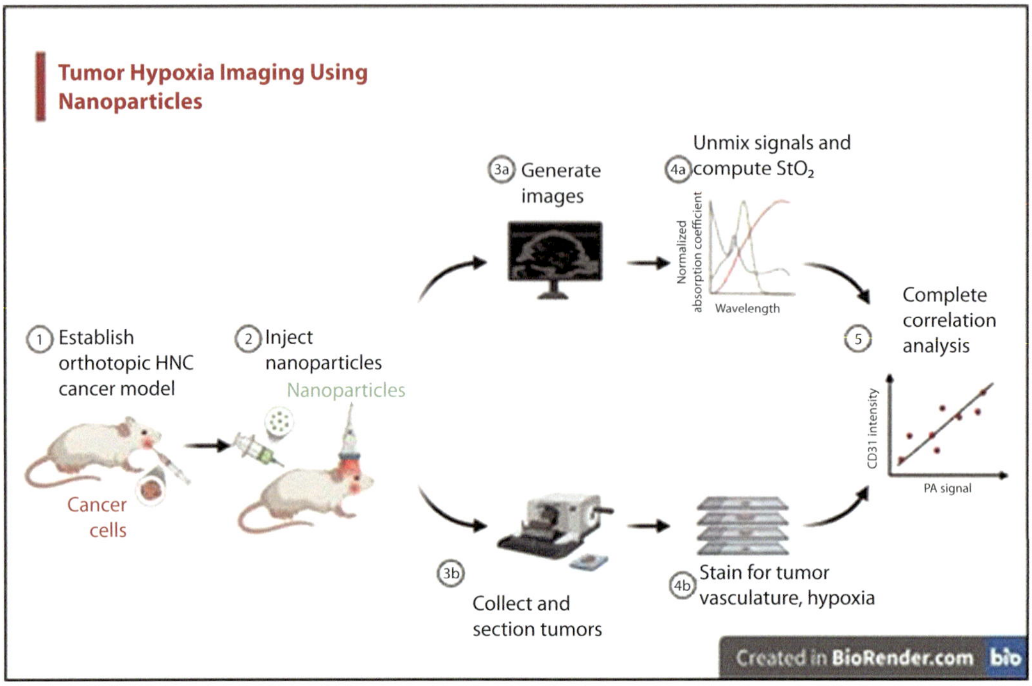

FIGURE 7.3 Diagrammatic representation of visualization of tumour hypoxia using nanoparticles.[43]

Porphyrin-based chemicals, for instance, can be included in certain nanoparticles to enable optical imaging of hypoxic tissues since they fluoresce in hypoxic environments.[55] Some nanomaterials use dyes that are sensitive to pH or redox, which alter their optical characteristics when exposed to low oxygen levels they allowing for the real-time, high-resolution monitoring of hypoxia dynamics in living animal models. These nanoparticles are especially helpful in preclinical research.[56] Table 7.2 is a compilation of such hypoxia-responsive nanomaterials.

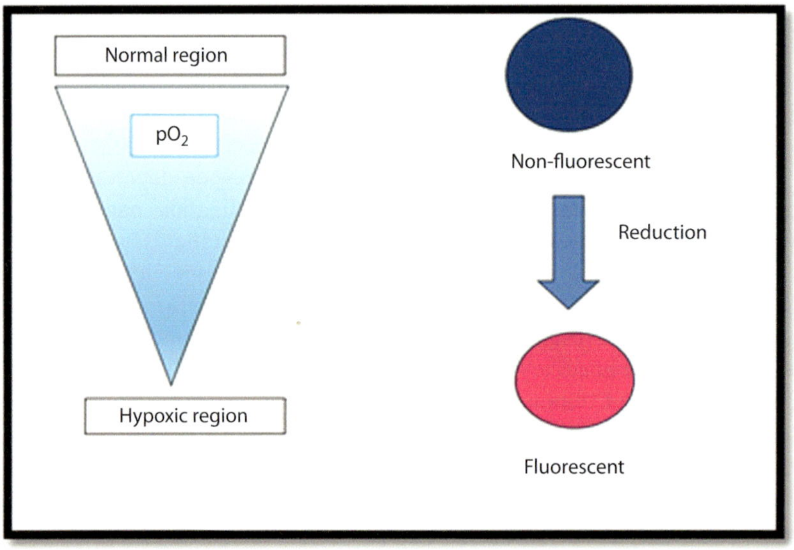

FIGURE 7.4 Schematics demonstrating smart nanomaterials with hypoxia-sensitive fluorescent properties.[43]

TABLE 7.2
Various Types of Oxygen and pH-Sensitive Nanoparticles[43]

	Nanoparticle Used	Composition	Sensitive Parameter	Sensitivity Mechanism	Applications	Ref
1.	Perfluorocarbon (PFC) nanoparticles	Perfluorocarbon core with fluorescent dyes	Oxygen	PFCs respond to varying oxygen levels by altering their fluorescence quenching properties	Tumour hypoxia imaging, oxygen delivery	57
2.	Metal-organic framework nanoparticles	Metal ions coordinated with organic linkers	Oxygen	MOFs modulate fluorescence or magnetic resonance under different oxygen concentrations	Hypoxia-responsive drug delivery, bioimaging	58
3.	pH-sensitive polymeric nanoparticles	Polymeric materials (e.g., PEG, Chitosan)	pH	Polymers undergo structural changes, swelling or degradation in acidic environments	Targeted drug release in acidic tumour microenvironment	59
4.	pH-responsive liposomes	Lipid bilayer with pH-sensitive lipids	pH	pH induced protonation causes lipid rearrangement, releasing encapsulated drugs	pH targeted drug delivery to cancer cells	60
5.	Quantum dots with pH-sensitive coating	CdSe QDs with polymer or dye coating	pH	pH changes influence fluorescence intensity and half-life of QDs	pH sensing in biological environments	61
6.	Metal nanoclusters	Gold or silver nanoclusters with responsive ligands	pH and Oxygen	Ligands respond to acidic pH and alter photoluminescence in hypoxic conditions	Hypoxia sensing in tumour tissues	62
7.	Nitroimidazole-conjugated nanoparticles	Polymeric or liposomal core with nitroimidazole	Oxygen	Nitroimidazole undergoes reduction under hypoxic conditions, making it selectively active	Hypoxia targeted drug delivery and imaging	63
8.	Polydopamine (PDA) nanoparticles	PDA coating	pH	pH-sensitive protonation of PDA allows systematic drug release in acidic environment	Controlled drug release at tumour sites	64
9	Hollow mesoporous silica nanoparticles	Silica shell with responsive inner core	pH and oxygen	Can be modified for dual sensitivity	Combination therapy in hypoxic solid tumours	65
10	Polymeric micelles with pH-sensitive linkers	Amphiphilic co-polymers with sensitive linkers	pH	Cleavage of linkers at low pH enables release of drug-loaded micelles	Targeted drug release in acidic TME	66

THE ROLE OF MULTI-OMICS TECHNOLOGIES

Multi-omics is the integrated research of various biological domains such as genomics, proteomics, metabolomics, and epigenomics together to better understand complicated biological systems, especially during diseases.[67]

One can explore cellular reactions and pathways by combining data from multiple omics fields to gain insight into various biological processes, such as the development of cancer.

In genomics, the complete DNA sequence undergoes assessment for identifying the mutations in genes and their impact on disease processes. Proteomics emphasizes the protein profile for a living system, evaluating its modification and alterations of gene expression levels to comprehend cellular functions and interactions in a cell. Furthermore, metabolomics analyses metabolites, showing the biochemical changes and cellular activities that occur in an organism. Lastly, epigenomics examines epigenetic modifications that affect gene expression without altering the sequence of DNA, thus helping us understand the environmental and lifestyle choices which affect gene function.

In cancer research, multi-omics techniques help in tumour subtyping, diagnosis, and prognosis through biomarkers and analysing the reaction to treatment (Figure 7.5).

By combining with data the research shows more genuine results and gives us a holistic view of tumour biology while helping in treatment.[68]

The following sections emphasize three significant studies that highlight innovative multi-omics techniques for understanding and visualizing cancer hypoxia and their implications for targeted therapies.

Multi-Omics Analysis of Acute Hypoxic Response

Andrysik et al.[69] presented the vitality of multi-omics by combining transcriptomic (gene expression) and proteomic data to investigate the acute hypoxic response in cancer. This integration is

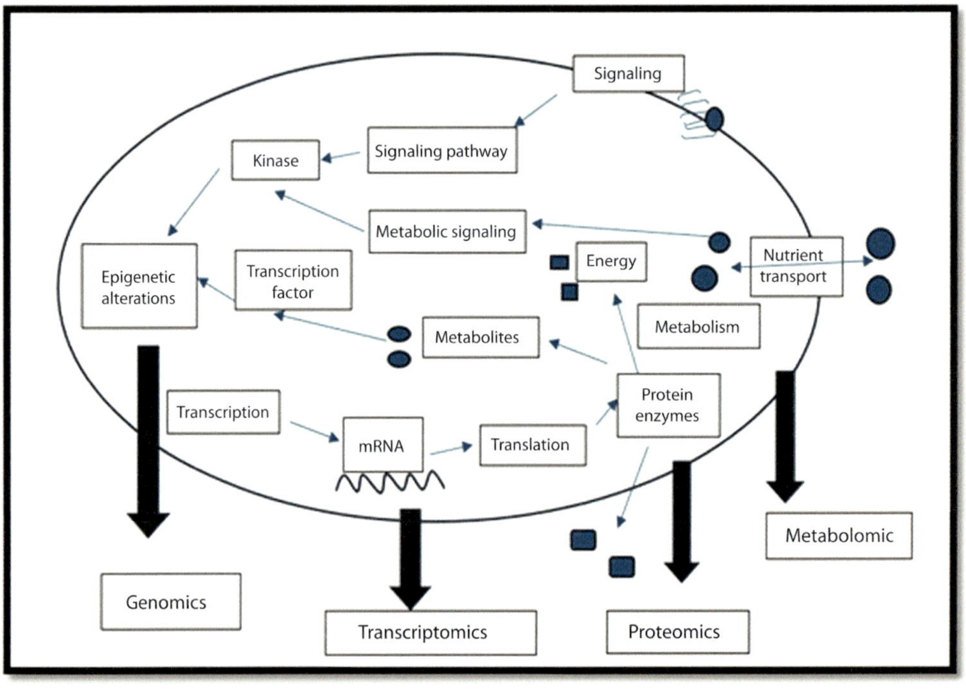

FIGURE 7.5 A snapshot of multi-omics technologies.[43]

important for revealing the signalling pathways and molecular networks under hypoxic tumours, which are critical for comprehension of cancer progression, metastasis, and resistance to treatment. These authors further elaborated on this by showing that hypoxia can activate oncogenic pathways as well as suppress tumour-suppressive pathways, providing a dual nature to hypoxia in cancers.

GENE EXPRESSION AND METABOLISM UNDER HYPOXIA

By combining transcriptomics (gene expression) and metabolomics (metabolic profiling). Schmidt et al. highlighted the different metabolic pathways of tumour, which are glycolysis and mitochondrial dysfunction.[67] This rewiring of the pathway is due to a hypoxic microenvironment. Hypoxia also suppresses some tumour suppressors while activating certain oncogenes. The multi-omics integration reveals how specific metabolic enzymes express themselves and how genes that are involved in angiogenesis and cell viability are changed due to hypoxic tumours.

It is reported that the cellular reactions are altered according to tumour type and thus show distinct expression of gene.[69] Therefore, it displays the different stages of tumour, which further explains its unique metabolic profile and the personalized treatment is designed accordingly.

Integration of Omics Technologies

The multiple omics technologies can provide a complete view of cancer.[70]

For example:

- Genomics helps in the identification of genetic mutations that may drive tumour formation.
- Transcriptomics explores gene expression patterns, offering knowledge into cellular responses to stressors like hypoxia.
- Proteomics maps out proteins that are involved in signalling and metabolic pathways.
- Metabolomics identifies shifts in metabolic pathways, including those altered by hypoxia, providing key insights into the tumour's ability to survive in low-oxygen conditions.[67]

By integrating this omics data, the studies can be used to reveal hidden signalling pathways and metabolic pathways. The integrated method helps in the complete comprehension of the molecular structure of cancer.

a. There are significant clinical applications of multi-omics for diagnosis and prognosis of hypoxic tumours. It can then help develop personalized treatment strategies. Therefore, metabolic data can be used for the identification of biomarkers for better diagnosis in patients. As in finding metabolites that are changed due to hypoxia in tumours and can lead to the evolution of biomarkers which are more sensitive than traditional diagnostic therapies. By using metabolomic insights with genomic and proteomic data, research can be used for precise models of cancer that assist in effective interventions and reduced side effects with better outcomes. It can be used to-Predict disease progression
b. Assess the likelihood of metastasis
c. Tailor treatments based on the specific metabolic needs and vulnerabilities of the tumour

The upcoming techniques that are changing the field of cancer research, such as spatial transcriptomics and single-cell omics. It allows for a more comprehensive assessment of TME, especially how each cell responds under hypoxic stress. Spatial transcriptomics helps in visualizing gene expression in tumours and how they act under hypoxic stress. This upcoming approach is regarding how metabolic shifts correlate with specific areas of tumours. The lactate production due to anaerobic respiration is due to altered metabolism. By combining spatial data with metabolomic profiles, it can also help to characterize the tumour and its resistance to therapies.

Furthermore, with single-cell omics, we can analyse even individual cells, therefore separating them from bulk tissue assessment. This is of utmost importance to understand the evolution of tumour and heterogeneity. Therefore, it can help us understand how hypoxic stress affects the single metabolic response at the cellular level, guiding the development of targeted therapies.

Multi-Omics Deep Learning for Hypoxia Phenotypes

The study[71] on multi-omics and deep learning (DL) models in predicting tumour aggressiveness and prognosis offered crucial information for the development of treatment of cancer. It combines the multi-omics findings with DL for addressing hypoxia, thus helping in designing better targeted therapies. It connects with metabolomics and informs the readers about application of data-driven approaches to obtain better patient outcomes.[67]

This work demonstrated the impact of multi-omics on DL models by combining genomic, transcriptomic, and clinical data to predict tumour development. This approach, along with different data, reveals complicated patterns that may not be as apparent through traditional methods. This provides a complete understanding of the molecular and clinical aspects of tumours. Integrating the metabolomic data with genomic and transcriptomic analysis shows a better comprehension of the metabolism of tumour, leading to better recognition of biomarkers related to hypoxia. This examination is critical to understanding tumour progression, especially in terms of hypoxia. In this context, DL models do better as they can produce vast and complex datasets from multiple omics platforms, offering greater predictive power and more accurate decision-making in clinical settings.

DL models enable predictive precision as these models help recognize patients who fall under the high-risk bracket. By using this method, one can predict the patient outcomes while assessing the stage of the tumour and assist in better therapeutic strategies. Integrating clinical data improves prediction ability. Patient data such as age, gender, and previous treatment history can be used for more accurate results, therefore leading to customizable treatments.

Role of AI in Visualization of Cancer Hypoxia

A programmed system with AI may identify patterns and relationships between inputs and outputs and utilize this information to make decisions on entirely fresh input data. DL and ML are the main techniques for implementing AI. DL is a subset of ML, which is a branch of AI in computer science that focuses on deep neural networks.[48,49]

Applications of AI in oncology include optimizing treatment choices, forecasting patient outcomes, and accurately diagnosing tumours from radiological imaging and pathology slides, along with measuring drug response. Therefore, AI has the potential to enhance cancer care and address the issue of the unequal distribution of medical resources[72] (Figure 7.6).

Within PM, a biomarker is data-utilized to identify a particular subgroup within a broader patient population for prognostic, predictive, or diagnostic purposes. Tissue biomarkers encode information in the tissue that only pathology can completely decipher. Classic tissue indicators for malignant tumours include histotype, grade, and stage.[73]

AI systems utilize details in hematoxylin and eosin stained (HE) images that humans may overlook and employ those details to anticipate specific outcomes. The predictions of therapy response, somatic mutations, or patient survival are some examples of these AI-based biomarkers. It has also been proposed to use DL to predict Microsatellite Instability (MSI) from HE pictures.[73]

The prognosis of cancer is significantly influenced by the dynamic interplay between immune cells and tumour cells within the TME. To quantitatively evaluate the spatial associations between tumour cells and immune cells, this study presents a novel method based on AI and IHC-stained whole-slide images (WSIs) of colorectal cancer (CRC) patients. This is achieved by using the Morisita-Horn ecological index (Mor-index), which enables a thorough analysis of the spatial

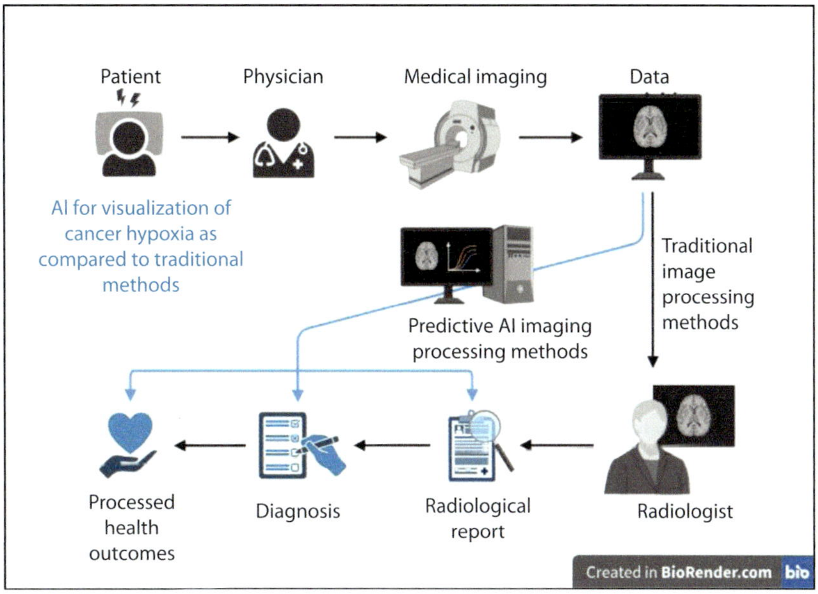

FIGURE 7.6 Illustration for traditional imaging techniques in comparison with artificial-intelligence-enabled imaging techniques. AI is much faster, convenient and generates higher resolution results as compared to traditional technique.[43]

distribution patterns between tumour cells and immune cells within the TME of CRC patients by obtaining the results of cell nuclei segmentation.[74] IHC-stained WSIs have been shown to be a useful predictive tool due to their ability to reveal information on immune cell location, type, and density.[75]

A high-quality HE-stained slide may typically confirm the diagnosis. DL can be used to quantify immune-related features found in HE-stained WSIs, such as Crohn's-like lymphoid reaction (CLR) and tumour-infiltrating lymphocytes (TILs).[76] Digital pathology in conjunction with DL has proven beneficial for treating prostate, lung, and CRC. DL can be used to quantify the tissue-level components of CRC, such as tumour-stroma ratio (TSR), hypoxia levels and CLR. Consequently, employing HE-stained WSIs, the AI-based approach may be able to quantify the tissue composition and immunological status.[39,40]

The spatial distribution of TILs is important for CRC prognosis. To produce tumour-killing immune cells for the defence of the organism, TILs can interact with the tumour directly or through cytokine signalling, primarily in the interstitial region. The lymphoid follicles around the tumour either produce the immune cells in the stroma or they migrate there from the circulation. The anti-tumour impact and the quantity of immune cells in the stroma diminish with increasing stroma. Thus, it can be postulated that a thorough analysis of the stroma percentage and immune cell infiltration in stroma would improve the CRC patient prognostic categorization considerably.[77]

The visualization of cancer hypoxia is revolutionized by AI, which provides previously unheard-of precision and efficiency in identifying and mapping oxygen-deficient areas within tumours. Hypoxia is a marker of aggressive tumour behaviour that worsens prognosis and resistance to treatment. Integrating multi-modal imaging data, including MRI, PET, and CT scans, is made possible by AI-driven models, especially those that use ML and DL techniques to assess hypoxic zones accurately. AI improves the spatial and temporal resolution of imaging by processing big datasets quickly, offering more in-depth insights into the TME. AI aids medical professionals in both the early detection of hypoxia-related cancer progression and the optimization of treatment plans, such as medication administration and radiation therapy.

Furthermore, by predicting hypoxic dynamics, AI can spot minuscule trends in imaging data that may escape human observation, supporting personalized treatment plans. Therefore, through improved visualization approaches, AI is critical in increasing our understanding of cancer hypoxia and improving patient outcomes.

CONCLUSIONS

Innovative imaging techniques for cancer hypoxia are advancing faster while also introducing various novel technologies, especially through enhancements in PET and MRI. These studies emphasize the importance of these modalities in obtaining crucial information regarding tumour biology and making personalized treatment approaches. As these visualization tools further upgrade their clinical practices, they will revolutionize cancer treatments, presenting better diagnosis as per the improved treatment. Application of multi-omics technologies in tandem with AI and ML holds a significant potential in enabling correct and early-stage diagnosis of hypoxia. In future research, it will likely focus on refining these technologies and detecting their use for various cancer types, making it easier for patients to get beneficial treatment and with better patient outcomes.

REFERENCES

1. Brown JM, Wilson WR. Exploiting tumor hypoxia in cancer treatment. *Nat Rev Cancer.* 2004;4:437–447.
2. Harris AL. Hypoxia-a key regulatory factor in tumor growth. *Nat Rev Cancer.* 2002; 2:38–47.
3. Ito K, Nakanishi M, Lee WC, Sasaki H, Zenno S, Saigo K, Kitade Y, Tanokura M. Three-dimensional structure of AzoR from *Escherichia coli*: An oxidoreductase conserved in microorganisms. *J Biol Chem.* 2006;281:20567–20576.
4. Hammond EM, Giaccia AJ. The role of p53 in hypoxia-induced apoptosis. *Biochem Biophys Res Commun.* 2005;331:718–725.
5. Blagosklonny MV. Hypoxia, mTOR and autophagy. *Autophagy.* 2013;9:260–262.
6. Chen Z, Siraj S, Liu L, Chen Q. MARCH5-FUNDC1 axis fine-tunes hypoxia induced mitophagy. *Autophagy.* 2017;13:1244–1245.
7. Carmeliet P, Dor Y, Herbert JM, et al. Role of HIF-1alpha in hypoxia-mediated apoptosis, cell proliferation and tumor angiogenesis. *Nature.* 1998;394:485–490.
8. Sørensen BS, Horsman MR. Tumor hypoxia: Impact on radiation therapy and molecular pathways. *Front Oncol.* 2020;10:562.
9. Zheng X, Wang X, Mao H, Wu W, Liu B, Jiang X. Hypoxia-specific ultrasensitive detection of tumours and cancer cells in vivo. *Nat Commun.* 2015, 8364.
10. Matsumoto K, English S, Yoo J, et al. Pharmacokinetics of a triarylmethyl-type paramagnetic spin probe used in EPR oximetry. *Magn Reson Med.* 2004;52:885–892.
11. Krohn KA, Link JM, Mason RP. Molecular imaging of hypoxia. *J Nucl Med.* 2008;49(Suppl 2):129S–148S.
12. Wang X, Xie X, Ku G, Wang LV, Stoica G. Noninvasive imaging of hemoglobin concentration and oxygenation in the rat brain using high resolution photoacoustic tomography. *J Biomed Opt.* 2006;11:024015.
13. Smith RC, McCarthy S. Physics of magnetic resonance. *J Reprod Med.* 1992;37:19–26.
14. Yan Y, Sun X, Shen B. Contrast agents in dynamic contrast-enhanced magnetic resonance imaging. *Oncotarget.* 2017;8:43491–43505.
15. Gaustad J-V, Hauge A, Wegner CS, Simonsen TG, Lund KV, Hansem LMK, Rofstad EK. DCE-MRI of tumor hypoxia and hypoxia-associated aggressiveness. *Cancers.* 2020;12:1979.
16. Colliez F, Gallez B, Jordan BF. Assessing tumor oxygenation for predicting outcome in radiation oncology: A review of studies correlating tumor hypoxic status and outcome in the preclinical and clinical settings. *Front Oncol.* 2017;7:10.
17. Baudelet C, Gallez B. How does blood oxygen level-dependent (BOLD) correlate with oxygen partial pressure (pO_2) inside tumors? *Magn Reson Med.* 2002;48:980–986.
18. Thomas SR, Pratt RG, Millard RW, et al. In vivo PO_2 imaging in the porcine model with perfluorocarbon F-19 NMR at low field. *Magn Reson Imaging.* 1996;14:103–114.
19. Mason RP, Shukla H, Antich PP. In vivo oxygen tension and temperature: Simultaneous determination using 19F NMR spectroscopy of perfluorocarbon. *Magn Reson Med.* 1993;29:296–302.

20. Yu JX, Kodibagkar VD, Cui W, Mason RP. 19F: A versatile reporter for non-invasive physiology and pharmacology using magnetic resonance. *Curr Med Chem*. 2005;12(7):819–848.
21. Chun Y, Kim J. AMPK-mTOR signaling and cellular adaptations in hypoxia. *Int J Mol Sci*. 2021;22:9765.
22. Pauken KE, Wherry EJ. Overcoming T cell exhaustion in infection and cancer. *Trends Immunol*. 2015;36:265–276.
23. Muz B, de la Puente P, Azab F, Azab AK. The role of hypoxia in cancer progression, angiogenesis, metastasis, and resistance to therapy. *Hypoxia*. 2015;3:83–92.
24. Semenza GL. Defining the role of hypoxia-inducible factor 1 in cancer biology and therapeutics. *Oncogene*. 2010;29:625–634.
25. Goggins E, Kakkad S, Mironchik Y, Jacob D, Wildes F, Krishnamachary B, Bhujwalla ZM. Hypoxia inducible factors modify collagen I fibers in MDA-MB-231 triple negative breast cancer xenografts. *Neoplasia*. 2018;20:131–139.
26. Kakkad SM, Solaiyappan M, O'rourke B, Stasinopoulos I, Ackerstaff E, Raman V, Bhujwalla ZM, Glunde K. Hypoxic tumor microenvironments reduce collagen I fiber density. *Neoplasia*. 2010;12:608–617.
27. Ni J, Wang X, Stojanovic A, et al. Single-cell RNA sequencing of tumor-infiltrating NK cells reveals that inhibition of transcription factor HIF 1_ unleashes NK cell activity. *Immunity*. 2020;52:1075 1087. e8.
28. Chiu DK, Tse A, Xu I, et al. Hypoxia inducible factor HIF-1 promotes myeloid-derived suppressor cells accumulation through ENTPD2/CD39L1 in hepatocellular carcinoma. *Nat Commun*. 2017;8:517.
29. Chiu DK-C, Xu IM-J, Lai RK-H, et al. Hypoxia induces myeloid-derived suppressor cell recruitment to hepatocellular carcinoma through chemokine (C-C motif) ligand 26. *Hepatology*. 2016;64:797–813.
30. Zhou CF, Han YD, Huiqing S, Zhou W. Hypoxic microenvironment in cancer. *Signal Transduct Target Ther*. 2023;8:70.
31. Brown JM. Tumor hypoxia in cancer therapy. *Methods Enzymol*. 2007;435:297–321.
32. Gouel P, Decaze P, Vera P, Gardin I, Thoreau S, Bohn P. Advances in PET and MRI imaging of tumor hypoxia. *Front Med*. 2023;10:1055022.
33. Weissleder R, Mahmood U. Molecular imaging. *Radiology*. 2001;219(2):316–333. doi: 10.1148/radiology.219.2.r01ma19316.
34. Kim SJ, Lee HY. In vivo molecular imaging in preclinical research. *Lab Anim Res*. 2022;38(1):31. doi: 10.1186/s42826-022-00142-3.
35. Sun T, Zhao H, Hu L, et al. Enhanced optical imaging and fluorescent labeling for visualizing drug molecules within living organisms. *Acta Pharm Sin B*. 2024;14(6):2428–2446. doi: 10.1016/j.apsb.2024.01.018.
36. Chen Z, Han F, Du Y, Shi H, Zhou W. Hypoxic microenvironment in cancer: Molecular mechanisms and therapeutic interventions. *Signal Transduct Target Ther*. 2023;8(1):70. doi: 10.1038/s41392-023-01332-8.
37. Papkovsky DB, Dmitriev RI. Imaging of oxygen and hypoxia in cell and tissue samples. *Cell Mol Life Sci*. 2018;75(16):2963–2980. doi: 10.1007/s00018-018-2840-x.
38. Emami Nejad A, Najafgholian S, Rostami A, et al. The role of hypoxia in the tumor microenvironment and development of cancer stem cell: A novel approach to developing treatment. *Cancer Cell Int*. 2021;21(1):62. doi: 10.1186/s12935-020-01719-5.
39. Huizing FJ, Hoeben BAW, Franssen GM, Boerman OC, Heskamp S, Bussink J. Quantitative imaging of the hypoxia-related marker CAIX in head and neck squamous cell carcinoma xenograft models. *Mol Pharm*. 2019;16(2):701–708. doi: 10.1021/acs.molpharmaceut.8b00950.
40. Huang M, Yang S, Tai WCS, et al. Bioinformatics identification of regulatory genes and mechanism related to hypoxia-induced PD-L1 inhibitor resistance in hepatocellular carcinoma. *Int J Mol Sci*. 2023;24(10):8720. doi: 10.3390/ijms24108720.
41. Bourigault P, Skwarski M, Macpherson RE, Higgins GS, McGowan DR. Timing of hypoxia PET/CT imaging after 18F-fluoromisonidazole injection in non-small cell lung cancer patients. *Sci Rep*. 2022;12(1):21746. doi: 10.1038/s41598-022-26199-7.
42. Godet I, Doctorman S, Wu F, Gilkes DM. Detection of hypoxia in cancer models: Significance, challenges, and advances. *Cells*. 2022;11(4):686. doi: 10.3390/cells11040686.
43. Pattarkine MV, Kamplikar P, Chauhan E. *Innovative Tools and Techniques for Visualization of Cancer Hypoxia*. Edited by S. Mukherjee, Elsevier;2025.
44. Masaki Y, Shimizu Y, Yoshioka T, et al. Imaging mass spectrometry revealed the accumulation characteristics of the 2-nitroimidazole-based agent "pimonidazole" in hypoxia. *PLOS ONE*. 2016;11(8):e0161639. doi: 10.1371/journal.pone.0161639.
45. Rashed FB, Stoica AC, MacDonald D, et al. Identification of proteins and cellular pathways targeted by 2-nitroimidazole hypoxic cytotoxins. *Redox Biol*. 2021;41:101905. doi: 10.1016/j.redox.2021.101905.

46. Wray R, Mauguen A, Michaud L, et al. Development of[18] F-fluoromisonidazole hypoxia PET/CT diagnostic interpretation criteria and validation of interreader reliability, reproducibility, and performance. *J Nucl Med.* 2024;65(10):1526–1532. doi: 10.2967/jnumed.124.267775.
47. Liu T, Karlsen M, Karlberg AM, Redalen KR. Hypoxia imaging and theranostic potential of [64Cu][Cu(ATSM)] and ionic Cu(II) salts: A review of current evidence and discussion of the retention mechanisms. *EJNMMI Res.* 2020;10(1):33. doi: 10.1186/s13550-020-00621-5.
48. Shang B, Yu Z, Wang Z. Recent advances and applications of nitroreductase activable agents for tumor theranostic. *Front Pharmacol.* 2024;15:1451517. doi: 10.3389/fphar.2024.1451517.
49. Mirabello V, Cortezon-Tamarit F, Pascu SI. Oxygen sensing, hypoxia tracing and in vivo imaging with functional metalloprobes for the early detection of non-communicable diseases. *Front Chem.* 2018;6:27. doi: 10.3389/fchem.2018.00027.
50. McDonald PC, Chafe SC, Supuran CT, Dedhar S. Cancer therapeutic targeting of hypoxia induced carbonic anhydrase IX: From bench to bedside. *Cancers.* 2022;14(14):3297. doi: 10.3390/cancers14143297.
51. Han X, Xu K, Taratula O, Farsad K. Applications of nanoparticles in biomedical imaging. *Nanoscale.* 2019;11(3):799–819. doi: 10.1039/C8NR07769J.
52. Fruhwirth GO, Kneilling M, De Vries IJM, Weigelin B, Srinivas M, Aarntzen EHJG. The potential of in vivo imaging for optimization of molecular and cellular anti-cancer immunotherapies. *Mol Imaging Biol.* 2018;20(5):696–704. doi: 10.1007/s11307-018-1254-3.
53. Pinto-Coelho L. How artificial intelligence is shaping medical imaging technology: A survey of innovations and applications. *Bioengineering.* 2023;10(12):1435. doi: 10.3390/bioengineering10121435.
54. Lan H, Jamil M, Ke G, Dong N. The role of nanoparticles and nanomaterials in cancer diagnosis and treatment: A comprehensive review. *Am J Cancer Res.* 2023;13(12):5751–5784.
55. Xia Y, Duan S, Han C, Jing C, Xiao Z, Li C. Hypoxia-responsive nanomaterials for tumor imaging and therapy. *Front Oncol.* 2022;12:1089446. doi: 10.3389/fonc.2022.1089446.
56. Huynh GT, Kesarwani V, Walker JA, Frith JE, Meagher L, Corrie SR. Review: Nanomaterials for reactive oxygen species detection and monitoring in biological environments. *Front Chem.* 2021;9:728717. doi: 10.3389/fchem.2021.728717.
57. Hoogendijk E, Swider E, Staal AHJ, et al. Continuous-flow production of perfluorocarbon-loaded polymeric nanoparticles: From the bench to clinic. *ACS Appl Mater Interfaces.* 2020;12(44):49335–49345. doi: 10.1021/acsami.0c12020.
58. Liu Y, Jiang T, Liu Z. Metal-organic frameworks for bioimaging: Strategies and challenges. *Nanotheranostics.* 2022;6(2):143–160. doi: 10.7150/ntno.63458.
59. Singh J, Nayak P. pH-responsive polymers for drug delivery: Trends and opportunities. *J Polym Sci.* 2023;61(22):2828–2850. doi: 10.1002/pol.20230403.
60. Shinn J, Kwon N, Lee SA, Lee Y. Smart pH-responsive nanomedicines for disease therapy. *J Pharm Investig.* 2022;52(4):427–441. doi: 10.1007/s40005-022-00573-z.
61. Yukawa H, Sato K, Baba Y. Theranostics applications of quantum dots in regenerative medicine, cancer medicine, and infectious diseases. *Adv Drug Deliv Rev.* 2023;200:114863. doi: 10.1016/j.addr.2023.114863.
62. Van De Looij SM, Hebels ER, Viola M, Hembury M, Oliveira S, Vermonden T. Gold nanoclusters: Imaging, therapy, and theranostic roles in biomedical applications. *Bioconjug Chem.* 2022;33(1):4–23. doi: 10.1021/acs.bioconjchem.1c00475.
63. Zhu M, Ren G, Guo J, et al. Hypoxia-responsive nanomicelle based on 2-nitroimidazole for tumor treatment through chemotherapy and modulation of the tumor redox microenvironment. *ACS Appl Nano Mater.* 2024;7(11):12452–12465. doi: 10.1021/acsanm.4c00826.
64. Ball V. Polydopamine nanomaterials: Recent advances in synthesis methods and applications. *Front Bioeng Biotechnol.* 2018;6:109. doi: 10.3389/fbioe.2018.00109.
65. Moodley T, Singh M. Current stimuli-responsive mesoporous silica nanoparticles for cancer therapy. *Pharmaceutics.* 2021;13(1):71. doi: 10.3390/pharmaceutics13010071.
66. Farhoudi L, Hosseinikhah SM, Kazemi-Beydokhti A, et al. pH-sensitive polymeric micelles enhance the co-delivery of doxorubicin and docetaxel: An emerging modality for treating breast cancer. *Cancer Nanotechnol.* 2024;15(1):37. doi: 10.1186/s12645-024-00275-1.
67. Schmidt DR, Patel R, Kirsch DG, et al. Metabolomics in cancer research and emerging applications in clinical oncology. *CA Cancer J Clin.* 2021;71(4), 333–358. doi: 10.3322/caac.21670.
68. Bhrugubanda M, T SRK. Role of deep learning in malware detection. In: T SRK, ASN Chakravarthy, eds. *Advances in Cyber Security and Digital Forensics.* Iterative International Publishers, Selfypage Developers Pvt Ltd;2024:103–110. doi: 10.58532/nbennurch262.

69. Andrysik Z, Bender H, Galbraith MD, et al. Multi-omics analysis reveals contextual tumor suppressive and oncogenic gene modules within the acute hypoxic response. *Nat Commun.* 2021;12:1375. doi: 10.1038/s41467-021-21687-2.
70. Zhang B, Shi H, Wang H. Machine learning and AI in cancer prognosis, Prediction, and treatment selection: A critical approach. *J Multidiscip Healthc.* 2023;16:1779–1791. doi: 10.2147/JMDH.S410301.
71. Bohr A, Memarzadeh K. The rise of artificial intelligence in healthcare applications. In: *Artificial Intelligence in Healthcare.* Elsevier; 2020:25–60. doi: 10.1016/B978-0-12-818438-7.00002-2.
72. Aad van der Lugt, Thomas B, Laure F, et al. Medical imaging in personalised medicine: A white paper of the research committee of the European Society of Radiology (ESR). *Insights Imaging.* 2015;6(2): 141–155. doi: 10.1007/s13244-015-0394-0.
73. Fröhlich H, Balling R, Beerenwinkel N, et al. From hype to reality: Data science enabling personalized medicine. *BMC Med.* 2018;16(1):150. doi: 10.1186/s12916-018-1122-7.
74. Dakal TC, George N, Xu C, Suravajhala P, Kumar A. Predictive and prognostic relevance of tumor-infiltrating immune cells: Tailoring personalized treatments against different cancer types. *Cancers.* 2024;16(9):1626. doi: 10.3390/cancers16091626.
75. Lancellotti C, Cancian P, Savevski V, et al. Artificial intelligence & tissue biomarkers: Advantages, risks and perspectives for pathology. *Cells.* 2021;10(4):787. doi: 10.3390/cells10040787.
76. Jiao P, Zheng Q, Yang R, et al. Prediction of HER2 status based on deep learning in H&E-stained histopathology images of bladder cancer. *Biomedicines.* 2024;12(7):1583. doi: 10.3390/biomedicines12071583.
77. Bai Z, Zhou Y, Ye Z, Xiong J, Lan H, Wang F. Tumor-infiltrating lymphocytes in colorectal cancer: The fundamental indication and application on immunotherapy. *Front Immunol.* 2022;12:808964. doi: 10.3389/fimmu.2021.808964.

8 *In Vivo* Models for Studying Hypoxic Cancer

Suman Kumar Ray and Sukhes Mukherjee
Department of Biochemistry, All India Institute of Medical Sciences, Bhopal, Madhya Pradesh, India

INTRODUCTION

One of the most important pathophysiological features of cancer growth is hypoxia (1). The main molecules that react to hypoxia are called hypoxia-inducible factors (HIFs). In low-oxygen environments, HIF-1α and the HIF-1β component form a dimer that activates target gene expression and has a role in angiogenesis, metabolism, cancer immune response, cell proliferation, and resistance to therapy (2,3). Thus, investigating the dynamic growth process of angiogenesis and hypoxia aids in a better understanding of the actual state of cancer progression and ultimately yields clinical data and theoretical models for treatment, prognosis, and recurrence. Theoretically, new blood arteries can ameliorate tissue hypoxia and provide tumor cells with oxygen and nutrients (4). In fact, the real situation *in vivo* is more convoluted. Researchers have discovered that the final blood vessel development is immature and deformed, and that the tumor-stimulated angiogenesis process is aberrant. Due to their inability to control vascular perfusion like mature blood arteries, these vessels can contribute to a tumor-hypoxic milieu, which can impact drug delivery and ultimately aid in metastasis (5,6).

According to this viewpoint, suitable animal models could hasten the integration of novel treatments, tailored strategies, and possibly even novel molecular imaging biomarkers into standard clinical practice. Being able to distinguish between a positive and a negative model for tumor hypoxia—that is, tumors that are poorly and highly oxygenated, respectively—is frequently essential in hypoxia research in particular. These models ought to appropriately depict human illness as well. According to this perspective, patient-derived xenografts, orthotopic models, or genetically modified models may be superior to cell-line-derived xenograft models (7). Nonetheless, subcutaneous models are still widely used in preclinical cancer studies, including hypoxia research, due to historical knowledge gained from subcutaneous xenograft models, the fact that tumors are externally visible and easily measurable, and the comparatively simple experimental procedures needed for their creation and follow-up. The availability of techniques to measure tumor oxygenation is a requirement for being able to distinguish between a positive and negative model for tumor hypoxia.

One effective way to address this issue is by molecular imaging. Imaging biomarkers, including radiolabeled substances from positron emission tomography (PET), provide noninvasive, long-term evaluation of a tumor's molecular and functional features, addressing intratumoral and inter-tumor heterogeneity. Therefore, imaging biomarkers have become much more significant over the last few decades. Tumor hypoxia or new blood vessels can be detected qualitatively and partially quantitatively using a variety of techniques, including optical imaging, photoacoustic imaging (PAI), magnetic resonance imaging (MRI), and PET/single-photon emission computed tomography (PET/SPECT). However, precise and simultaneous monitoring of hypoxia and tumor angiogenesis is lacking. According to a recent review by Fleming and his colleagues (8), blood O_2 level dependent (BOLD) MRI, oxygen (O_2) electrodes like OxyLite, electron paramagnetic resonance

 DOI: 10.1201/9781003477419-8

(EPR), histological evaluation using extrinsic biomarkers, primarily pimonidazole, and intrinsic biomarkers, like carbonic anhydrase IX (CAIX), SPECT or PET with, for example, hypoxia-targeting 2-nitroimidazole-based radiotracers (8,9). However, since each measurement method provides information on a different site inside the tumor, such as intracellular hypoxia, interstitial hypoxia, or blood oxygenation (8), correlations between the various methods are frequently lacking (10,11). Furthermore, certain methods, like Oxy Lite, invariably harm the tumor tissue. Therefore, it is still unclear whether of these methods may be regarded as the gold standard for determining tumor hypoxia. A number of 2-nitroimidazole derivatives have been created for hypoxic PET imaging in recent decades. Considered the prototype tracer, [^{18}F]fluoromisonidazole ([^{18}F]FMISO) is a lipophilic substance that undergoes significant hepatobiliary and gastrointestinal metabolism. For example, [^{18}F]flortanidazole ([^{18}F]HX4) and other more hydrophilic next-generation 2-nitroimidazole derivatives have improved pharmacokinetic characteristics, leading to mostly renal excretion of the intact molecule and only little (<20%) hepatobiliary clearance. In other words, it produces better hypoxia-to-normoxia tissue ratios and, consequently, pictures with greater contrast than [^{18}F]FMISO (8,12–14).

In vivo monitoring of tumor hypoxia and angiogenesis in mouse models of breast cancer and hepatocellular carcinoma has been tried by two research groups. Tang et al. created the Ca761-HRE-GFP cell line and used contrast-enhanced ultrasound imaging to detect angiogenesis in Ca761 HRE-GFP subcutaneous allografted tumors and analyze fluorescence imaging to identify HRE-driven GFP signals (15). The Ca761-HRE-GFP tumor models can only be used for superficial tissue imaging because of the high background and limited spectral range in animal tissues. In a hepatocellular carcinoma subcutaneous tumor, Kis et al. employed hypoxia-specific 68Ga-DOTA-nitroimidazole to monitor hypoxia and aminopeptidase N-specific 68Ga-NOTA-c(NGR) to trace angiogenesis using PET imaging (16).

Given the inherent challenges of different techniques in *in vivo* hypoxic cancer research, in this book chapter, we present an overview of the various strategies and study designs that might be useful for modifying the tumor oxygenation state for *in vivo* hypoxia research.

GENERATING DIFFERENTIAL HYPOXIA IN TUMOR MODELS

One independent predictive factor linked to poor patient survival is tumor hypoxia. There is growing evidence that hypoxia may sustain cancer cells. It is yet unknown, though, if the hypoxic tumor microenvironment (TME) controls cell fate *in vivo*. Crucially, tumor cells treated by hypoxia alone do not exhibit the varied cell fates between hypoxic and non-hypoxic tumor cells; rather, these differences are only observed in tumor cells recovered from the hypoxic TME *in vivo*. Different hypoxias in tumor models for *in vivo* experiments are shown in Table 8.1.

PHARMACOLOGICAL INTERVENTIONS AND DETECTION OF HYPOXIA *IN VIVO*

Numerous prospective pharmacological strategies to combat tumor hypoxia have been developed in recent decades as a result of the quest for radiosensitizers and hypoxia-targeting medicines. The administration of erythropoietin (EPO), a chemical that the body naturally produces, appears to be necessary to boost the delivery of oxygen to tumors. For example, EPO therapy led to significantly decreased hypoxia in glioblastoma and carboplatin-treated non-small cell lung cancer (NSCLC) xenograft tumors, as measured polarographically or with HIF-1α immune fluorescence, respectively (55).

EPO may have harmful tumor effects through mechanisms unrelated to hypoxia because it also functions as a stimulatory growth factor (56). Metformin, a reasonably safe antidiabetic with a good pharmacokinetic profile, might be a more promising medication. Metformin's inhibitory action on

TABLE 8.1
Generating Differential Hypoxia in Tumor Model (*In Vivo*)

Parameters	Description
Animal physiological parameters	
Tumor location	• Absorption of pimonidazole, [^{18}F]FAZA, and the glucose analog 2-deoxy-2-[^{18}F]fluoro-D-glucose ([^{18}F]FDG) in genetically produced lung tumors in situ, subcutaneous, and orthotopic A549 xenograft models (17). • Decrease tumor hypoxia in an orthotopic CRC xenograft models, may be determined by CAIX immunohistochemistry (18). • Proliferation and differentiation of HIF-1α-deficient astrocytomas are also influenced by the inoculation site and its associated microenvironment (19).
Caloric restriction	• Intermittent fasting, short-term fasting, or chronic daily energy restriction are methods that can be used to accomplish caloric restriction (20). • Since the Warburg effect and tumor hypoxia are closely related, CR might offer yet another clear method of experimentally affecting tumor oxygenation. • In fact, EF5 immunostaining demonstrated that daily dietary restriction significantly reduced tumor hypoxia in A549 lung cancer xenograft models, in addition to significantly inhibiting tumor growth. Accordingly, there was a decrease in microvessel density (MVD), VEGF expression, and HIF-1α expression (21). • Similar findings of reductions in HIF-1α, VEGF, and MVD were noted in brain tumor models from rats, mice, and humans (22). • Accordingly, it was demonstrated that CR and radiation therapy functioned in concert in orthotopic allograft breast cancer models (23). • Because VEGF suppression by CR may lead to vascular normalization and consequent increases in O_2 tension, it was proposed that this could explain its reported radiosensitizing capabilities in the context of tumor hypoxia (20).
Tumor physiological parameters	
Inherent variation without manipulations	• The ideal paradigm for *in vivo* cancer hypoxia research is the capacity to identify differential hypoxia in a single xenograft animal without the need for underlying external modification. • The characteristics of hypoxia PET as a prognostic biomarker were demonstrated in certain xenograft models due to the observed intertumoral fluctuation in tumor oxygenation. For example, strong associations between [^{18}F]EF5 uptake and response to single-dose radiation were detected because of the large intertumoral variation in oxygenation reported in 9L glioma tumors (24). • These findings are supported by Beck et al.'s [^{18}F]fluoroazomycin arabinoside ([^{18}F]FAZA) imaging of 67 EMT6 breast tumor-bearing mice, which distinguished between hypoxic and normoxic tumors using the median tumor-to-background ratio. • The predictive nature of hypoxia PET has been successfully validated by these encouraging results; however, there are still some drawbacks to this strategy. For example, it is typically necessary to use fairly large animal cohorts to detect differential hypoxia, which is not desirable from an ethical perspective.
Inoculation of different cell lines	• Animal models of osteosarcoma, fibrosarcoma, glioma, head and neck cancer, lung cancer, melanoma, and prostate cancer that were all derived from different cell lines, as well as a panel of colorectal cancer (CRC) patient-derived xenograft tumors, were found to exhibit differential tumor hypoxia using pimonidazole immunostaining and [^{18}F]FMISO, [^{18}F]-2-nitroimidazol trifluoropropyl acetamide ([^{18}F]EF3), and [^{18}F]EF5 PET (17). • The Shionogi prostate cancer tumor model's various stages of castration responsiveness could be differentiated using [^{18}F]EF5 PET (25). • HIF-1α knockdown promoted tumor growth in gastric and subcutaneous lung xenograft tumors (26,27). • Additionally, in the instance of gastric cancer, knockdown led to greater sensitivity to 5-FU chemotherapy through higher vulnerability to apoptosis and downregulation of drug efflux transporters, as well as aggressive peritoneal spread through overexpression of matrix metallopeptidase-1 (28). • Pimonidazole labeling revealed that HIF-1α deficiency led to increased tumor hypoxia, reduced perfusion, and faster tumor growth in subcutaneous xenografts made from HIF-1α-deficient embryonic stem cells (29). • In addition to decreasing vascularity and tumor volume in a range of tumors, genetic ablation of vascular endothelial growth factor (VEGF), a proangiogenic signal protein that is one of the downstream targets of HIF-1 and consequently tumor hypoxia (30). • Remarkably, compared to VEGF disruption alone, genetic disruption of both HIF-1 and VEGF substantially suppressed the growth of CRC xenograft tumors; however, no synergistic effect on the hypoxic tumor compartments could be observed (31).

Tumor volume	• It was found that when the tumor volume in rat rhabdomyosarcoma tumors rose, so did the hypoxic volume measured by pimonidazole staining and [^{18}F]FMISO autoradiography (32). • In contrast, auto-radiographically determined [18F]fluoro erythronitroimidazole ([^{18}F]FETNIM) and tumor volume were found to be inversely correlated in murine sarcoma models (33). • Only in ex vivo tissue samples can the extent of tumor necrosis be easily and accurately quantified with autoradiographs. It is more difficult to adjust for the impact of necrosis on *in vivo* hypoxia. • In fact, macroscopically necrotic regions without tracer uptake may be excluded by the automatic thresholding method utilized in this investigation to identify tumors on PET scans (10). • However, the polarographic approach is unable to differentiate between tumor fractions that are necrotic and those that are alive. • However, it is interesting to note that when necrosis correction was applied to murine rhabdomyosarcoma tumors, it was found that polarographically determined pO_2 values did not correlate with the degree of necrosis and did not significantly change as tumors grew larger, unless the tumors weighed more than two grams (34). • In order to address these issues, parametric pictures based on distinct tracer uptake patterns over time across normoxic, hypoxic, and necrotic regions also appeared promising (35).
External interventions	
Breathing	• Intertumoral oxygenation heterogeneity was increased by exposing some of the animals to carbogen breathing prior to [^{18}F]FAZA scanning and radiotherapy (11). • Several hypoxia PET tracers, such as [^{18}F]FMISO, [^{18}F]EF3, [^{18}F]FETNIM, [^{18}F]FAZA, [^{18}F]fluoroetanidazole ([^{18}F]FETA), and [^{18}F]HX4 have shown great utility in detecting varying degrees of hypoxia in a number of cancer xenograft models (17). • It has been noted that breathing in carbogen or hypoxic gas considerably changed the uptake of [^{18}F]FMISO in adipose tissue as well as [^{18}F]FETNIM and [^{18}F]FAZA in muscle (17). • Similar findings were reported by Cairns et al., who observed increases in pO_2 upon reintroducing ambient air and decreases in pO_2 in normal muscle tissue when animals breathed 5–7% O_2 (36). • Acute hypoxia may not be visible with PET due to the extended absorption duration needed for 2-nitroimidazole-based tracers and the comparatively low temporal resolution of PET (37). • Numerous studies that looked into hypoxia-evoked therapeutic resistance have also demonstrated the efficacy of breathing models. For example, when a single dosage of 5-FU was given during short-term carbogen breathing, tumor growth was considerably reduced in models of fibrosarcoma, colon cancer, and hepatoma (17,38–40). • Mice and rats with lung tumors and rhabdomyosarcoma were exposed to altered O_2 concentrations for 4 hours a day for five days in a row. By employing this method, the researchers demonstrated that the hypoxic prodrug TH 302's effectiveness as a treatment was reliant on tumor oxygenation: daily brief exposure to carbogen eliminated TH 302's effect in the xenograft models (41). • Therefore, animals exposed to a hypoxic atmosphere had better results in inducing the hypoxia prodrug CEN-209 in subcutaneous HCT116 tumors, while hyperbaric O_2 breathing inhibited CEN-209 activation when the drug was given after irradiation (42).
Clamping	• By physically cutting off the tumor's blood supply, the O_2 status of tumors can be momentarily decreased; nevertheless, this clamping procedure results in severe hypoxia. Clamping causes HIF-1α to be expressed (43). • In an orthotopic liver tumor model, where hepatic artery ligation could cause severe hypoxia, this clamping approach has also been successfully used (44). • The clamping technique's one disadvantage is that ischemia, rather than hypoxia, can happen, resulting in irreparable damage and cell death. • During clamping and reperfusion, the occluded artery may clot (44).

(Continued)

TABLE 8.1 *(Continued)*

Generating Differential Hypoxia in Tumor Model (*In Vivo*)

Parameters	Description
Temperature modification	• Numerous studies in a range of xenograft models demonstrate that tumor oxygenation improves both during and after heating at 39–42°C, as reviewed excellently by Song and his colleagues (45). • Hyperthermic cytotoxicity, which is advantageous from a therapeutic perspective, but it could make therapy response evaluation trials that focus on tumor hypoxia more difficult. • In practice, animals that are confined or under anesthesia have their tumor-bearing leg submerged in warm water. According to the extrinsic hypoxia markers pimonidazole and EF5, this caused an instantaneous drop in the hypoxic percentage in a subcutaneous colorectal cancer model; however, the effect vanished 24 hours after heating (46). • After 1 hour of heat treatment, HIF-1α rose in a breast cancer model and returned 48 hours later. However, up to 48 hours after therapy, VEGF was boosted, which in turn caused angiogenesis to be induced, tumor perfusion to increase, and tumor hypoxia to decrease (47). • In a CRC xenograft model, pimonidazole staining demonstrated a decrease in hypoxia after 6 hours of whole-body heating, which may have been caused by an increase in vascular volume. However, after heating, hypoxia marginally rose once more (48). • The importance of HIF-1 in therapy resistance is undeniable, and its upregulation via heating may most likely be harmful, notwithstanding the suggestion that transient elevations in HIF-1α may result in tumor reoxygenation and may therefore be advantageous in specific situations (47). • Long-term usage of hyperthermia may be challenging due to its temporary nature. Tumor heating might not be a simple method for developing a differential hypoxic tumor model.
Exercise	• Exercise might increase the amount of oxygen delivered to the heart and muscle tissue, which might reroute the oxygen supply from tumors to these metabolically active tissues (49). • In order to maintain local homeostasis, exercise may trigger the HIF-1 cascade within the tumor, potentially resulting in angiogenesis (49,50). • Daily treadmill running has been shown to boost orthotopic breast tumor perfusion without impacting tumor oxygenation (51). • Crucially, these findings were consistent with additional preclinical information gathered in a model of orthotopic prostate cancer in rats (52).
Other approaches	
Matrigel and electrical stimulation	• The use of matrigel during tumor inoculations (53) and electrical stimulation (54) are two further, less researched external interventions to reduce tumor hypoxia. • Electrical stimulation of the sciatic nerve in intramuscularly implanted liver and rhabdomyosarcoma tumors was studied. In both models, tumor pO_2 and tumor blood flow significantly increased, while the O_2 consumption rate decreased (54).

complex I of the mitochondrial electron transport chain is thought to increase tumor oxygenation, among other anticancer effects (57).

Using [^{18}F]FAZA PET, Zannella et al. demonstrated in HCT116 CRC models that a single dose of metformin did, in fact, reduce tumor hypoxia and improve radiotherapy response (58).

Vascular-targeting drugs can also be used to affect tumor oxygenation. Hydralazine, a vasodilator that relaxes arterial smooth muscle, is a well-researched example of such a medication. Through the 'steal' effect, hydralazine reduces tumor perfusion at high doses, increasing tumor hypoxia (59).

[^{18}F]FMISO PET in patient-derived pancreas xenograft models following dovitinib treatment (60), it is generally accepted that the proper dosage of angiogenesis inhibitors causes vascular normalization and, as a result, decreases in tumor hypoxia (61).

Nimorazole and other O_2 mimetics are in the first class. This medication is used in Denmark to treat head and neck cancer with regular radiation (62). Hypoxic prodrugs like TH-302 belong to a second class (63). For example, it was demonstrated that TH-302 markedly reduced the hypoxic percentage in rhabdomyosarcoma and NSCLC xenograft tumors, as measured with [^{18}F]HX4 PET. Different methods for the detection of hypoxia *in vivo* are shown in Figure 8.1.

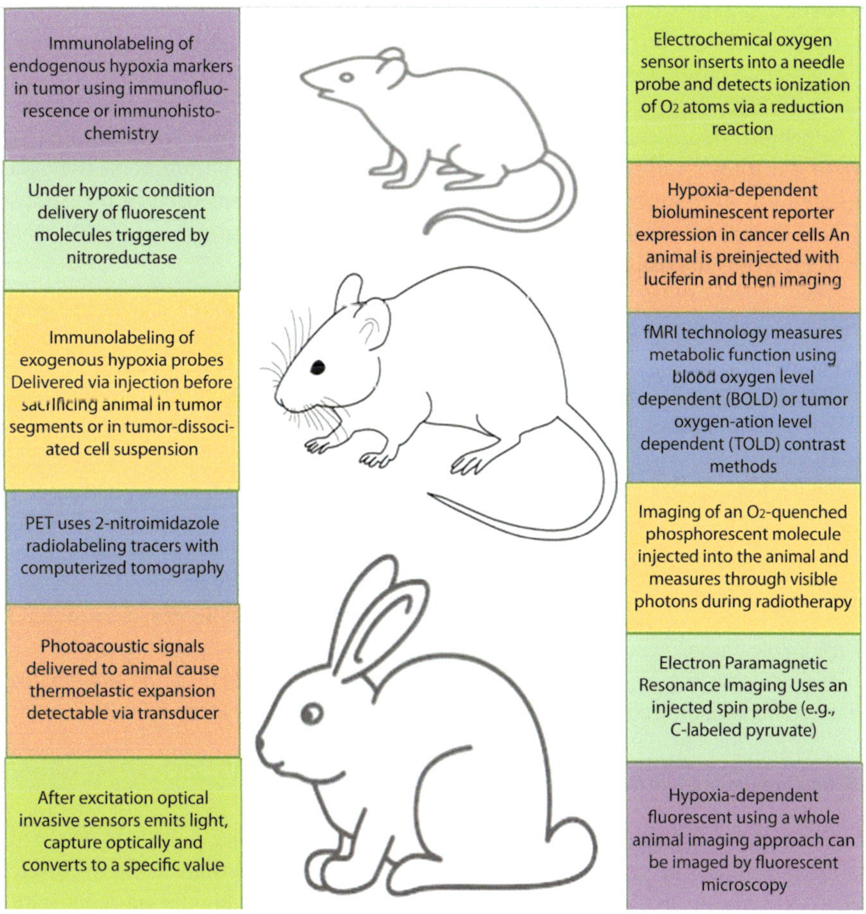
Immunolabeling of endogenous hypoxia markers in tumor using immunofluo-rescence or immunohisto-chemistry
Under hypoxic condition delivery of fluorescent molecules triggered by nitroreductase
Immunolabeling of exogenous hypoxia probes Delivered via injection before sacrificing animal in tumor segments or in tumor-dissoci-ated cell suspension
PET uses 2-nitroimidazole radiolabeling tracers with computerized tomography
Photoacoustic signals delivered to animal cause thermoelastic expansion detectable via transducer
After excitation optical invasive sensors emits light, capture optically and converts to a specific value
Electrochemical oxygen sensor inserts into a needle probe and detects ionization of O2 atoms via a reduction reaction
Hypoxia-dependent bioluminescent reporter expression in cancer cells An animal is preinjected with luciferin and then imaging
fMRI technology measures metabolic function using blood oxygen level dependent (BOLD) or tumor oxygen-ation level dependent (TOLD) contrast methods
Imaging of an O2-quenched phosphorescent molecule injected into the animal and measures through visible photons during radiotherapy
Electron Paramagnetic Resonance Imaging Uses an injected spin probe (e.g., C-labeled pyruvate)
Hypoxia-dependent fluorescent using a whole animal imaging approach can be imaged by fluorescent microscopy

FIGURE 8.1 *In vivo* detection of hypoxia. (From Zheng J, Shen Y, Xu Z, Yuan Z, He Y, Wei C, Er M, Yin J, Chen H. Near-infrared off-on fluorescence probe activated by NTR for *in vivo* hypoxia imaging. Biosens Bioelectron. 2018;119:141–148.)

FLUORESCENT REPORTERS

It is also possible to create tumors in mice that allow for the imaging of spontaneous hypoxic regions using cell lines that have been modified to express a fluorescent reporter during hypoxic exposure. The study demonstrated that UnaG expression may be detected at single-cell resolution in the brain of living mice by orthotopically introducing Gli36 reporter cells into SCID mice (64). Vermeer et al. employed a different fate mapping strategy that involved delivering an HIF-1-GFP-Cre-ER fusion protein via a LoxP-flanked-STOP tdTomato cassette. This method is tamoxifen-inducible, meaning that it permanently triggers tdTomato expression once the Cre-ER fusion protein is stable under hypoxia (65).

However, fluorescent reporters can be observed live over long periods of time utilizing small animal fluorescent imaging or improved intravital imaging, but immunolabeling techniques will only detect cells when they are hypoxic. Furthermore, they can be designed to identify hypoxic cells even after they have been reoxygenated. The drawback of the technique is that it usually takes the delivery of two different reporters to differentiate between hypoxic and reoxygenated cells within the tumor (64)

NITROREDUCTASE-SENSITIVE FLUORESCENT PROBES

Experimental murine models can receive intravenous delivery of fluorescent substrates triggered by nitroreductase enzymes under hypoxia. For example, Zheng and his colleagues (2018) created a Cy-NO_2 fluorescent near-infrared (NIR) substrate that can be activated by nitroreductases. They injected Cy-NO_2 into mouse tumors made from H22 cells to test it. A whole animal imaging system could capture the NIR fluorescence (66). A CRi Maestro spectrum fluorescent small animal imager was used to achieve fluorescence imaging after NO_2-Rosol was injected straight into the tumor. According to the study's findings, NO_2-Rosol successfully reported intratumoral hypoxia, and its signal persisted for 90 minutes—much longer than prior constructions used in this situation (67). All things considered, NTR-sensitive substrates with fluorescent imaging have a great sensitivity to variations in O_2 levels and can be employed for real-time monitoring (68).

IMMUNOLABELING OF EXOGENOUS MARKERS

Exogenous probes can be utilized to identify hypoxic areas in cells, tissue, 3D organoids, or fixed spheroids. Exogenous probes like pimonidazole must be injected or given orally to a human or experimental animal model in order to be used *in vivo*. After the tissue has been preserved and sectioned for staining, the probe produces hypoxia adducts, which can subsequently be identified by IHC or IF using a probe-specific antibody (69). Additionally, probes that do not require antibody labeling have recently been produced. Mice were given pimonidazole intravenously for each probe after two weeks, and tissue samples were taken, immunolabeled for Hypoxyprobe, and then photographed. Pimonidazole-Hypoxyprobe™ staining colocalized with the fluorescence signal from the two nitroimidazole fluorescent derivatives. The conjugated derivatives can be directly identified using fluorescence imaging ex vivo, which eliminates the need for further immunolabeling procedures and could be a viable substitute for Hypoxyprobe™ immunolabeling (70).

IMMUNOLABELING OF ENDOGENOUS MARKERS

The well-established techniques of immunolabeling HIF-1 and HIF-2 and their downstream targets are employed to detect intratumoral hypoxic areas in tissue sections using both IHC and IF techniques (71). Staining for HIFs and HIF-target gene expression should be done with caution because HIFs can also be controlled by a variety of non-canonical mechanisms, including oxidative phosphorylation inhibitors, dietary deprivation, and von Hippel-Lindau (VHL) gene mutations (72).

PHOTOACOUSTIC IMAGING (PAI)

Photoacoustic (PA) signals are produced by the absorption of near-infrared photons, whereas low tissue penetration and light dispersion can impede fluorescence imaging.

In order to identify hypoxia through spectral absorbance variations, PAI uses O_2-sensitive dyes that cause fast thermoelastic expansion. This causes sound waves to propagate and be recordable by a transducer (73).

With the development of ratiometric PA probes more recently, it is now possible to evaluate the ratio of reacted to unreacted probes. Knox and his colleagues (2018) created a reaction-based ratiometric PA probe with an N-oxide activity that, in hypoxic environments, is selectively bioreduced by heme proteins (74). The maximum absorbance of the probe is shifted by this irreversible chemical reaction, which also strengthens the PA signal for better detection.

The scientists tested this method by subcutaneously implanting 4T1 cells into BALB/c mice to create tumors that were 300–400 mm^3 in size. They were able to identify hypoxic gradients at centimeter depths and with good precision (74).

Deep tissue imaging with PAI is still difficult, despite the fact that it can detect hypoxia at a deeper tissue depth than fluorescent reporters and other optical imaging modalities. The fact that this technology has so far been used to identify human breast cancers based on their hypoxic state indicates that PAI O_2 probes may eventually be developed for clinical usage and offer O_2 readouts (75).

BIOLUMINESCENCE IMAGING (BLI) REPORTERS

A live cell containing a vector encoding a luciferase gene emits light, which is measured by bioluminescence imaging (BLI). When the substrate luciferin is present, luciferase converts it to oxyluciferin, which emits light that can be picked up by a detector.

Since the luciferase enzyme was rapidly degraded by the oxygen-dependent degradation (ODD) domain upon reoxygenation, the bioluminescence signal was utilized to track acute hypoxia. However, because of its longer half-life and slower rate of degradation following reoxygenation, eGFP made it possible to image hypoxic cells even after reoxygenation. Because the half-lives of the bioluminescent and fluorescent reporters differed—34 minutes and 15 hours, respectively—it was possible to distinguish between hypoxic and post-hypoxic cells using this combination. Nevertheless, in contrast to BLI, changes in tissue thickness during excitation and emission can weaken the eGFP signal (76).

CHERENKOV-EXCITED LUMINESCENCE IMAGING (CELI)

Phosphorescent compounds like Ru(II) and Ir(III) complexes and Pt(II) and Pd(II) porphyrins can dynamically monitor hypoxia by O_2-quenching. Using a phosphorescent probe and visible photons generated during radiation, CELI is a new imaging technique that measures PO_2 (64). The O_2-quenched dendritic molecule PtG4 is among the most widely used probes for CELI imaging. The phosphorescence of PtG4 is excited by Cherenkov light produced by radiation-exposed tissue, and the decay period of the phosphorescence is a direct measure of tissue PO_2 (77).

A few challenges remain before CELI can be applied clinically to map intratumoral hypoxia, including the toxicity of O_2 probes. Nonetheless, hypoxia in murine tumors could be seen using implantable PtG4 gel probes given at a dosage allowed by the FDA and recommended for mice (77). Thus, the most likely application for this technology would be to include it in the protocols for radiotherapy, which certain cancer patients undergo as a therapy to track intratumoral hypoxia in order to assess the effectiveness of treatment.

INVASIVE OPTICAL OXYGEN SENSORS

Invasive optical O_2 sensors are another needle-based technique for determining hypoxia in solid tumors. These sensors have an optical fiber coated with an O_2-specific phosphorescent dye at the tip. Because of their great spatial resolution of 300 m and 0.1 mmHg, invasive optical sensors are often employed as an accurate way to validate local O_2 concentrations (78). For instance, PO_2 levels in mouse models of sarcoma (79) and pancreas (80) have been measured using fiberoptic needle microsensors. Furthermore, limiting variables may include variations in heart rate, poor blood circulation, and outside light. However, because of their accuracy and precision, invasive optical O_2 sensors have been effectively employed to analyze O_2 gradients across tumors, albeit with some room for improvement (64).

ELECTROCHEMICAL OXYGEN SENSORS

The gold standard for O_2 detection has been the 'Clark electrode' O_2 sensor, which was created in 1956 (81). A detectable current that is precisely proportional to the O_2 concentration is produced when a voltage is given to the platinum electrode, which reduces the amount of O_2 on the electrode's surface (82). A wireless, implantable Clark-type electrochemical O_2 sensor was recently tested by Rivas and his colleagues (2020) in rabbits with the sensor placed in the right femoral quadricep muscle (83). By changing the fraction of inspired oxygen (FiO_2) that the rabbits could breathe, the sensors were able to differentiate between induced hyperoxia and hypoxic states (83). Gray et al. investigated changes in O_2 concentrations and visceral tissue O_2 tension during intestinal surgery using a comparable Clark-like sensor applied to the rats' serosal surface (84). All things considered, these sensors offer a precise way to immediately identify hypoxia; yet, their clinical usefulness is still restricted to needle probes.

POSITRON EMISSION TOMOGRAPHY (PET)

PET is an imaging technique that can indirectly and noninvasively detect hypoxia in live animals when combined with computerized tomography (CT) with 2-nitroimidazole radiolabeling tracers (64). PET agents are radioactive substances that may be measured quantitatively by their beta-decay, which is then transformed into a three-dimensional image.

Recent research by Hirata and his colleagues revealed that ^{18}F-FMISO offers useful predictive information on tumor necrosis, vascularization, and permeability as well as survival and response to treatment for patients with gliomas (85). Peeters and his research group discovered that ^{18}F-FMISO and ^{18}F-HX4 exhibited good spatial repeatability, but in rat tumors, ^{18}F-FAZA and ^{18}F-HX4 showed greater sensitivity to acute hypoxia (86).

Similarly, due to its better tumor-to-background ratio and biodistribution, ^{18}F-FAZA has been described as a more promising tracer than ^{18}F-FMISO (87). Moreover, ^{18}F-HX4 has been shown in clinical trials involving patients with head and neck malignancies to have superior sensitivity and specificity, quicker clearance, and a shorter injection acquisition time than ^{18}F-FMISO (88).

More and his colleagues (2018) created an ^{18}F-PET radiotracer using acetazolamide, a medication that inhibits carbonic anhydrase. The authors used the HT-29 and 4T1 BALB/c skin xenograft models to test this strategy. Regretfully, tracer uptake in the tumors was minimal, despite its potential viability (89). PET is a tried-and-true technique that has been effectively applied in the clinic to measure intratumoral hypoxia in a variety of solid tumor types, despite certain drawbacks (90).

MAGNETIC RESONANCE IMAGING (MRI)

MRI is a noninvasive technique that was initially used in the latter half of the 20th century to assess hypoxia *in vivo* (91). Protons, or hydrogen nuclei, are excited by a magnetic field produced by a collection of magnets pointed in various directions in an MRI. Hypoxia in animal models of cancer has been successfully mapped using BOLD fMRI (92). However, a number of biological variables, including diverse tumor tissue, poor blood flow regulation, and differences in blood vessel size, can complicate the assessment.

A second MRI technique that has been used to study hypoxia is tumor oxygenation level-dependent (TOLD) MRI, which measures the amount of free O_2 molecules in the tissue (93,94). In order to get accurate measurements of PO_2 in animal models, recent research has combined siloxane injections with TOLD MRI techniques. This technique is known as proton imaging of siloxanes to map tissue oxygen levels (PISTOL) (95). In order to create greater resolution and quicker MRI readouts, Kodibagkar and his colleagues (2008) created PISTOL and tested it *in vivo* to monitor O_2 in the rat thigh muscle (95). Magnetic resonance contrast amplification nanoprobes have also been used in MRI scans to enhance the detection of hypoxia in xenograft models by increasing resolution (64).

ELECTRON PARAMAGNETIC RESONANCE IMAGING (EPRI)

An imaging system that is comparable to MRI is called EPRI. However, EPRI uses an injected spin probe to monitor the unpaired electron spins of diffusible O_2 in order to directly assess relaxation, whereas MRI maps the distribution of protons (64). Direct PO_2 measurements are therefore possible since the energy generated when the two unpaired electrons of molecular O_2 collide with the unpaired electron of the probe is linearly proportional to the O_2 concentration (96). EPRI probes can detect hypoxic areas in a live animal since they endure repetitive imaging (over a few hours) and remain in the site for several months after injection (64).

Orthotopic and transgenic mouse models of breast cancer have both been used to assess the applicability of EPRI (97). Additionally, EPRI's viability for hypoxia detection was effectively evaluated in animal models of colon adenocarcinomas and glioblastoma (64). EPRI's accuracy for tissue O_2 imaging is generally good, although it is constrained by its 10-mm penetration depth and need for tracer injections. EPRI is a new technique that has shown promise in preclinical studies but has not yet received FDA approval.

CONCLUSIONS

Ideally, it would be possible to identify naturally occurring differential hypoxia in a single group of lab animals with tumors. External modifications, however, might be essential, particularly for the research and validation of innovative hypoxia-targeting treatments. Because tumor hypoxia is such a delicate, intricate, and fleeting process, it is highly vulnerable to numerous internal and external affecting variables. Unpredictable, unanticipated, unreliable, or unreproducible experimental results can result from even the slightest alteration in any of the previously described variables, either alone or in combination. However, there are still other influences that can affect implementation in a clinical environment. In this regard, using mouse models has significant benefits over clinical research, including the ease of collecting biopsy specimens, the elimination of the need for time-consuming patient recruitment, the potential for goal failure, and the reduction of patient heterogeneity, among other benefits. In fact, mouse models have shown their value; for example, [^{18}F]FMISO has been successfully used in patients following thorough preclinical *in vivo* validation. Other hypoxia tracers are still being validated, though.

Larger animals, like rats or rabbits, more closely mimic human size and physiology and have been employed to evaluate O_2 detection techniques, even though mouse models are the norm in cancer research. Additionally, non-human primate models have been used to evaluate biosafety factors such as the effect of BOLD signal on brain activity or the biodistribution of radioactive hypoxia tracers for PET imaging. The need for techniques to measure O_2 levels both in vitro and *in vivo* grew as intratumoral hypoxia became more significant.

To examine dynamic changes in hypoxia, phosphorescent and nitroreductase-regulated fluorescent probes are a simple substitute. For instant measurement, these probes can be injected into the animal, and they are easily marketable because of this property, and there are a number of commercially available variations. To track the dynamics of hypoxic and reoxygenated cancer cells, basic scientists have used transcriptionally driven fluorescent and luminescent reporters. These methods necessitate a great deal of design and optimization, which can take time.

Recent developments in medical imaging have made it possible to precisely identify O_2 levels in a tumor using imaging modalities like MRI and PET. By applying these techniques in preclinical models, basic scientists have stayed up to date with these developments. Additionally, whole-body imaging has been widely used in murine models by employing BLI and PAI to facilitate time course research in living animals. Single-cell tracing is not possible due to the limited spatial resolution of whole-body imaging, despite the fact that it better mimics clinical techniques and enables dynamic monitoring of intratumoral hypoxia across extended time-course investigations.

ABBREVIATIONS

^{18}F-FAZA	^{18}F-fluoroazomycin arabinoside
^{18}F-FMISO	^{18}F-fluoromisonidazole
AuNR	gold nanorod
BLI	bioluminescence imaging
BOLD	blood-oxygen-level dependent
CAIX	carbonic anhydrase IX
CELI	Cherenkov-excited luminescence imaging
EPRI	electron paramagnetic resonance imaging
fMRI-	functional magnetic resonance imaging
GLUT-1	glucose transporter 1
HIF	hypoxia-inducible factor
HRE	hypoxia-responsive element
IF	immunofluorescent
IHC	immunohistochemical
MCT-1	monocarboxylate transporter 1
MR-CA	magnetic resonance contrast amplification
MRI	magnetic resonance imaging
NIR	near-infrared
NITP	A2-nitroimidazole
NTR	nitroreductase
ODD	oxygen-dependent degradation
PA	photoacoustic
PAI	photoacoustic imaging
PET	positron emission tomography
PISTOL	proton imaging of siloxanes to map tissue oxygen levels
PLIM	phosphorescence lifetime imaging
PO_2	O_2 partial pressure
TOLD	tumor oxygenation level-dependent
VHL	von Hippel–Lindau

CONSENT FOR PUBLICATION

Not applicable.

FUNDING

None.

CONFLICT OF INTEREST

The authors declare no conflict of interest, financial or otherwise.

ACKNOWLEDGMENTS

Declared none.

REFERENCES

1. Li Y, Zhao L, Li XF. Hypoxia and the tumor microenvironment. Technol Cancer Res Treat. 2021 Jan-Dec;20. doi: 10.1177/15330338211036304.
2. You L, Wu W, Wang X, Fang L, Adam V, Nepovimova E, Wu Q, Kuca K. The role of hypoxia-inducible factor 1 in tumor immune evasion. Med Res Rev. 2021 May;41(3):1622–1643.
3. Tang W, Zhao G. Small molecules targeting HIF-1α pathway for cancer therapy in recent years. Bioorg Med Chem. 2020 Jan 15;28(2):115235.
4. Potente M, Gerhardt H, Carmeliet P. Basic and therapeutic aspects of angiogenesis. Cell. 2011Sep 16;146(6):873–887.
5. Rodriguez D, Watts D, Gaete D, Sormendi S, Wielockx B. Hypoxia pathway proteins and their impact on the blood vasculature. Int J Mol Sci. 2021 Aug 25;22(17):9191.
6. Jászai J, Schmidt MHH. Trends and challenges in tumor anti-angiogenic therapies. Cells. 2019 Sep 18;8(9):1102.
7. de Jong M, Essers J, Van Weerden WM. Imaging preclinical: Improving translational power. Nat Rev Cancer. 2014;14(7):481–493.
8. Fleming IN, Manavaki R, Blower PJ, et al. Imaging tumour hypoxia with positron emission tomography. Br. J. Cancer. 2014;112(2):238–250.
9. Wack LJ, M onnich D, Van Elmpt W, et al. Comparison of [18F]-FMISO, [18F]-FAZA and [18F]-HX4 for PET imaging of hypoxia – A simulation study. Acta Oncologica. 2015;54(9):1370–1377.
10. Bentzen L, Keiding S, Horsman MR, et al. Assessment of hypoxia in experimental mice tumours by [18F]fluoromisonidazole PET and pO_2 electrode measurements. Acta Oncologica. 2002;41(3):304–312.
11. Mortensen LS, Busk M, Nordsmark M, et al. Accessing radiation response using hypoxia PET imaging and oxygen sensitive electrodes: A preclinical study. Radiother Oncol. 2011;99(3):418–423.
12. Mahy P, De Bast M, De Groot T, et al. Comparative pharmacokinetics, biodistribution, metabolism and hypoxiadependent uptake of [18F]-EF3 and [18F]-MISO in rodent tumor models. Radiother Oncol. 2008;89(3):353–360.
13. Dubois LJ, Lieuwes NG, Janssen MHM, et al. Preclinical evaluation and validation of [18F]HX4, a promising hypoxia marker for PET imaging. PNAS. 2011;108(35):14620–14625.
14. Doss M, Zhang JJ, B´elanger M-J, et al. Biodistribution and radiation dosimetry of the hypoxia marker 18F–HX4 in monkeys and humans determined by using whole-body PET/CT. Nucl. Med. Commun. 2010;31:1016–1024.
15. Tang HW, Feng HL, Wang M, Zhu QL, Liu YQ, Jiang YX. *In vivo* longitudinal and multimodal imaging of hypoxia-inducible factor 1α and angiogenesis in breast cancer. Chin Med J (Engl). 2020 Jan 20;133(2):205–211.
16. Kis A, Szabó JP, Dénes N, Vágner A, Nagy G, Garai I, Fekete A, Szikra D, Hajdu I, Matolay O, Méhes G, Mező G, Kertész I, Trencsényi G. *In vivo* imaging of hypoxia and neoangiogenesis in experimental syngeneic hepatocellular carcinoma tumor model using positron emission tomography. Biomed Res Int. 2020 Aug 7;2020:4952372.
17. De Bruycker S, Vangestel C, Staelens S, Van den Wyngaert T, Stroobants S. How to modulate tumor hypoxia for preclinical *in vivo* imaging research. Contrast Media Mol Imaging. 2018 Oct 18; 2018:4608186. doi: 10.1155/2018/4608186.
18. Rapic S, Vangestel C, Verhaeghe J, et al. Characterization of an orthotopic colorectal cancer mouse model and its feasibility for accurate quantification in positron emission tomography. Mol. Imaging Biol. 2017;19(5):762–771.

19. Blouw B, Song H, Tihan T, et al. The hypoxic response of tumors is dependent on their microenvironment. Cancer Cell. 2003;4(2):133–146.
20. Klement RJ, Champ CE. Calories, carbohydrates, and cancer therapy with radiation: Exploiting the five-R's through dietary manipulation. Cancer Metastasis Rev. 2014;33(1):217–229.
21. Lin B-Q, Zeng Z-Y, Yang S-S, Zhuang C-W. Dietary restriction suppresses tumor growth, reduces angiogenesis, and improves tumor microenvironment in human non-small-cell lung cancer xenografts. Lung Cancer. 2013;79(2):111–117.
22. Mukherjee P. Antiangiogenic and proapoptotic effects of dietary restriction on experimental mouse and human brain tumors. Clin Cancer Res. 2004;10(16):5622–5629.
23. Saleh A, Simone B, Palazzo J, et al. Caloric restriction augments radiation efficacy in breast cancer. Cell Cycle. 2014;12(12):1955–1963.
24. Koch CJ, Shuman AL, Jenkins WT, et al. The radiation response of cells from 9L gliosarcoma tumours is correlated with [F18]-EF5 uptake. Int J Radiat Biol. 2010;85(12):1137–1147.
25. Yapp DTT, Woo J, Kartono A, et al. Non-invasive evaluation of tumour hypoxia in the Shionogi tumour model for prostate cancer with 18F-EF5 and positron emission tomography. BJU Int. 2007;99(5):1154–1160.
26. Nakamura J, Kitajima Y, Kai K, et al. HIF-1α is an unfavorable determinant of relapse in gastric cancer patients who underwent curative surgery followed by adjuvant 5-FU chemotherapy. Int J Cancer. 2009;127(5):1158–1171.
27. Li W, Chen Y-Q, Shen Y-B, et al. HIF-1α knockdown by miRNA decreases survivin expression and inhibits A549 cell growth in vitro and *in vivo*. Int J Mol Med. 2013;32(2):271–280.
28. Hiraki M, Kitajima Y, Kai K, et al. Knockdown of hypoxiainducible factor-1α accelerates peritoneal dissemination via the upregulation of MMP-1 expression in gastric cancer cell lines. Exp Ther Med. 2012;4(3):355–362.
29. Carmeliet P, Dor Y, Herbert J-M, et al. Role of HIF-1α in hypoxia-mediated apoptosis, cell proliferation and tumour angiogenesis. Nature. 1998;394(6692):485–490.
30. Takeda T, Okuyama H, Nishizawa Y, et al. Hypoxia inducible factor-1α is necessary for invasive phenotype in Vegf-deleted islet cell tumors. Sci Rep. 2012;2(1):494.
31. Dang DT, Chen F, Gardner LB, et al. Hypoxia-inducible factor-1 promotes nonhypoxia-mediated proliferation in colon cancer cells and xenografts. Cancer Res. 2006;66(3):1684–1936.
32. Dubois L, Landuyt W, Haustermans K, et al. Evaluation of hypoxia in an experimental rat tumour model by [18F]Fluoromisonidazole PET and immunohistochemistry. Br J Cancer. 2004;91(11):1947–1954.
33. Chung J-K, Chang YS, Lee YJ, et al. The effect of tumor size on F-18-labeled fluorodeoxyglucose and fluoroerythronitroimidazole uptake in a murine sarcoma model. Ann Nucl Med. 1999;13(5):303–308.
34. De Jaeger K, Merlo FM, Kavanagh M-C, et al. Heterogeneity of tumor oxygenation: Relationship to tumor necrosis, tumor size, and metastasis. Int J Radiat Oncol Biol Phys. 1998;42(4):717–721.
35. Torwarth D, Eschmann SM, Paulsen F, Alber M. A kinetic model for dynamic [18F]-Fmiso PET data to analyse tumour hypoxia. Phys Med Biol. 2005;50(10):2209–2224.
36. Cairns RA, Kalliomaki T, Hill RP. Acute (cyclic) hypoxia enhances spontaneous metastasis of KHT murine tumors. Cancer Res. 2001;61:8903–8908.
37. Busk M, Horsman MR, Kristjansen PEG, et al. Aerobic glycolysis in cancers: Implications for the usability of oxygenresponsive genes and fluorodeoxyglucose-PET as markers of tissue hypoxia. Int J Cancer. 2008;122(12):2726–2734.
38. McSheehy PMJ, Port RE, Rodrigues LM, et al. Investigations *in vivo* of the effects of carbogen breathing on 5-fluorouracil pharmacokinetics and physiology of solid rodent tumours. Cancer Chemother Pharmacol. 2004;55(2):117–128.
39. Kamm YJL, Peters GJ, Hull WE, et al. Correlation between 5-fluorouracil metabolism and treatment response in two variants of C26 murine colon carcinoma. Br J Cancer. 2003;89(4):754–762.
40. Van Laarhoven HWM, Gambarota G, Lok J, et al. Carbogen breathing differentially enhances blood plasma volume and 5-fluorouracil uptake in two murine colon tumor models with a distinct vascular structure. Neoplasia. 2006;8(6):477–487.
41. Peeters SGJA, Zegers CML, Biemans R, et al. TH-302 in combination with radiotherapy enhances the therapeutic outcome and is associated with pretreatment [18F]HX4 hypoxia PET imaging. Clin Cancer Res. 2015;21(13):2984–2992.
42. Wang J, Foehrenbacher A, Su J, et al. The 2-nitroimidazole EF5 is a biomarker for oxidoreductases that activate the bioreductive prodrug CEN-209 under hypoxia. Clin Cancer Res. 2012;18(6):1684–1695.
43. Ferrario A, Tiehl Von KF, Rucker N, et al. Antiangiogenic treatment enhances photodynamic therapy responsiveness in a mouse mammary carcinoma. Cancer Res. 2000;60:4066–4069.

44. Brader P, Riedl CC, Woo Y, et al. Imaging of hypoxiadriven gene expression in an orthotopic liver tumor model. Mol. Cancer Ther. 2007;6(11):2900–2908.
45. Song CW, Park H, Griffin RJ. Improvement of tumor oxygenation by mild hyperthermia. Radiation Res. 2001;155(4):515–528.
46. Sun X, Li X-F, Russell J, et al. Changes in tumor hypoxia induced by mild temperature hyperthermia as assessed by dual-tracer immunohistochemistry. Radiother Oncol. 2008;88(2):269–276.
47. Moon EJ, Sonveaux P, Porporato PE, et al. NADPH oxidase-mediated reactive oxygen species production activates hypoxia-inducible factor-1 (HIF-1) via the ERK pathway after hyperthermia treatment. PNAS. 2010;107(47):20477–20482.
48. Sen A, Capitano ML, Spernyak JA, et al. Mild elevation of body temperature reduces tumor interstitial fluid pressure and hypoxia and enhances efficacy of radiotherapy in murine tumor models. Cancer Res. 2011;71(11):3872–3880.
49. Jones LW, Viglianti BL, Tashjian JA, et al. Effect of aerobic exercise on tumor physiology in an animal model of human breast cancer. J. Appl. Physiol. 2010;108(2):343–348.
50. Jones LW, Antonelli J, Masko EM, et al. Exercise modulation of the host-tumor interaction in an orthotopic model of murine prostate cancer. J. Appl. Physiol. 2012;113(2):263–272.
51. Wiggins JM, Rice L, Lepler S, et al. "The impact of daily exercise on tumor perfusion," in Proceedings of the 110th Annual Meeting of the American Association for Cancer Research (AACR), Abstract nr 5913, AACR, Philadelphia, PA, USA, April 2017.
52. McCullough DJ, Stabley JN, Siemann DW, Behnke BJ. Modulation of blood flow, hypoxia, and vascular function in orthotopic prostate tumors during exercise. J Natl Cancer Inst. 2014;106(4):dju036.
53. Fliedner FP, Hansen AE, Jørgensen JT, Kjær A. The use of matrigel has no influence on tumor development or PET imaging in FaDu human head and neck cancer xenografts. BMC Med Imaging. 2016;16(1):5.
54. Jordan BF, Sonveaux P, Feron O, et al. Nitric oxide–mediated increase in tumor blood flow and oxygenation of tumors implanted in muscles stimulated by electric pulses. Int. J. Radiat. Oncol. Biol. Phys. 2003;55(4):1066–1073.
55. Doleschel D, Rix A, Arns S, et al. Erythropoietin improves the accumulation and therapeutic effects of carboplatin by enhancing tumor vascularization and perfusion. Theranostics. 2015;5(8):905–918.
56. Horsman MR, Overgaard J. The impact of hypoxia and its modification of the outcome of radiotherapy. J Radiat Res. 2016;57(S1):i90–i98.
57. Wheaton WW, Weinberg SE, Hamanaka RB, et al. Metformin inhitibs mitochondrial complex I of cancer cells to reduce tumorigenesis. eLife. 2014;3:e02242.
58. Zannella VE, Dal Pra A, Muaddi H, et al. Reprogramming metabolism with metformin improves tumor oxygenation and radiotherapy response. Clin Cancer Res. 2013;19(24):6741–6750.
59. Sonveaux P. Provascular strategy: Targeting functional adaptations of mature blood vessels in tumors to selectively influence the tumor vascular reactivity and improve cancer treatment. Radiother Oncol. 2008;86(3):300–313.
60. Hern´andez-Agudo E, Mondejar T, Soto-Montenegro ML, et al. Monitoring vascular normalization induced by antiangiogenic treatment with 18F-fluoromisonidazole-PET. Mol Oncol. 2016;10(5):704–718.
61. Jain RK. Normalization of tumor vasculature: An emerging concept in antiangiogenic therapy. Science. 2005;307(5706):58–62.
62. Siemann DW, Horsman MR. Modulation of the tumor vasculature and oxygenation to improve therapy. Pharmacol. Ther. 2015;153:107–124.
63. Horsman MR, Overgaard J. The impact of hypoxia and its modification of the outcome of radiotherapy. J Radiat. Res. 2016;57(S1):i90–i98.
64. Godet I, Doctorman S, Wu F, Gilkes DM. Detection of hypoxia in cancer models: Significance, challenges, and advances. Cells. 2022 Feb 16;11(4):686. doi: 10.3390/cells11040686.
65. Vermeer JAF, Ient J, Markelc B, Kaeppler J, Barbeau LMO, Groot AJ, Muschel RJ, Vooijs MA. A lineage-tracing tool to map the fate of hypoxic tumour cells. Dis Model Mech. 2020;13:044768.
66. Zheng J, Shen Y, Xu Z, Yuan Z, He Y, Wei C, Er M, Yin J, Chen H. Near-infrared off-on fluorescence probe activated by NTR for *in vivo* hypoxia imaging. Biosens Bioelectron. 2018;119:141–148.
67. Hettie KS, Klockow JL, Moon EJ, Giaccia AJ, Chin FT. A NIR fluorescent smart probe for imaging tumor hypoxia. Cancer Rep. 2021;4:e1384.
68. Li X, Kim J, Yoon J, Chen X. Cancer-associated, stimuli-driven, turn on theranostics for multimodality imaging and therapy. Adv Mater. 2017;29:1606857.
69. Varia MA, Calkins-Adams DP, Rinker LH, Kennedy AS, Novotny DB, Fowler WC, Raleigh JA. Pimonidazole: A novel hypoxia marker for complementary study of tumor hypoxia and cell proliferation in cervical carcinoma. Gynecol Oncol. 1998;71:270–277.

70. Seelam SR, Hong MK, Lee Y-S, Jeong JM. Comparative study of 2-nitroimidazole-fluorophore-conjugated derivatives with pimonidazole for imaging tumor hypoxia. J Radiopharm Mol Probes. 2019;5:101–112.
71. Talks KL, Turley H, Gatter KC, Maxwell P, Pugh C, Ratcliffe P, Harris AL. The expression and distribution of the hypoxia-inducible factors HIF-1 and HIF-2 in normal human tissues, cancers, and tumor-associated macrophages. Am J Pathol. 2000;157:411–421.
72. Iommarini L, Porcelli AM, Gasparre G, Kurelac I. Non-canonical mechanisms regulating hypoxia-inducible factor 1 alpha in cancer. Front Oncol. 2017;7:286.
73. Cheng MHY, Mo Y, Zheng G. Nano versus molecular: Optical imaging approaches to detect and monitor tumor hypoxia. Adv Health Mater. 2021;10:e2001549.
74. Knox HJ, Kim TW, Zhu Z, Chan J. Photophysical tuning of N-oxide-based probes enables ratiometric photoacoustic imaging of tumor hypoxia. ACS Chem Biol. 2018;13:1838–1843.
75. Nyayapathi N, Xia J. Photoacoustic imaging of breast cancer: A mini review of system design and image features. J Biomed Opt. 2019;24:1–13.
76. Danhier P, Krishnamachary B, Bharti S, Kakkad S, Mironchik Y, Bhujwalla ZM. Combining optical reporter proteins with different half-lives to detect temporal evolution of hypoxia and reoxygenation in tumors. Neoplasia. 2015;17:871–881.
77. Cao X, Gunn JR, Allu SR, Bruza P, Jiang S, Vinogradov SA, Pogue BW. Implantable sensor for local Cherenkov-excited luminescence imaging of tumor pO2 during radiotherapy. J Biomed Opt. 2020;25:112704.
78. Springett R, Swartz HM. Measurements of oxygen *In vivo*: Overview and perspectives on methods to measure oxygen within cells and tissues. Antioxid. Redox Signal. 2007;9:1295–1302.
79. Lewis DM, Park KM, Tang V, Xu Y, Pak K, Eisinger-Mathason TSK, Simon MC, Gerecht S. Intratumoral oxygen gradients mediate sarcoma cell invasion. PNAS USA. 2016;113:9292–9297.
80. Owen J, Logan K, Nesbitt H, et al. Orally administered oxygen nanobubbles enhance tumor response to sonodynamic therapy. Nano Sel. 2022;3:394–401.
81. Qlark LC. Monitor and control of blood and tissue oxygen tensions. Trans—Am Soc Artif Intern Organs. 1956;2:41–48.
82. Marland JR, Gray ME, Dunare C, et al. Real-time measurement of tumour hypoxia using an implantable microfabricated oxygen sensor. Sens Bio-Sensing Res. 2020;30:100375.
83. Rivas L, Dulay S, Miserere S, et al. Micro-needle implantable electrochemical oxygen sensor: Ex-vivo and in-vivo studies. Biosens Bioelectron. 2020;153:112028.
84. Gray ME, Marland J, Dunare C, et al. *In vivo* validation of a miniaturized electrochemical oxygen sensor for measuring intestinal oxygen tension. Am J Physiol Liver Physiol. 2019;317:G242–G252.
85. Hirata K, Yamaguchi S, Shiga T, Kuge Y, Tamaki N. The roles of hypoxia imaging using 18F-fluoromisonidazole positron emission tomography in glioma treatment. J Clin Med. 2019;8:1088.
86. Peeters SG, Zegers CM, Lieuwes NG, van Elmpt W, Eriksson J, van Dongen GA, Dubois L, Lambin P. A comparative study of the hypoxia PET tracers [18F]HX4, [18F]FAZA, and [18F]FMISO in a preclinical tumor model. Int J Radiat Oncol. 2015;91:351–359.
87. Quartuccio N, Young AIMN Working Group, Laudicella R, Mapelli P, Guglielmo P, Pizzuto DA, Boero M, Arnone G, Picchio M. Hypoxia PET imaging beyond 18F-FMISO in patients with high-grade glioma: 18F-FAZA and other hypoxia radiotracers. Clin Transl Imaging. 2020;8:11–20.
88. Chen L, Zhang Z, Kolb HC, Walsh JC, Zhang J, Guan Y. 18F-HX4 hypoxia imaging with PET/CT in head and neck cancer: A comparison with 18F-FMISO. Nucl Med Commun. 2012;33:1096–1102.
89. More KN, Lee JY, Kim D-Y, et al. Acetazolamide-based [18F]-PET tracer: *In vivo* validation of carbonic anhydrase IX as a sole target for imaging of CA-IX expressing hypoxic solid tumors. Bioorganic Med Chem Lett. 2018;28:915–921.
90. Lopci E, Grassi I, Chiti A, Nanni C, Cicoria G, Toschi L, Fonti C, Lodi F, Mattioli S, Fanti S. PET radiopharmaceuticals for imaging of tumor hypoxia: A review of the evidence. Am J Nucl Med Mol Imaging. 2014;4:365–384.
91. Wyatt JS, Edwards AD, Azzopardi D, Reynolds EO. Magnetic resonance and near infrared spectroscopy for investigation of perinatal hypoxic-ischaemic brain injury. Arch Dis Child. 1989;64:953–963.
92. Virani N, Kwon J, Zhou H, Mason R, Berbeco R, Protti A. *In vivo* hypoxia characterization using blood oxygen level dependent magnetic resonance imaging in a preclinical glioblastoma mouse model. Magn Reson Imaging. 2021;76:52–60.
93. O'Connor JPB, Robinson SP, Waterton JC. Imaging tumour hypoxia with oxygen-enhanced MRI and BOLD MRI. Br J Radiol. 2019;92:20180642.

94. White DA, Zhang Z, Li L, Gerberich J, Stojadinovic S, Peschke P, Mason RP. Developing oxygen-enhanced magnetic resonance imaging as a prognostic biomarker of radiation response. Cancer Lett. 2016;380:69–77.
95. Kodibagkar VD, Wang X, Torres JP, Gulaka P, Mason RP. Proton imaging of siloxanes to map tissue oxygenation levels (PISTOL): A tool for quantitative tissue oximetry. NMR Biomed. 2008;21:899–907.
96. Krishna MC, Matsumoto S, Yasui H, Saito K, Devasahayam N, Subramanian S, Mitchell JB. Electron paramagnetic resonance imaging of tumor pO2. Radiat Res. 2012;177:376–386.
97. Bobko AA, Eubank TD, Driesschaert B, Khramtsov VV. *In vivo* EPR assessment of pH, pO2, redox status, and concentrations of phosphate and glutathione in the tumor microenvironment. J Vis Exp. 2018;133:e56624.

9 Hypoxia-Driven Angiogenesis in Cancer

Adityaraj Patidar, Debprosit Karmakar, Aditya Khatri, Divyansh Jain, and Sukhes Mukherjee
Department of Biochemistry, All India Institute of Medical Sciences, Bhopal, Madhya Pradesh, India

INTRODUCTION

Angiogenesis, as the name suggests, refers to the formation of new blood vessels, which occurs through the proliferation and movement of endothelial cells (ECs) originating from existing blood vessels (La Mendola et al., 2022). The word "angiogenesis" came from the Greek word *Angeion* and it was first used by John Hunter, a British surgeon in the year 1787. However, it was Judah Folkman in 1971, who hypothesized the dependence of tumor growth on angiogenesis that laid the basis for most of its modern understanding (Folkman, 1974). We now know that tumor angiogenesis is essentially a four-step process. It begins with local damage to the basement membrane, leading to hypoxia. This hypoxic environment triggers the release of angiogenic factors such as vascular endothelial growth factor (VEGF)-A. Next, these factors activate ECs, causing them to migrate. In the third step, the ECs proliferate and stabilize. Finally, mature blood vessel tubes are formed (Nishida et al., 2006). However, there is a period during the initial stages of malignant progression where the tumor remains dormant, and it is only after an "Angiogenic switch" that the tumor goes from a non-angiogenic state to active blood vessel formation (Krock et al., 2011).

THE VASCULAR NETWORK

Our body has an extensive vascular network of arteries, veins, and capillaries that ensure proper nutrient and oxygen supply, as well as the removal of metabolic waste. Internally, these blood vessels are composed of a single layer of ECs, which are interconnected by VE-cadherins and claudins. These ECs are bound to a basal membrane and are surrounded by mural cells, which maintain cohesion between the ECs and the basal membrane. This also limits hyperpermeability and vascular leakage (Viallard and Larrivée, 2017).

Arteries contain multiple concentric layers of vascular smooth muscle cells, enabling them to withstand high blood pressure. Veins, on the other hand, are exposed to lower blood pressure and are thus surrounded by thin layers of smooth muscle cells. Capillaries lack any smooth muscle cell layer and are instead covered by specialized cells called pericytes, which are involved in the maturation and stabilization of blood vessels (Pugsley and Tabrizchi, 2000).

The blood vessels associated with tumors differ from normal vessels both morphologically and functionally. In normal tissues, blood vessels are organized hierarchically and evenly distributed. Their effective lining of smooth muscle cells and pericytes allows for efficient nutrient delivery to the surrounding tissue. In contrast, tumor blood vessels are often inefficient due to structural changes caused by paracrine signaling and interactions between tumor cells and ECs. Tumor vasculature is typically unevenly distributed, creating chaotic, twisted networks

 DOI: 10.1201/9781003477419-9

with irregular branching patterns. Tumor vessels display bidirectional blood flow and are not continuously perfused, which further diminishes their efficiency (Ziyad and Iruela-Arispe, 2011).

ANGIOGENESIS

The vascular network forms during embryogenesis through a combination of two processes: vasculogenesis, which is the *de novo* formation of blood vessels from endothelial progenitor cells, and angiogenesis, which is the formation of new vessels from the existing vascular network. Angiogenesis begins with the sprouting, migration, and proliferation of ECs and is regulated by factors such as VEGF (Gerhardt et al., 2003). During this process, some ECs differentiate into "tip cells," which are highly motile and invasive, extending numerous filopodia that respond to growth factors, the extracellular matrix (ECM), and other signals. The remaining ECs, known as "stalk cells," proliferate and contribute to the formation and structural integrity of the new blood vessels. This differentiation between tip and stalk cells is governed by the Delta-Notch signaling pathway (Phng and Gerhardt, 2009). This type of angiogenesis, known as "sprouting angiogenesis," is particularly common in tissues that are poorly perfused and in need of oxygen (Carmeliet and Jain, 2011).

The endothelial tip cell directs the developing capillary sprout through the ECM toward an angiogenic stimulus, such as VEGF-A. Tip cells extend numerous filopodia that not only guide sprout formation but also influence the patterning of the vascular network. These filopodia are responsive to pro-angiogenic signals, promoting cell motility, and they secrete proteolytic enzymes that create a path through the ECM for the sprout to follow. Meanwhile, the stalk cells proliferate and contribute to the elongation of the capillary sprout. As the sprout grows longer, vacuoles form within the stalk cells and coalesce, creating a lumen within the developing vessel. When the tip cells of two or more capillary sprouts meet at the source of VEGF-A secretion, they fuse, forming a continuous lumen through which oxygenated blood can flow. Once the tissue's oxygen needs are met, VEGF-A levels decrease, halting angiogenesis. Pericytes are then recruited, and ECM deposition occurs, leading to the maturation and stabilization of the newly formed capillary (Hillen and Griffioen, 2007) (Table 9.1; Figure 9.1).

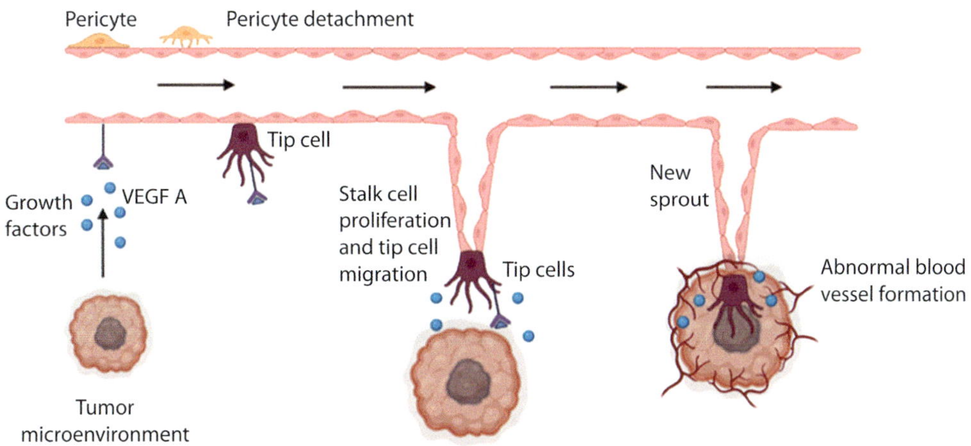

FIGURE 9.1 Schematic diagram of sprouting angiogenesis.

TABLE 9.1
Endogenous Regulators of Angiogenesis

Activators	Inhibitors
Growth factors:	
Vascular endothelial growth factor family	
Acidic and basic fibroblast growth factor	
Angiogenin	
Angiostatin	
Transforming growth factor	
Tumor necrosis factor-α	
Plated-delivered endothelial growth factor	
Hepatocyte growth factor	
Epidermal growth factor	
Placental growth factor	
Granulocyte colony stimulating factor	
Cytokines:	
Interleukin-1	Interleukin-10
Interleukin-6	Interleukin-12
Interleukin-8	
Proteases and protease inhibitors:	
Cathepsin	Tissue inhibitor metalloprotease
Gelatinase A, B	Plasminogen activator-inhibitor-1
Stromelysin	
Urokinase-type plasminogen activator	
Trace elements:	
Copper	Zinc
Oncogenes:	
c-myc	p53
Ras	Rb
c-src	
v-raf	
c-jun	
Endogenous modulators:	
Alpha v beta 3 integrin	Angiotensin
Angiopoietin-I	Angiopoietin 2
Angiotensin II (AT1 Receptor)	Angiostatin II (AT2 Receptor)
Endothelin	Caveolin 1,2
Erythropoietin	Endostatin
Hypoxia	Interferon alpha
Nitric oxide synthase	Isoflavones
Platelet activating factor 4	
Prostaglandin E	
Prolactin (16kd fragment)	

ROLE OF HYPOXIA IN ANGIOGENESIS

Hypoxia occurs due to a combination of elevated metabolic and proliferative rates, along with abnormal tumor vascularization that leads to inadequate oxygen delivery. As solid tumors reach a certain growth stage, they encounter a hypoxic environment, which is recognized as a key characteristic of tumor development. Prolyl hydroxylases (PHDs) enable both tumor and stromal cells to detect the oxygen levels in their surroundings. Under these hypoxic conditions, solid tumors produce substantial levels of hypoxia-inducible factor 1 (HIF-1), which is essential for tumor progression, metastasis, and poor prognosis (Semenza, 2014). HIF-1 is part of the basic helix-loop-helix-Per-ARNT-Sim (bHLH-PAS) transcription factor family, which forms αβ-heterodimers consisting of subunits like HIF-1α, HIF-2α, HIF-3α, and HIF-1β. Unlike the oxygen-sensitive HIF-α subunits, HIF-1β is consistently expressed and does not respond to oxygen changes. Among the HIF-α subunits, HIF-1α is widely expressed across various cell types and is key to maintaining oxygen balance. HIF-2α primarily appears in ECs and induces expression of VEGF A. On the other hand, integrated phospho-AKT (protein kinase B (serine/threonine kinase)) signaling (iPAS), a splice variant of HIF-3α, acts as a negative regulator of HIF-1α activity and is found in tissues like the cornea, cerebellum, and cerebrum (Liao and Johnson, 2007).

HIFs control the transcription of genes that influence cell growth, blood vessel formation, metabolism, and the consumption and supply of oxygen, adjusting their effects based on the surrounding conditions. Hypoxia influences the expression of genes that are regulated by HIF-1α and HIF-2α. These factors form heterodimers with HIF-1β and attach to the hypoxia response element (HRE) located in the promoters of numerous genes. When activated, these HREs trigger the overproduction of various factors that encourage angiogenesis (Zhang et al., 2024).

At the level of protein stability, hypoxic regulation of HIF-1α occurs. In normal oxygen conditions, oxygen facilitates the posttranslational hydroxylation of two proline residues within the oxygen-dependent degradation (ODD) domain of HIF-1α. This hydroxylation process is carried out by three prolyl hydroxylase domain proteins (PHD 1–3) and enables the binding of the tumor suppressor protein von Hippel-Lindau (VHL) to the N-terminal transactivation domain (TAD-N) of HIF-1α. When VHL, an E3 ubiquitin-protein ligase, binds to HIF-1α, it marks it for swift degradation by the proteasome. In low-oxygen (hypoxic) conditions, however, HIF-1α evades this degradation, allowing it to form a heterodimer with HIF-1β. This complex can then bind to HREs in the promoter regions of specific target genes (Semenza, 2004).

The activity of HIF-1α protein is further regulated by factor inhibiting HIF-1 (FIH). In normal oxygen conditions, FIH mediates the hydroxylation of an asparagine residue within the C terminal transactivation domain (TAD-C) of HIF-1α. This hydroxylation inhibits HIF-1α's ability to bind to the transcriptional co-activators p300/CREB-binding protein (CBP). Besides FIH, the activation of the p42/p44 mitogen-activated protein kinase (MAPK) pathway also enhances HIF-1α's transcriptional function by promoting its accumulation in the nucleus. Unlike FIH, which is directly oxygen-dependent, the p42/p44 MAPK pathway involves the phosphorylation of HIF-1α, which does not require oxygen but is dependent on the protein's availability, making it indirectly influenced by hypoxic conditions (Mahon et al., 2001).

HIF-1α protein is also regulated at the mRNA level through the PI3K/AKT signaling pathway. Alterations in growth factors and their receptor tyrosine kinases—often due to mutations causing either loss of function in tumor suppressor genes or gain of function in oncogenes—can lead to PI3K pathway activation, which, in turn, influences tumor cell growth. Activation of the PI3K/AKT pathway by growth factors, as well as downstream signaling molecules, has been shown to enhance HIF-1α activity. Moreover, loss of function of the tumor suppressor phosphatase and tensin homolog (PTEN), which normally inhibits AKT activation by PI3K, can also lead to increased HIF-1α activity. Additionally, insulin-like growth factor 1 (IGF-1) can stimulate HIF-1α activity by activating the PI3K/AKT pathway (Shaw and Cantley, 2006).

The upregulation of HIF-1 in response to hypoxia is crucial for coordinating the molecular processes that lead to the formation of new blood vessels, which are vital for supplying oxygen and nutrients necessary for tumor survival and growth. In hypoxic conditions, HIF-1 increases the expression of growth factors like VEGF and FGF, enhancing EC permeability, growth, and proliferation. Additionally, it can stimulate other growth factors such as platelet-derived growth factor (PDGF) and transforming growth factor (TGF), as well as the transcription of angiopoietins (Ang), which aid in the release of angiogenic factors from cancer cells (McIntyre and Harris, 2015) (Figure 9.2).

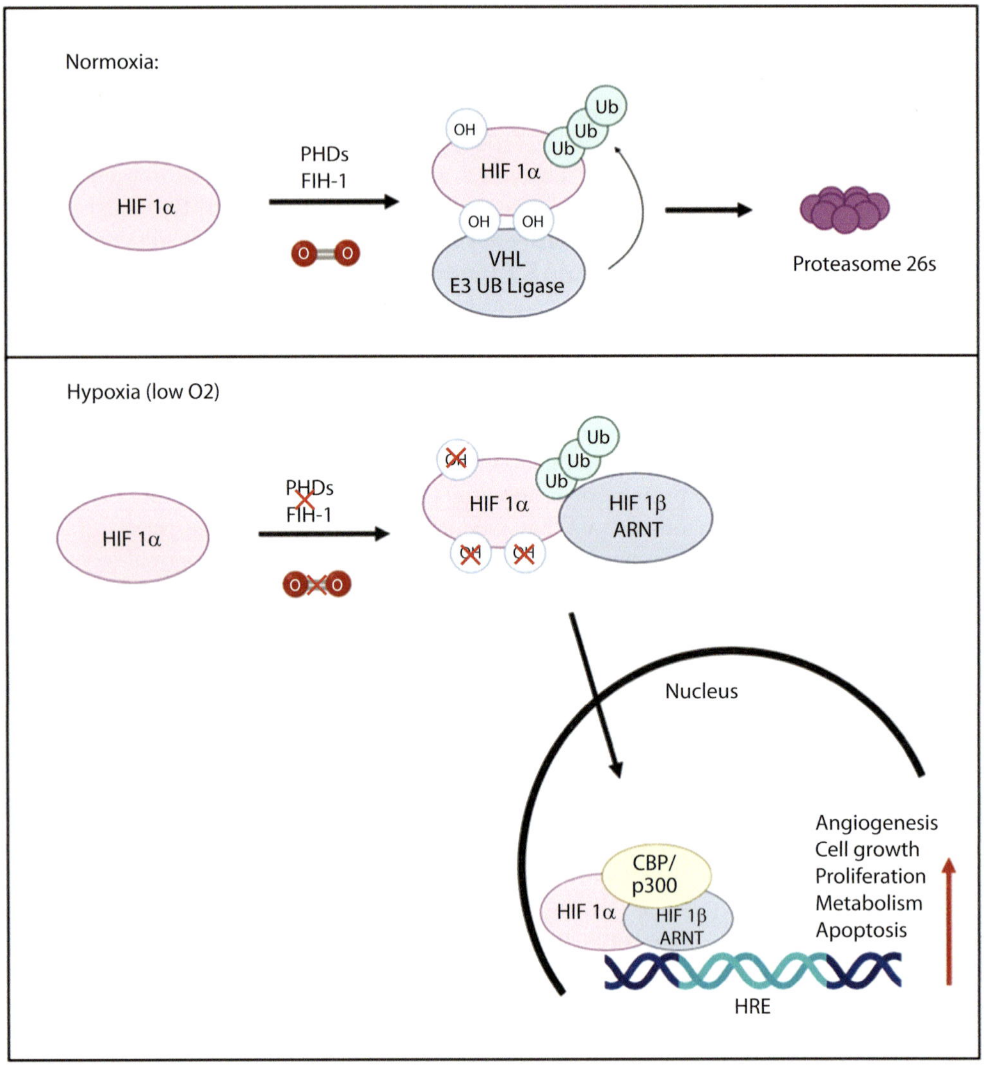

FIGURE 9.2 Regulation of HIF activity.

MOLECULAR MECHANISMS OF ANGIOGENESIS

So far, several ligand-receptor signaling networks have been identified as contributors to tumor angiogenesis: (1) the VEGF ligand with its receptors VEGFR-1, VEGFR-2, and NRP1; (2) angiopoietin ligands with Tie receptors; (3) Delta-like and Jagged ligands with Notch receptors; (4) ephrin ligands with Eph receptors; and (5) the Slit ligand with Robo receptors.

VEGF Pathway

VEGF is a key pro-angiogenic factor that specifically influences vascular ECs and plays a crucial role in processes such as tumor growth, invasion, and angiogenesis. The VEGF family includes VEGF-A, VEGF-B, VEGF-C, VEGF-D, and placental growth factor (PIGF). VEGF-A binds to VEGFR-2, leading to the upregulation of VEGFR-3 and Delta-like 4 (DLL4) in the tip cells, along with activation of the Notch pathway in neighboring stalk cells. This signaling cascade downregulates VEGFR-2 and VEGFR-3 while upregulating VEGFR-1, thereby balancing the roles of tip and stalk cells. Upon VEGF-A's interaction with VEGFR-2 on EC surfaces, it activates downstream pathways, including p38-mitogen-activated protein kinase (p38/MAPK) and AKT-phosphatidylinositol 3-kinase (PI3K/AKT). This activation promotes EC proliferation and migration, leading to the release of numerous pro-angiogenic proteases that increase the permeability of the vascular barrier (Apte et al., 2019).

Alternate splicing of a single gene (most commonly VEGF164) results in expression of multiple isoforms of VEGF. These isoforms differ in their carboxy terminal end (encoded by exons 6a, 6b, 7, and 8). These differences affect their respective capacities to bind to the ECM and to the non-enzymatic single-pass transmembrane proteins, Neuropilin-1 and Neuropilin-2 (NRP1 and NRP2). ECs respond to the VEGF ligand through two receptor tyrosine kinases, VEGFR-1 and VEGFR-2 (also known as VEGF receptor-1 and -2). VEGFR-2 primarily mediates pro-angiogenic responses, while VEGFR-1 is thought to function as a decoy regulator. When VEGF binds as a dimer, VEGFR-2 undergoes homodimerization and initiates cross-phosphorylation. This activated VEGFR-2 then triggers downstream signaling that promotes EC proliferation, migration, and increases vascular permeability. Soluble VEGF is mainly responsible for increasing vessel diameter, whereas signaling from bound VEGF promotes vessel branching (Grünewald et al., 2010). Neuropilin-1 and -2 are transmembrane glycoproteins found in various cell types, including neurons, cancer cells, smooth muscle cells, and ECs. NRPs can bind to at least two different ligands: semaphorins, which inhibit cell migration, and growth factors such as VEGF, PDGF, and hepatocyte growth factor (HGF), which promote cell migration. Small-molecule inhibitors targeting NRP1, along with antibodies designed to target NRP1, have demonstrated promise in cancer treatment (Pellet-Many et al., 2008).

PDGF Pathway

PDGF plays a critical role in tumor angiogenesis. The PDGF family comprises PDGF-A, PDGF-B, PDGF-C, and PDGF-D. When PDGF binds to PDGFR, it induces receptor dimerization, which activates signaling pathways such as Ras-mitogen-activated protein kinase (RAS/MAPK) and PI3K. PDGF-AB aids in stabilizing the newly formed tumor vasculature by recruiting pericytes, while PDGF-BB modulates VEGFR2 signaling and EC proliferation, helping to prevent vascular irregularities caused by elevated VEGF level (Gianni-Barrera et al., 2018).

Notch Signaling Pathway

Notch signaling orchestrates the early stages of vascular sprouting by defining key differences between leading tip cells and trailing stalk cells. Known for its role in regulating cell fate and maintaining homeostasis, the Notch pathway operates across multiple contexts, such as morphogenesis in tracheal branching and determining neuronal cell fate. Notch receptors and ligands are single-pass transmembrane proteins found on cell surfaces, capable of engaging in autocrine or juxtacrine signaling interactions to drive these processes (Ghabrial and Krasnow, 2006). Activation of Notch by DLL4 initiates the formation of an angiogenic sprout composed of two distinct EC types: tip and stalk cells. Tip cells, which do not engage in Notch signaling, detect environmental signals through filopodia equipped with VEGFR-2 receptors. When VEGF binds to VEGFR-2, DLL4 expression is increased in arterial ECs in vitro via the PI3K/Akt pathway (Liu et al., 2003).

Angiopoietin Ligands with Tie Receptors

Ang promotes interactions between tumor and ECs, playing a regulatory role in tumor angiogenesis. The Ang family consists of Ang-1, Ang-2, Ang-3, and Ang-4, which interact with their respective tyrosine kinase receptors, Tiel and Tie2. Ang-1 activates signaling pathways through Tie2 phosphorylation, helping maintain strong EC connections. Inhibiting Tie/Ang-2 can reduce vascular sprouting and foster tumor neovascularization. Furthermore, the Ang-2/Tie signaling pathway works together with VEGF signaling to enhance tumor neo-angiogenesis, while blocking both Ang-2 and VEGF slows tumor growth, promotes survival benefits, and reprograms tumor-associated macrophages (TAMs) to adopt an antitumor role, as well as trimming immature tumor vessels. Pericytes release Ang-1, which binds to Tie2 receptors on ECs, suppressing their proliferation and stabilizing angiogenesis through downstream pathways, including calpain, protein kinase B, and forkhead box O3A (Kloepper et al., 2016).

TUMOR VASCULATURE

As previously mentioned, the body's blood supply is maintained by an orderly and efficient vascular network. This network is regulated by a balance between pro-angiogenic and anti-angiogenic factors, driven by the metabolic demands of the tissues. However, in tumors, the rapid proliferation of cancerous cells results in an overproduction of pro-angiogenic factors. This causes the tumor's vascular network to become disorganized and fundamentally different from normal blood vessels. The vessels in tumors are often immature, tortuous, and highly permeable. Unlike normal blood vessels, tumor vasculature lacks the distinct structure of arterioles, capillaries, and venules (Lugano et al., 2020).

Due to this abnormal nature, the ability of these abnormal tumor blood vessels to supply nutrients is significantly impaired, resulting in hypoxic microenvironments (Chen et al., 2023). Tumor vessels are poorly developed, with inadequate smooth muscle coverage and frequently disrupted endothelial linings and basement membranes, contributing to their leaky nature (Siemann, 2011). These aberrant characteristics of tumor vasculature create abnormal microenvironments that can hinder the effectiveness of traditional anti-cancer therapies. However, the unique properties of tumor blood vessels also provide opportunities for developing targeted therapeutic interventions, which will be discussed later in this chapter (Tzeng and Huang, 2023).

DIFFERENT FORMS OF TUMOR ANGIOGENESIS

Tumor angiogenesis is a complex and dynamic process that involves multiple cell types and intricate signaling pathways. Current research on angiogenesis has primarily concentrated on the mechanisms of sprouting angiogenesis, while other forms of angiogenesis remain less well understood. Six major cellular mechanisms of tumor angiogenesis are (1) sprouting angiogenesis (SA), (2) vasculogenic mimicry (VM), (3) vessel intussusception, (4) vascular co-option, (5) angiogenesis driven by cancer stem cells, and (6) angiogenesis originating from bone marrow-derived cells (Zhang et al., 2024).

The presence of various angiogenesis mechanisms offers a new approach to hindering tumor cell spread. While certain small-molecule drugs that target vascular co-option and vascular mimicry have been developed, further investigation into these diverse mechanisms may help researchers pinpoint crucial molecular targets to create more specific therapies. Moreover, considering the broad application and clinical importance of anti-angiogenic treatment, it's essential to advance the development of innovative, more effective combination therapies to improve outcomes (Figure 9.3).

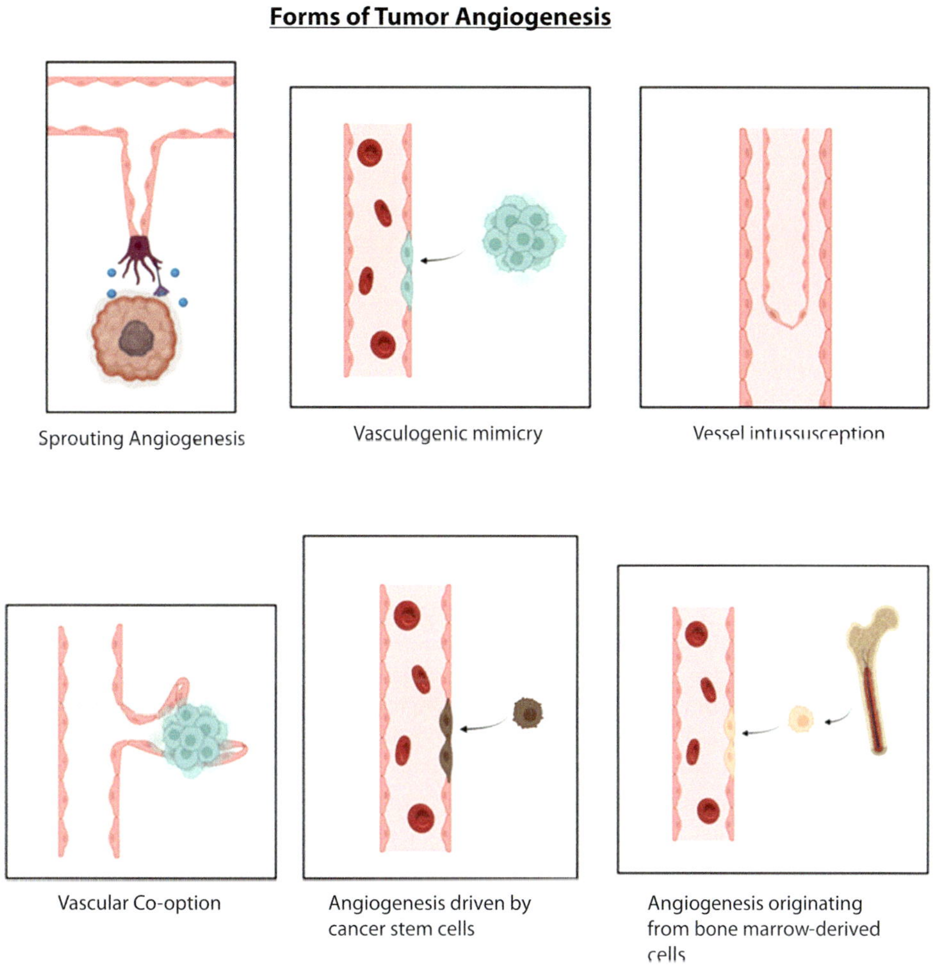

FIGURE 9.3 Different forms of tumor angiogenesis.

ANTI-ANGIOGENIC THERAPY

Pro-angiogenic factors or the receptors expressed by ECs, such as VEGF, VEGFR1, VEGFR2, and VEGFR3, as well as ANG 1 and 2, Tie2, FGF2, FGFR, c-Met, and HGF, are targeted in most anti-angiogenic therapies (Bridges and Harris, 2011). Food and Drug Administration (FDA) approved initial anti-angiogenic therapy, Avastin (bevacizumab), in 2003. This treatment works by blocking VEGFA, the primary factor driving angiogenesis. Receptor tyrosine kinase (RTK)-based inhibitors used in anti-angiogenic therapy likely also impact tumor RTK signaling pathways, which control tumor cell proliferation, survival, metabolism, and HIF regulation (McIntyre and Harris, 2015).

Another class of inhibitors, known as vascular disrupting agents (VDAs) like Zybrestat (combretastatin A-4 phosphate; CA4P), function by selectively targeting immature, rapidly dividing ECs. This results in apoptosis or disruption of the endothelial cytoskeleton, leading to vascular collapse. CA4P has also been tested in combination with bevacizumab in both pre-clinical and clinical trials, though it has shown significant toxicity (Nathan et al., 2012).

Clinically, MRI has identified three primary vascular responses to anti-angiogenic therapy: decreased perfusion, no change in perfusion, and increased perfusion, the latter also known as

TABLE 9.2
A List of All FDA-Approved Anti-Angiogenic Therapies (2014)

Compound	Target
Bevacizumab (Avastin)	Anti-VEGF antibody
Aflibercept (Eylea)	VEGF-trap recombinant fusion protein of VEGF-binding domains from VEGFR
Ramucirumab (Cyramza)	Human monoclonal VEGFR2 antibody inhibits VEGF binding
Axitinib (Inlyta)	VEGFR1-3, PDGFR-β, and c-KIT
Cabozantinib (Cometriq)	VEGFR1-3, MET
Everolimus (Afinitor)	mTOR
Pazopanib (Votrient)	VEGFR1-3, PDGFR, c-KIT
Regorafenib (Stivarga)	VEGFR1-3, PDGFR-β, Tie2
Sorafenib (Nexavar)	VEGFR1-3, PDGFR, RAF
Sunitinib (Sutent)	VEGFR1-3, PDGFR, c-KIT, FLT3, RET, CSF-1R
Vandetanib (Caprelsa)	VEGFR1-3, EGFR, RET

vascular normalization (Mehta et al., 2011). Numerous mechanisms have been identified to explain the lack of improvement in overall patient survival with anti-angiogenic therapy, as tumors can still maintain vascularization despite treatment. Two primary types of resistance to anti-angiogenic therapy have been proposed: intrinsic and adaptive resistance. Intrinsic resistance arises from inherent molecular characteristics of the tumor and its blood vessels. Possible causes include differential expression of pro- and anti-angiogenic VEGF isoforms, VEGF and VEGFR polymorphisms, limited antibody penetration into the tumor mass, and a pre-existing tumor microenvironment (TME) that reduces treatment efficacy. Tumors that rely on vessel co-option, have well-differentiated vessels, or use VEGF-independent pathways are also likely to be resistant. Additionally, Notch signaling may reduce VEGF signaling, contributing to resistance (Bergers and Hanahan, 2008).

Adaptive resistance develops in response to the therapy's effects on the tumor and its vascular structure. Causes may include tumor metabolic reprogramming and expression changes induced by HIF due to hypoxia, increased invasion or vessel co-option driven by hypoxia, and upregulation of alternative pro-angiogenic factors from the tumor or hypoxia-recruited stromal cells like TAM. Enhanced recruitment of protective pericyte coverage may also occur (Bergers and Hanahan, 2008) (Table 9.2).

CONCLUSION

In conclusion, hypoxia plays a crucial role in driving angiogenesis within tumors, significantly impacting tumor progression and metastasis. By promoting the accumulation of HIFs and the activation of angiogenic genes like VEGF, hypoxia facilitates the formation of a dysfunctional vascular network that supports tumor growth. The TME, through components such as cancer-associated fibroblasts (CAFs) and TAMs, further promotes angiogenesis, while also creating an immunosuppressive environment that contributes to tumor progression. Despite the promise of anti-angiogenic therapies like VEGF inhibitors, tumors often develop resistance by maintaining hypoxic conditions and abnormal vasculature. Therefore, targeting hypoxia-driven angiogenesis through novel strategies such as HIF inhibition, blood vessel normalization, and combination therapies may offer more effective treatments. Understanding the intricate mechanisms of tumor angiogenesis opens the door to potential therapeutic advancements, providing hope for improved precision oncology strategies in cancer treatment.

REFERENCES

Apte RS, Chen DS, Ferrara N. VEGF in signaling and disease: Beyond discovery and development. Cell. 2019;176(6):1248–1264. doi: 10.1016/j.cell.2019.01.021.

Bergers G, Hanahan D. Modes of resistance to anti-angiogenic therapy. Nat Rev Cancer. 2008;8(8):592–603. doi: 10.1038/nrc2442.

Bridges EM, Harris AL. The angiogenic process as a therapeutic target in cancer. Biochem Pharmacol. 2011;81(10):1183–1191. doi: 10.1016/j.bcp.2011.02.016.

Carmeliet P, Jain RK. Molecular mechanisms and clinical applications of angiogenesis. Nature. 2011;473(7347):298–307. doi: 10.1038/nature10144.

Chen Z, Han F, Du Y, Shi H, Zhou W. Hypoxic microenvironment in cancer: Molecular mechanisms and therapeutic interventions. Signal Transduct Target Ther. 2023;8(1):70. doi: 10.1038/s41392-023-01332-8.

Folkman J. Tumor angiogenesis. Adv Cancer Res. 1974;19(0):331–358. doi: 10.1016/s0065-230x(08)60058-5.

Gerhardt H, Golding M, Fruttiger M, Ruhrberg C, Lundkvist A, Abramsson A, et al VEGF guides angiogenic sprouting utilizing endothelial tip cell filopodia. J Cell Biol. 2003;161:1163–1177. doi: 10.1083/jcb.200302047.

Ghabrial AS, Krasnow MA. Social interactions among epithelial cells during tracheal branching morphogenesis. Nature. 2006;441:746–749.

Gianni-Barrera R, Butschkau A, Uccelli A, Certelli A, Valente P, Bartolomeo M, et al. PDGF-BB regulates splitting angiogenesis in skeletal muscle by limiting VEGF-induced endothelial proliferation. Angiogenesis. 2018;21(4):883–900. doi: 10.1007/s10456-018-9634-5.

Grünewald FS, Prota AE, Giese A, Ballmer-Hofer K. Structure-function analysis of VEGF receptor activation and the role of coreceptors in angiogenic signaling. Biochim Biophys Acta. 2010;1804(3):567–580. doi: 10.1016/j.bbapap.2009.09.002.

Hillen F, Griffioen AW. Tumour vascularization: Sprouting angiogenesis and beyond. Cancer Metastasis Rev. 2007;26(3–4):489–502. doi: 10.1007/s10555-007-9094-7.

Kloepper J, Riedemann L, Amoozgar Z, Seano G, Susek K, Yu V, et al. Ang-2/VEGF bispecific antibody reprograms macrophages and resident microglia to antitumor phenotype and prolongs glioblastoma survival. Proc Natl Acad Sci U S A. 2016;113:4476–4481. doi: 10.1073/pnas.1525360113.

Krock BL, Skuli N, Simon MC. Hypoxia-induced angiogenesis: Good and evil. Genes Cancer. 2011;2(12):1117–1133.

La Mendola D, Trincavelli ML, Martini C. Angiogenesis in disease. Int J Mol Sci. 2022;23(18):10962. doi: 10.3390/ijms231810962.

Liao D, Johnson RS. Hypoxia: A key regulator of angiogenesis in cancer. Cancer Metastasis Rev. 2007;26: 281–290. doi: 10.1007/s10555-007-9066-y.

Liu ZJ, Shirakawa T, Li Y, Soma A, Oka M, Dotto GP, et al. Regulation of Notch1 and Dll4 by vascular endothelial growth factor in arterial endothelial cells: Implications for modulating arteriogenesis and angiogenesis. Mol Cell Biol. 2003;23(1):14–25. doi: 10.1128/MCB.23.1.14-25.2003.

Lugano R, Ramachandran M, Dimberg A. Tumor angiogenesis: Causes, consequences, challenges and opportunities. Cell Mol Life Sci. 2020;77(9), 1745–1770. doi: 10.1007/s00018-019-03351-7.

Mahon PC, Hirota K, Semenza GL. FIH-1: A novel protein that interacts with HIF-1alpha and VHL to mediate repression of HIF-1 transcriptional activity. Genes Dev. 2001 15;15(20):2675–2686. doi: 10.1101/gad.924501.

McIntyre A, Harris AL. Metabolic and hypoxic adaptation to anti-angiogenic therapy: A target for induced essentiality. EMBO Mol Med. 2015;7(4):368–379. doi: 10.15252/emmm.201404271.

Mehta S, Hughes NP, Buffa FM, Li SP, Adams RF, Adwani A, et al. Assessing early therapeutic response to bevacizumab in primary breast cancer using magnetic resonance imaging and gene expression profiles. J Natl Cancer Inst Monogr. 2011;2011(43):71–74. doi: 10.1093/jncimonographs/lgr027.

Nathan P, Zweifel M, Padhani AR, Koh DM, Ng M, Collins DJ, et al. Phase I trial of combretastatin A4 phosphate (CA4P) in combination with bevacizumab in patients with advanced cancer. Clin Cancer Res. 2012;18(12):3428–3439. doi: 10.1158/1078-0432.CCR-11-3376.

Nishida N, Yano H, Nishida T, Kamura T, Kojiro M. Angiogenesis in cancer. Vasc Health Risk Manag. 2006;2(3):213–219. doi: 10.2147/vhrm.2006.2.3.213.

Pellet-Many C, Frankel P, Jia H, Zachary I. Neuropilins: Structure, function and role in disease. Biochem J. 2008;411(2):211–226. doi: 10.1042/BJ20071639.

Phng L-K, Gerhardt H. Angiogenesis: A team effort coordinated by notch. Dev Cell. 2009;16:196–208. doi: 10.1016/j.devcel.2009.01.015.

Pugsley MK, Tabrizchi R. The vascular system. An overview of structure and function. J Pharmacol Toxicol Methods. 2000;44(2):333–340. doi: 10.1016/s1056-8719(00)00125-8.

Semenza GL. Hydroxylation of HIF-1: Oxygen sensing at the molecular level. Physiology (Bethesda). 2004;19:176–182. doi: 10.1152/physiol.00001.2004.

Semenza GL. Oxygen sensing, hypoxia-inducible factors, and disease pathophysiology. Annu Rev Pathol. 2014;9:47–71. doi: 10.1146/annurev-pathol-012513-104720.

Shaw RJ, Cantley LC. Ras, PI(3)K and mTOR signalling controls tumour cell growth. Nature. 2006;441(7092):424–430. doi: 10.1038/nature04869.

Siemann DW. The unique characteristics of tumor vasculature and preclinical evidence for its selective disruption by tumor-vascular disrupting agents. Cancer Treat Rev. 2011;37(1), 63–74. doi: 10.1016/j.ctrv.2010.05.001.

Tzeng H-T, Huang Y-J. Tumor vasculature as an emerging pharmacological target to promote anti-tumor immunity. Int J Mol Sci. 2023;24(5):4422. doi: 10.3390/ijms24054422.

Viallard C, Larrivée B. Tumor angiogenesis and vascular normalization: Alternative therapeutic targets. Angiogenesis. 2017;20(4):409–426. doi: 10.1007/s10456-017-9562-9.

Zhang R, Yao Y, Gao H, Hu X. Mechanisms of angiogenesis in tumour. Front Oncol. 2024;14:1359069. doi: 10.3389/fonc.2024.1359069.

Ziyad S, Iruela-Arispe ML. Molecular mechanisms of tumor angiogenesis. Genes Cancer. 2011;2(12): 1085–1096.

10 Therapeutic Approaches Targeting Hypoxic Tumor Vasculature

Suman Kumar Ray and Sukhes Mukherjee
Department of Biochemistry, All India Institute of Medical Sciences, Bhopal, Madhya Pradesh, India

INTRODUCTION

Angiogenesis refers to the intricate and controlled process by which new blood vessels develop from old ones in various parts of the body. It is common practice to maintain a steady state by balancing growth factors and inhibitors. Some examples of normal adult processes that need angiogenesis include: the development of the endometrium during menstruation, the formation of the mammary gland in preparation for nursing, and the construction of the placenta during pregnancy (1, 2).

Angiogenesis is a process that occurs in all of these contexts and involves a series of events such as vascular stabilization, nascent tube formation, migration and proliferation of the endothelial cells (ECs) that make up the new sprout, degradation of the capillary basement membrane, and removal of structural pericytes in the area of the developing sprout (3).

The release of growth factors occurs in response to angiogenic stimuli, including inflammation, mechanical stress, or hypoxia. Cellular effectors are activated by these signaling events, and their ultimate goal is to shape the developing vasculature (3). The process begins with the removal of pericytes, which are smooth muscle cells situated at regular intervals along the capillary wall, from the sprouting area of a mother artery in response to effector activation.

ECs are able to be selected for a specific function—a process known as tip cell selection—through complex calcium oscillations triggered by vascular endothelial growth factors (VEGFs) activation (4). Following angiogenic signals released by the target tissue that needs more blood flow, the tip cell directs the growing sprout through chemotaxis (4). Disorganized vasculature may result from an imbalance in growth factor signaling, since even little changes in this system have a significant impact on tip cells. Matrix metalloproteases (MMPs) released by the tip cell break down components of the basement membrane that they cross (5).

In order to lengthen the developing sprout, a second type of specialized ECs known as stalk cells communicate with tip cells via delta-notch signaling; these cells are extremely proliferative (6). Junctional adhesion proteins are placed at the contact location of two tip cells at an anastomosis between other nascent or stable vessels. A functioning vascular network is generated when a lumen is formed through the invagination of cell membranes or the hollowing out of cords (7). The newly formed vessels are branched in an unorganized fashion (Figure 10.1) and receive support from circulating endothelial progenitor cells. Poorly perfused branches are either removed (pruning) or the ECs that make them up are recycled to places with high blood flow because of local pressure and flow variations (8, 9). Basement membrane deposition, decreased EC activity, tightened cell junctions, and recruitment of pericytes maintain highly perfused sprouts, on the other hand (9).

DOI: 10.1201/9781003477419-10

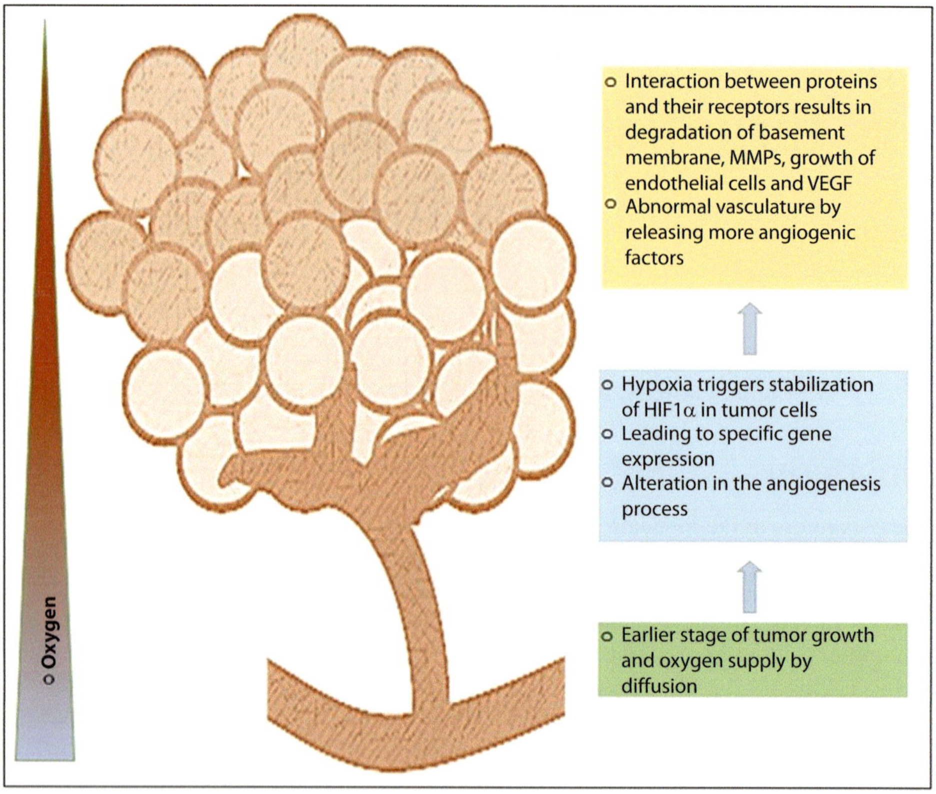

FIGURE 10.1 A fundamental form of angiogenesis is produced when hypoxia brought on by an expanding tumor mass sets off an angiogenic switch in the tumor microenvironment (10).

In the early 1980s, Juliana Denekamp articulated the principles underlying vascular targeting agents (VTAs) as cancer treatments (10). The idea for VTAs that pharmacologically block tumor vasculature originated from the finding that physical blockage of solid tumor blood channels caused tumor regressions in mice (10). The idea was later confirmed when it was demonstrated that anti-tubulin medications have intrinsic VTA activity and that a toxin targeted by an antibody specific for tumor blood vessels caused tumor regressions in mice (11). It is believed that the high interstitial pressure in tumor interiors contributes to vascular collapse, which is why VTAs work best against these arteries. The fast-dividing tumor cells in the tumor's well-oxygenated periphery, on the other hand, are the primary targets of many direct-acting anticancer treatments. Particularly potent against tumor cells are angiogenesis inhibitors in the tumor periphery, the site of the most intense angiogenesis (12, 13).

Synergistic or additive effects have been observed in experimental solid tumors when VTAs are used with antiproliferative anticancer treatments or angiogenesis inhibitors (14, 15).

Small molecular weight VTAs and ligand-directed VTAs are the two main categories into which VTAs fall (14, 16). Although small molecule VTAs are unable to localize to tumor arteries with any degree of selectivity, they are able to selectively occlude tumor vasculature by capitalizing on pathophysiological distinctions between tumor and normal tissue endothelium. Increased proliferation, permeability, and dependence on a tubulin cytoskeleton to sustain cell shape are some of the ways in which tumor ECs differ from normal tissue ECs (17, 18). Alternatively, tumor vasculature can be selectively bound and occluded by ligand-based VTAs, which employ a targeted ligand.

TUMOR CONTROL OF ANGIOGENESIS

Rather than just a collection of defective cells, tumors might be seen as functioning organs. In an uneven pattern that the tumor has altered to suit its life requirements, the tumor stroma contains cells originating from mesenchymal tissue, cells that cause inflammation, and cells that provide blood flow (19, 20). Thus, tumors can induce angiogenesis by hijacking the same pathway that promotes blood vessel growth. Small solid tumors that lack vasculature can get the nutrients and oxygen they need through passive diffusion from surrounding blood vessels (21). The tumor core becomes hypoxic, and the process of angiogenesis begins to feed oxygen and nutritional demands (22, 23). When oxygen supply drops too low, tumor cells undergo what is known as "the angiogenic switch" and secrete a plethora of angiogenic factors (24, 25). Hypoxia-inducible factors (HIFs) are DNA-binding transcription factors that mainly control cellular reactions to low oxygen levels. A constitutively produced HIF-1ß subunit and an oxygen-regulating subunit (HIF-1 or HIF-2) make up heterodimers, which are known as HIFs (26). These alpha subunits include an oxygen-dependent degradation domain (ODDD), PAS-A and PAS-B domains for protein-protein dimerization, a DNA-binding amino terminal basic helix-loop-helix (bHLH) that is essential for hypoxia response element (HRE) activation, and transactivation domains (N-TAD and C-TAD) that are critical for heat shock factor (HSF) target gene activation (27, 28).

An acetyl transferase enzyme known as arrest-defective-1 (ARD-1) can acetylate a secondary lysine residue inside the ODDD, which promotes HIF-1 degradation, demonstrating redundancy in HIF-1 stability (27). Because hypoxia reduces ARD-1 expression, HIF-1 is stabilized in this environment (27).

Using oxygen as a substrate and iron as a cofactor, the prolyl hydroxylase domain (PHD) hydroxylates two proline residues inside the ODDD under normoxic circumstances (27). In order to create a complex with E3 ubiquitin ligase activity, hydroxylated HIF-1 associates with pVHL, elongins B and C, cullin-2 (cul-2), and rbx1 cofactors (HIF-1-VBC complex) (29). Nevertheless, HIF-1 is stabilized in hypoxic environments by means of limited PHD activity. A buildup of non-hydroxylated HIF-1 can be facilitated by this. In addition, pVHL-interacting deubiquitinating enzyme (VDU2) destabilizes ubiquitin ligases on HIF-1, and ubiquitin ligases, which are PHD enzymes in and of themselves, regulate HIF-1 stability (30). Considering that HIF-1 has a very short half-life (less than 1 minute in a perfused lung), it undergoes continuous degradation in normal cells at physiological oxygen levels and is tightly controlled when oxygen levels decrease (31). Untreated tumors often have median oxygen levels below 2%, while the range for treated tumors is around 0.3%–4.2% (32). At this low oxygen level, HIF-1 is released and stabilized, and cancer-causing processes are induced, which further disrupt the HIF pathway and reduce the oxygen dependence of tumors (32). Evidence suggests that tumor-induced changes in the pVHL binding pocket can destabilize the E3 ubiquitin ligase (VEC) complex by interfering with HIF-1 interactions (33, 34). To be more specific, TP53 mutations increase the expression of hypoxia-response genes in lung cancer by gaining function from HIF-1 (35). While mutations or knockouts of TP53 prevent HIF-1 from interacting with the tumor suppressor, HIF-1 can bind directly to Mdm2, facilitating its ubiquitination and proteosomal destruction (36). Multiple investigations have demonstrated that inhibition of the phosphoinositide 3-kinase (PI3K) pathway abolishes HIF expression independent of oxygen levels (37). Likewise, protein kinase B (serine/threonine kinase) (AKT) upregulates HIF-1 in human gastric, breast, and non-small-cell lung cancers (38).

FACTORS CONTRIBUTING TO TUMOR VASCULAR DYSFUNCTION

Multiple substances, including the most important angiogenic ligand, VEGFs, and its receptors, such as vascular endothelial growth factor receptor (VEGFR2), are activated by tumors to start the angiogenic process (39). Proteins such as VEGF-A, VEGF-B, VEGF-C, VEGF-D, VEGF-E, and placenta growth factor (PIGF) are all members of the VEGF family (40, 41). While VEGF-A is more popularly known as VEGF because of its main involvement in angiogenesis, VEGF-C and VEGF-D are explored as regulators of lymphangiogenesis. Multiple isoforms of VEGF that differ in heparin binding affinity, extracellular matrix location, and diffusive potential result from alternative splicing. In order to avoid abnormal angiogenesis, it is crucial to strictly manage the levels of VEGF, which is transcriptionally regulated in response to HIF (41). Tumor cells respond to hypoxia by secreting increased amounts of VEGF into the extracellular space, a process facilitated by their control over HIF (42). Irregular branching and convoluted vascular networks are contributed to by an overabundance of tip cells selected for by high concentrations of VEGF surrounding ECs. Because of chemical breakdown by tumor-derived proteases, the basement membrane of tumor arteries is often weak or nonexistent (43), despite its physical role as a barrier for cancer cell spread to neighboring tissues. Disorganization in the EC monolayer, as well as karyotypic abnormalities, chromosomal instability, and aberrant gene expression profiles, are common (44).

The ECs lining tumors are more receptive to VEGF activation because they express higher VEGFR-1 and VEGFR-2 (45, 46). Angiogenesis and stemness markers, including CD61, CD105, Sca-1, CD34, CD90, and ALDH, are highly expressed by tumor ECs, according to recent research (47). Tumor ECs have an increased angiogenic capacity compared to normal ECs, which helps to explain the abnormal vascular arrangement observed in tumors (48). In the tumor microenvironment (TME), extracellular factors like VEGF, PMA, TGF-ß, and cytochalasin B are overexpressed. Downregulation of connexin expression results from abnormal VEGF signaling in tumor ECs, which in turn causes gap junction dysfunction, increased vascular fenestrations, and increased vascular permeability (49). The fact that VEGF can enhance vascular permeability and the extravasation of plasma proteins like fibrinogen led to its original identification (50).

When ECs release PDGF-ß, they attract specialized smooth muscle cells called pericytes to develop and establish blood arteries. The significance of pericytes for normal vascular function is demonstrated by the fact that mice defective in PDGF-ß signaling do not have any and die from micro hemorrhaging (51). By increasing the production of the antiapoptotic protein BCL-w, signals released by pericytes ensure the survival of ECs (52). Thus, pericytes also protect normal arteries from antiangiogenic treatments, enabling these drugs to target tumors specifically. In order for the nascent vascular sprout to emerge, pericytes are detached from ECs by hypoxia and downstream angiogenic substances secreted by tumor cells. This results in an immature vascular phenotype and the maintenance of angiogenesis in tumor-associated arteries, which are either completely pericyte-free or have poor linkages between pericytes and ECs (53).

ABNORMAL VASCULATURE RESULTS IN LIMITED TREATMENT DELIVERY

A physical obstacle to the administration of therapy to tumors is the poor tissue perfusion caused by the anomalies of the tumor vasculature. The greatest obstacle to therapeutic access to the tumor, among the many delivery and uptake barriers, is high interstitial fluid pressure (IFP) (54). Excessive vascular permeability and mechanical compression of lymphatic blood vessels are two of the many factors that contribute to the development of elevated IFP levels (55). The loss of integrity at the EC junction and an active endothelium are linked to disrupted vascular shape and reduced pericyte coverage. This leads to leaky arteries that extravasate fluid into the tumor environment, which in turn increases the pressure within the tumor (56). Intratumoral pressure (ITP) rises dramatically when coupled with solid stress, a condition in which tumors accumulate cancer cells, stromal cells, cancer-associated fibroblasts (CAFs), and the extracellular matrix that surrounds them, resulting in substantial mechanical pressure inside the tumor (57).

Compared to systemic administration, intratumoral treatment delivery has not improved survival rates and does not take metastatic disease into consideration, but it does reduce off-target toxicity (58). Some tumor subtypes, like ovarian and pancreatic tumors, are unreachable through transdermal injection, making the clinical use of intratumoral medicines difficult. Systemic medications have a formidable therapeutic hurdle when trying to reach the tumor vasculature from the injection site; furthermore, they encounter numerous obstacles on their way and must disseminate throughout the tumor for their effects to be felt (59).

An oxygen gradient forms inside a tumor when its size exceeds its vascular supply, which is caused by factors such as an uneven oxygen supply and demand, as well as a heterogeneous blood supply. Rapidly dividing cells in the periphery use all the oxygen that is available from the blood vessels, cutting off oxygen from reaching the center. There has been a lot of review on the topic of how this uneven oxygen distribution and resultant hypoxic areas promote treatment resistance, fuel metastasis, and an aggressive phenotype (60).

In tumor cells, hypoxia can change metabolic pathways, which can decrease ATP synthesis through oxygen-dependent mitochondrial oxidative phosphorylation. This causes tumor cells to undergo the Warburg Effect, which is a metabolic rewiring from oxidative phosphorylation to aerobic glycolysis. In order to help them grow at a quicker pace than normal cells, tumor cells develop an addiction to glucose intake and are able to create ATP at a considerably faster rate through glycolysis.

An excess of lactate builds up as a result of the tumor cells' massive glucose consumption for survival and proliferation. Normoxic tumor cells, found closest to the vasculature, can feed their metabolic processes with either glucose or lactate, but hypoxic tumor cells prefer glucose consumption. The hypoxic tumor cells generate lactate waste, which is recycled and utilized by the normoxic tumor cells. This metabolic symbiosis fuels the tumor cells and their surroundings (61). It is interesting to note that these normoxic cells prefer lactate over glucose.

Since glutamine is essential for the fast proliferation of tumor cells, its production by oxidative tumor cells in response to low glucose levels triggers glutaminolysis, another metabolic pathway that tumor cells depend substantially on for energy (62). Since nicotinamide adenine dinucleotide phosphate (reduced form) (NADPH) and other biosynthetic precursors are in high demand in cancer cells, glutaminolysis provides an ideal means of restoring ATP levels and keeping the tricarboxylic acid (TCA) cycle running smoothly. The metabolic synergy in the TME is further enhanced by the generation of lactate in addition to ATP (63).

Tumor aerobic glycolysis and glutaminolysis produce extracellular lactate buildup, which creates an acidic TME and influences the possibility of more aggressive and invasive tumor cells. Research has demonstrated that gene expression, G1 cell cycle arrest, and necrotic cell death can be influenced by extracellular acidic environments (64). The acidity can make tumor cells more aggressive, mostly by influencing their ability to invade and spread to other areas (65). Keeping the pH low allows tumor cells to avoid detection and killing by immune cells, just like in hypoxic settings (66). Aggressive tumor characteristics and chemoresistance are both known to be exacerbated by a TME with a low pH (67).

TUMOR-ASSOCIATED BLOOD VASCULATURE FAVORS AN IMMUNORESISTANT TUMOR MICROENVIRONMENT

To meet their high energy demands and continue growing, solid tumors that have expanded beyond a few cubic millimeters in volume must initiate tumor angiogenesis in order to obtain nutrients like glucose and oxygen (23, 68). Tumor angiogenesis differs from vasculogenesis and vasculogenic mimicry in that it involves the development of new blood vessels from preexisting vascular beds, rather than the creation of vessels from the ground up using endothelial precursor cells derived from bone marrow (68).

The process of forming a new vascular sprout is complex and well-coordinated. It begins with the highly invasive and motile tip cells at the leading edge, which migrate toward proangiogenic cues and are guided by the VEGFR-2 axis. Then, the proliferating stalk cells underlying the tip cells elongate the sprout and generate the lumen. The recruitment of pericytes and vascular smooth muscle cells into a fully developed artery improves its stability, integrity, and blood perfusion (69).

In the TME, an imbalance between pro- and antiangiogenic signals is the primary driver of pathological angiogenesis. The list of important factors that promote angiogenesis is vast and includes VEGF-A, bFGF, and interleukin (IL). When these cytokines accumulate at toxic levels in the TME, they suppress angiostatin and endostatin, two angiostatic signals, and trigger a proangiogenic switch (70). Not only do cancer cells secrete a lot of VEGF and can help with angiogenesis that doesn't involve VEGF, but they can also react autocrinally or paracrinally to VEGF signaling that promotes survival or metastasis. Despite its intended purpose, tumor angiogenesis produces a network of vessels that are poorly perfused, thin-walled, immature, leaky, and disorderly. Cancer cells are able to evade anticancer immunosurveillance, spread, and react to immunotherapy in large part because of this extremely abnormal and inefficient angiogenesis, which also helps to sustain the protumorigenic and immunosuppressive TME (71).

The presence of structurally immature, unstable, leaky, and tortuous arteries is linked to a chaotic vascular network, which in turn causes blunt-ended vessels and erratic blood flow (72). Nutrient transport is hindered by diffusion limits when perfusion is not well covered, since cells are located too far from a functioning vessel. In addition, the tumor's high IFP is a consequence of the leakiness of the tumor's arteries, which makes these veins vulnerable to collapse and reduces the area of the tumor that is perfused. Importantly, acidosis and hypoxia (73) promote the development of immune cells that suppress the immune system, decrease the cytotoxic activity of effector T cells that infiltrate tumors, and impede the delivery of chemotherapeutics and immunotherapeutic entities, as well as the killing of cancer cells in response to radiotherapy, chemotherapy, and immunotherapy.

ANTIANGIOGENIC TREATMENT, VESSEL NORMALIZATION AND IMMUNOTHERAPY

Research into immunotherapy has mostly relied on combinatorial approaches that target the VEGF/VEGFR axis (74). It was once believed that monotherapy with antiangiogenic medicines, like the anti-VEGF antibody bevacizumab, would starve the tumor, stopping tumor progression and improving patient survival. This was due to the fact that the drug blocked the VEGF/VEGFR-dependent survival and growth of the blood vasculature. This vessel-targeting treatment, known as vascular blocking, did not produce the anticipated effects in cancer patients and did not demonstrate significant improvements in response rates or survival benefits (75), despite encouraging early preclinical findings. In subsequent preclinical investigations, it was demonstrated that vascular pruning causes an increase in hypoxic tumor areas (76), as opposed to ischemic ones, which fosters tumor development and metastasis. In fact, different immunosuppressive immune-cell populations, such as Grl+CD11b+ and tumor-associated macrophages (TAMs) (77), may be involved in the angiogenic relapse and treatment resistance seen after vascular blockage tactics, which may be caused, in part, by hypoxia caused by anti-VEGF/VEGFR therapy. The angiostatic chemokine CXCL14, which originates in cancer cells, recruited these myeloid cells and activated PI3K signaling, according to a recent study (78). Similarly, antiangiogenic treatment's long-term benefits necessitated blocking this pathway.

Avastin, a recombinant humanized antibody that binds VEGF isoforms, causes a temporary remodeling of the tumor vasculature in experimental mouse models (79). This remodeling includes an increase in the number of mature (i.e., pericyte-covered) vessels, a decrease in permeability, a reduction in IFP, and an increase in perfusion in neuroblastoma xenografts. There was only a temporary improvement in the intratumoral penetration of topotecan and etoposide in the first few days following Bevacizumab treatment, suggesting that this vascular "normalizing" effect was temporary. When administered to glioma xenografts, DC-101 (a monoclonal antibody specific to mouse VEGFR-2) improved vascular normalization, which coincides with a window of opportunity for the synergistic effect of radiation therapy, an inducer of immunogenic cell death (ICD) (76), according to another study.

Therefore, these results point to a potential opening for a synergistic effect between immunotherapy (80) and tumor vessel normalizing therapies.

Additionally, they imply that a better treatment result may be achieved by "normalizing" or "healing" the abnormal tumor vasculature instead of eliminating it. This would involve restoring the normal anatomical and functional features of the arteries. Consistent with this, "vessel normalization" enhances tumor perfusion and drug delivery by increasing the transport capacity of vessels, which in turn improves therapy responses, which are highly dependent on an adequate blood supply to the tumor (81). On top of that, immunotherapy may work better as a result of better tumor oxygenation. Hypoxia and inadequate intratumoral infiltration of T cells, brought on by inadequate blood flow to the abnormal tumor arteries, reduce the effectiveness of immunotherapy based on immune checkpoint inhibitor (ICIs), as previously stated (82).

In contrast, hyperoxygenation is associated with enhanced cytotoxic T lymphocyte (CTL) activation and better clinical responses to ICIs (83).

There was an increase in the infiltration of adoptively transferred T cells into B16-F10 melanoma and an improvement in the delay of tumor growth in the setting of immunotherapy when DC-101 was used. And while modest doses (10–20 mg/kg) of DC-101 were associated with reduced tumor hypoxia and normalization of tumor vessels, high doses (40 mg/kg) had no such effect (84). In addition, significant alterations occurred in the TME, including a transition to tumor-suppressing Th1-mediated immune responses, an increase in tumor infiltration of CD4+ and CD8+ T cells, and polarization of TAM to an M1-like phenotype. As a result of these alterations in the TME, vaccine-based immunotherapy (84) was also able to work better. Bevacizumab may also impair the phagocytic activity of DCs and macrophages (82), whereas temporary targeting of the VEGF/VEGFR axis may restore DC maturation defects (81) and lower VEGF-A-induced PD-1, TIM3, and CTLA-4 expression on CD8+ T cells (85).

Activation of the Notch-signaling pathway in blood ECs (4/85), leading to a more quiescent EC phenotype (86), was discovered to induce in vivo vascular normalization by the antimalarial drug and first-generation autophagy inhibitor chloroquine (CQ). Inserting melanoma cells into mice deficient in Notch1 in ECs rendered CQ's tumor vasculature-normalizing and antimetastatic actions utterly ineffective. To reduce tumor hypoxia and promote the formation of a more EC solid barrier, which inhibited the intravasation and spread of cancer cells, CQ normalized the aberrant tumor vasculature. Curiously, a recent preclinical investigation demonstrated that CQ can complement immunotherapy and does not hinder anticancer immunity in vivo, despite its minor immunosuppressant effects (87). Reprogramming the glycolytic nature of the ECs is another potential therapeutic approach. Glycolysis is the primary pathway for ECs to produce ATP, according to recent studies.

Additionally, vascular dysfunction is contributed to by this glycolytic phenotype, which is worsened in the TME by the elevated VEGF signaling (88).

There was a correlation between a tightened vascular barrier (fewer metastases) and higher perfusion (better chemotherapy efficacy) (89), as demonstrated in a recent study that normalized blood vessels after blocking the major glycolytic activator 6-phosphofructo-2-kinase/fructose-2,6-bisphosphatase-3.

Therefore, additional experimental and clinical validation is needed to confirm that pharmacological inhibitors that target EC glycolytic metabolism could reverse tumor-induced changes in ECs, resulting in a vascular normalization phenotype (90).

Hypoxia can trigger proangiogenic microRNAs (miR-210 and miR-494) (91) or, conversely, specific miRNAs can influence angiogenesis by influencing the VEGF/VEGFR pathway (miR-16, for instance, which also disrupts TGF-β signaling) (92).

Vesicles containing miR-494 released by cancer cells have the interesting property of promoting angiogenesis in ECs (93). Antiangiogenic and vessel-normalizing strategies may target miRNAs because tumor-associated circumstances might enhance their expression (either cell-autonomously or by cross-communication), therefore supporting the highly angiogenic TME. Still, more study is needed in this developing area before we can know for sure how (targeted) miRNAs may improve the effectiveness of immunotherapy.

Possible additional targets to consider beyond VEGF-A include other proteins involved in immunosuppression and angiogenesis. In addition to generating immunosuppressive events (tryptophan depletion), indoleamine 2,3-dioxygenase (IDO) can stimulate angiogenic events (94). Intriguingly, preclinical models show that IDO inhibition and ICI methods work together in the context of immunotherapy; this may be due to IDO-mediated effects on tumor vasculature (95). In addition, hypoxia and starvation trigger the production of galectin-3, which in turn suppresses CD8+ T-cell effector function and enhances VEGF and bFGF-induced angiogenesis in ECs (68). Thus, future research and validation in preclinical models are required to explore the possibility that targeting these cross-talks and signaling axes could influence a TME in a way that promotes antitumor immunity.

Curiously, while normalizing blood vessels can lead to better lymphocyte infiltration and a less therapy-resistant TME, CD4+ T-cell infiltration can also cause normalization of blood vessels. A recent and well-executed investigation found that while CD4 depletion decreased vascular pericyte coverage, adoptive CD4+ T-cell transfer enhanced perfusion and decreased hypoxia and leakiness (68, 96).

Taken as a whole, these findings point to a virtuous cycle wherein improving the vasculature's integrity leads to a lymphocyte-admissible TME through vascular normalization. Using a B16-F10-OVA model, researchers found that protecting against the antitumor immune response induced by OVA vaccination was possible through VEGF-C overexpression. The effectiveness of a vaccination strategy was diminished in a transgenic model that removed dermal lymphatic capillaries (perhaps because of reduced immunosuppressive TME), whereas an adoptive cell transfer (ACT) strategy (OT-1 cells activated with OVA-peptide-loaded DCs) was more effective (68). The aforementioned findings provide strong evidence that immunotherapies can be more effective when they target angiogenesis, namely, through vessel-normalizing techniques.

HYPOXIA AND DRUG RESISTANCE

The presence of oxygen is crucial for the antitumor effects of several cancer treatment techniques. The production of reactive oxygen species is the fundamental process in radiotherapy (97). These species damage the DNA of tumor cells, leading to cell death. Once oxygen combines with the free radical's electron, the reaction becomes permanent. A long time ago, Gray and his colleagues (1953) showed in a ground-breaking study that cancers become more radiation sensitive when oxygen is present. Radiation doses needed to kill hypoxic tumor cells are three times higher than those needed to kill normoxic tumor cells (98). Because normal tissues have a limited radiation tolerance, it is not possible to safely raise the radiation dose to compensate for this disparity, which is problematic for the outcome of the treatment. Radiation treatment is more likely to be effective against normoxic malignancies. Hypoxic tumors are characterized by a lack of oxygen, which makes photodynamic treatment (PDT) ineffective (99).

An increase in HIF synthesis, which in turn increases the expression of membrane efflux pumps, is a well-documented response to hypoxia and its function in chemoresistance. The ABC family of transporters, which decreases intracellular accumulation of chemotherapy to sub-therapeutic levels, is the most prevalent efflux pump associated with multidrug resistance (100). Despite their continual expression, HIFs are stabilized under hypoxia and destroyed in normal oxygen tension. Hypoxia activated HIF-1, leading to upregulation of multidrug resistance 1 (MDR1; P-glycoprotein) in colon cancer cells (101). One of the main reasons why chemotherapy doesn't work is because of MDR1, an ATP-dependent efflux pump that may get chemotherapy medications out of the cell (102). In triple-negative breast tumors, HIF-1 upregulation of MDR1 is linked to chemoresistance, an enriched stem cell population, and an aggressive phenotype. Research has demonstrated that inhibiting HIF-1 in colon cancer cells helps alleviate multidrug resistance by reducing P-glycoprotein levels (103).

When hypoxia is present, HIF-1 enhances the activity of transcription factors Snail and Twist, which are involved in promoting epithelial-to-mesenchymal transition (EMT) and are linked to chemotherapy resistance (104). Since chemotherapy only kills cells with a high proliferation rate, this becomes an issue since it favors the aggressive hypoxic cells. Chemotherapy, according to Saggar and his colleagues (2015) repopulates hypoxic cells that cause treatment failure, perhaps because nutrients are more easily available after quickly growing cells are cleared out (105). One possible explanation for hyperbaric oxygen therapy's (HBOT) positive effects on chemotherapy outcomes is the correlation between normoxia and treatment success (106). Reducing the therapeutic dose and reducing side effects, HBOT increases chemotherapy-induced oxidative stress with its extra oxygen molecules (106).

THERAPEUTIC USE OF VASCULAR-TARGETING AGENTS

Research into determining tumor oxygenation status as a predictor of therapeutic efficacy has been motivated by the poor prognosis of treatment regimens in hypoxic malignancies (107).

The therapeutic potential of hypoxia has been explored through a number of approaches (108, 109). One example is the production of harmful species by the enzymatic reduction of hypoxia-activated prodrugs (HAPs) in environments with low oxygen levels (110). Some methods aim to restore oxygen levels in tumors, such as HBOT, which increases the plasma's oxygen-carrying capacity (111). Combination treatments, including compounds that increase the rate of oxygen diffusion from red blood cells (RBCs) to the vascular wall and modified molecules that transport oxygen, have also shown promise in preclinical trials (97). The tumor vasculature, which is the origin of tumor hypoxia, is the target of subsequent efforts. Finding that VEGF monoclonal antibodies (mAbs) inhibited tumor growth in 1993, Kim and his colleagues established mouse tumor models of rhabdomyosarcoma, glioblastoma, and leiomyosarcoma (112). By modifying tumor vasculature, this groundbreaking study showed that stopping the actions of an angiogenic mediator directly affects tumor growth, even though the antibodies had no effect on these cells in vitro (Figures 10.2 and 10.3).

The original goal of researching antiangiogenic medications was to starve the tumor by causing the tumor's arteries to burst. This well-reviewed approach does not result in long-term tumor suppression, despite the fact that vascular disruption produces immediate antitumor effects (112, 113). Clinical approval has been granted for multiple antiangiogenic medicines; nonetheless, the overall survival effect has been minimal, most likely because cancer cells adapt aggressively to environments with lower oxygen levels (114). Changes in p53 and e-cadherin are part of the gene profile that hypoxic cells create, which helps them survive oxidative stress and fuels metastasis (115).

The cells showed "hypoxic memory" and kept their aggressive phenotype even after they were re-oxygenated (115). In addition to causing tumor perfusion impairment and additional vascular

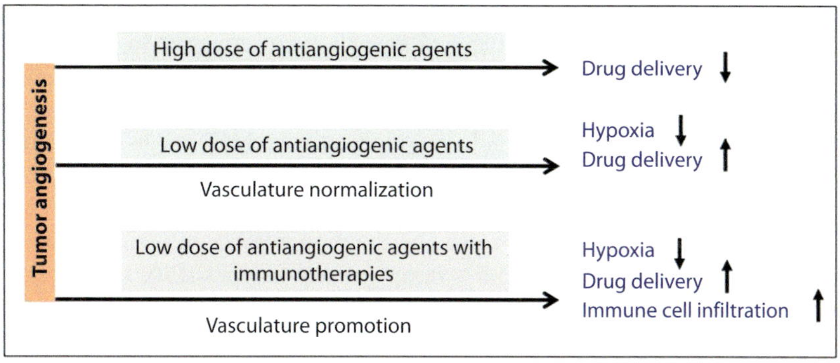

FIGURE 10.2 Therapeutic approaches targeting hypoxic tumor vasculature through antiangiogenic agents.

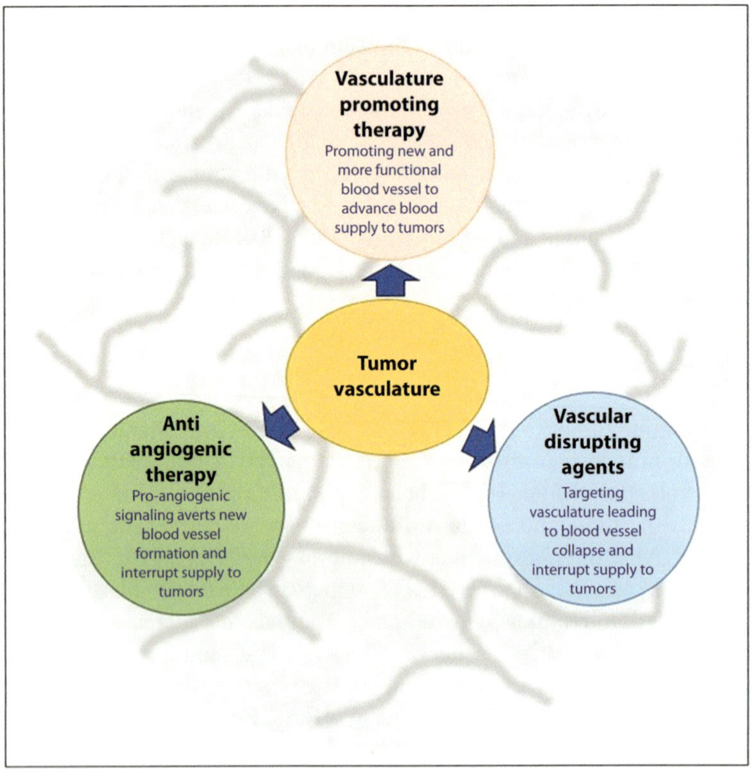

FIGURE 10.3 Tumor growth depends on nutrient and oxygen supply, and tumor vasculature is aberrant due to a high concentration of proangiogenic chemicals. Various techniques have been used to prevent tumor development and progression, like (a) antiangiogenic therapy, (b) vascular disrupting drugs target, and (c) vascular boosting therapy.

damage, high-dose antiangiogenic treatments have the unintended consequence of reducing oxygen levels and decreasing chemotherapeutic delivery to tumors.

Clinical success has been achieved with these medicines when tested at modest dosages as adjuvants to chemotherapy, as shown in Table 10.1. Reducing HIF-1, which is caused by the decreased demand for blood supply due to dependable circulation, restores the balance between factors that promote and those that inhibit angiogenesis. A great deal of the survival of immature vasculature depends on circulating angiogenic factors; these include vessels that are twisted with enlarged lumens, have less pericyte coverage, and need VEGF (116). The process of vascular normalization involves pruning them because of their reliance, which renders them sensitive to antiangiogenic chemicals. In a similar vein, antiangiogenic treatment is more effective in vasculature that has minimal pericyte investment. The paracrine communication that occurs between pericytes and ECs is probably responsible for this, as it keeps mature arteries stable (117).

Treatments with cytokines/immunomodulatory medications, ACT, mAbs, and anticancer vaccines, such as DC vaccines, are all part of immunotherapy, which tries to modify the host immune system to enhance antitumor immunity (118, 119). But ICIs are currently ruling the cancer immunotherapy field, thanks to their widespread use and the high number of patients who have shown significant and long-lasting responses across a variety of tumor types (120, 121). Major interferon (IFN-γ) inhibitors include mAbs that inhibit CTLA-4, PD-1, and PD-L1 action. Furthermore, new data suggest that antitumor immunity and the efficacy of ICIs in combinatorial regimens are influenced by the kind of cancer cell death (122). By stimulating ICD in cancer cells, which functions as a kind of "in situ" vaccination, antitumor immunity can be enhanced (123).

TABLE 10.1
Clinical Approved of FDA-Approved Antiangiogenic Drugs for Different Cancer Treatment (97)

Types of Cancer	Antiangiogenic Drug	Drug Combination/Placebo	FDA Approval Year
Breast	Everolimus (Afinitor®, Zortress®)	Exemestane	2009
Colorectal carcinoma	Bevacizumab (Avastin®)	5-Fluorouracil	2004
	Regorafenib (Stivarga®)	Placebo	2012
	Ziv-aflibercept	FOLFIRIchemo (Folinic Acid, Fluorouracil, irinotecan)	2012
Cervical	Bevacizumab (Avastin®)	Paclitaxel+ Topotecan Paclitaxel+ Cisplatin	2004
Renal cell carcinoma	Axitinib (Inlyta®)	Pembrolizumab	2012
	Bevacizumab (Avastin®)	Interferon alfa	2004
	Sorafenib (Nexavar®)	Placebo	2005
	Pazopanib (votrient®)	placebo	2009
NSCLC	Ramucirumab	Docetaxel	2014
Medullary thyroid	Vandetanib	Placebo	2011
Advanced thyroid	Sorafenib (Nexavar®)	Placebo	2005
Gastric	Ramucirumab	Paclitaxel	2014
Gastrointestinal	Sunitinib (Sutent®)	Placebo	2006
	Regorafenib (Stivarga®)	Placebo	2012
Hepatocellular	Sorafenib (Nexavar®)	Placebo	2005
	Regorafenib (Stivarga®)	Placebo	2012
	Cabozantinib (Cometriq®)	Placebo	2012
Ovarian, Fallopian tube	Bevacizumab (Avastin®)	Carboplatin+Paclitaxel	2004

The main characteristics of ICD include the spatially and temporally specified emission of danger signals that are regulated by endoplasmic reticulin stress. These signals include surface calreticulin, secreted ATP, nucleic acids, double-stranded RNA, and double-stranded DNA, among others (124). In addition, CXCL-1, CCL-2, CXCL-10, or their homologs are part of a pathogen response-like chemokine profile, and type I IFN cytokines (IFN-α and IFN-β) are specifically linked to "altered-self mimicry" in ICD (125, 126) years. Importantly, next-generation DC-based vaccines (64) can be made from cancer cells that have succumbed to ICD.

A number of recent FDA approvals attest to immunotherapy's ability to extend patients' lives despite their cancer diagnosis; however, the treatment isn't without its drawbacks (127). The TME and cancer cells' inherent immunoevasion mechanisms (such as decreased tumor-associated antigen (TAA) or major histocompatibility complex (MHC) expression levels, abnormalities in IFN signaling, abnormalities in danger signaling, and immunogenic phagocytosis) are major contributors to these (127). As mentioned earlier, the abnormal tumor vasculature can impede immunotherapy by preventing the delivery of mAbs and by promoting the presence of immunosuppressive immune cells (e.g., MDSCs, M2 TAMs, and Treg cells) rather than immunostimulatory immune cells (mainly CD8+ T cells). There is strong evidence that T-cell density, functional orientation, and spatial proximity inside the tumor are linked to a favorable prognosis for patients with breast cancer (128).

We hypothesize that targeting tumor vasculature may enhance the efficacy of cancer immunotherapy based on these new lines of evidence. Indeed, this is a key rationale for the new push to combine cancer immunotherapy with targeting the tumor vascular.

The following section details and discusses a number of possible immunotherapy and antiangiogenic combination techniques.

CONCLUSIONS

Dysregulated tumor vasculature leads to tumor hypoxia, which encourages aggressive tumor cell adaptations, impedes immune surveillance, fuels metastasis, and promotes resistance to current treatments. Tumor stabilizations are commonly seen in preclinical models, and in combination with antiproliferative modalities, lasting tumor regressions are obtained. Future directions lie in understanding the molecular basis of the mechanism of action of drugs currently undergoing clinical evaluation, developing second-generation small molecule VTAs with enhanced specificity for tumor endothelium, and evaluating noninvasive imaging methods for routine clinical use. Tumor vasculature-induced effects on both the blood and lymph endothelium are crucial in the generation and maintenance of an immunosuppressive TME. Antiangiogenic therapies have the potential to normalize the TME, allowing for better antitumor results when used in combination with other therapeutics. Future studies should focus on optimal timing and dosing of these agents in candidate solid tumors to prevent over-normalizing or pruning back tumor vasculature. Vessel targeting as a cancer therapeutic approach has been established in experimental studies, leading to rapid reductions in tumor blood flow and extensive necrosis. Targeting abnormal tumor vasculature to induce vessel normalization may provide a promising strategy to optimize the efficacy of currently employed immunotherapies, but it is clear that to exploit the full potential of the immune system to cure cancer, multiple levels must be addressed.

CONSENT FOR PUBLICATION

Not applicable.

FUNDING

None.

CONFLICT OF INTEREST

The authors declare no conflict of interest, financial or otherwise.

ACKNOWLEDGMENTS

Declared none.

REFERENCES

1. Pereira, R.D.; de Long, N.E.; Wang, R.C.; Yazdi, F.T.; Holloway, A.C.; Raha, S. Angiogenesis in the Placenta: The Role of Reactive Oxygen Species Signaling. BioMed Res Int. 2015, 2015, 814543.
2. Dangat, K.; Khaire, A.; Joshi, S. Cross Talk of Vascular Endothelial Growth Factor and Neurotrophins in Mammary Gland Development. Growth Factors. 2020, 38, 16–24.
3. Ucuzian, A.A.; Gassman, A.A.; East, A.T.; Greisler, H.P. Molecular Mediators of Angiogenesis. J Burn Care Res. 2010, 31, 158–175.
4. Yokota, Y.; Nakajima, H.; Wakayama, Y.; Muto, A.; Kawakami, K.; Fukuhara, S.; Mochizuki, N. Endothelial Ca2+ Oscillations Reflect VEGFR Signaling-Regulated Angiogenic Capacity In Vivo. eLife. 2015, 4, e08817.
5. Ghajar, C.M.; George, S.C.; Putnam, A.J. Matrix Metalloproteinase Control of Capillary Morphogenesis. Crit Rev Eukaryot Gene Expr. 2008, 18, 251–278.

6. Sauteur, L.; Krudewig, A.; Herwig, L.; Ehrenfeuchter, N.; Lenard, A.; Affolter, M.; Belting, H.G. Cdh5/VE-Cadherin Promotes Endothelial Cell Interface Elongation via Cortical Actin Polymerization during Angiogenic Sprouting. Cell Rep. 2014, 9, 504–513.
7. Franco, C.A.; Jones, M.L.; Bernabeu, M.O.; Vion, A.C.; Barbacena, P.; Fan, J.; Mathivet, T.; Fonseca, C.G.; Ragab, A.; Yamaguchi, T.P.; et al. Non-Canonical Wnt Signalling Modulates the Endothelial Shear Stress Flow Sensor in Vascular Remodelling. eLife. 2016, 5, e07727.
8. Chen, Q.; Jiang, L.; Li, C.; Hu, D.; Bu, J.W.; Cai, D.; Du, J.L. Haemodynamics-Driven Developmental Pruning of Brain Vasculature in Zebrafish. PLoS Biol. 2012, 10, e1001374.
9. Murakami, M. Signaling Required for Blood Vessel Maintenance: Molecular Basis and Pathological Manifestations. Int J Vasc Med. 2012, 2012, 293641.
10. Denekamp, J. Endothelial Cell Proliferation as a Novel Approach to Targeting Tumour Therapy. Br J Cancer. 1982, 45, 136–139.
11. Burrows, F.J.; Thorpe, P.E. Vascular Targeting–A New Approach to the Therapy of Solid Tumors. Pharmacol Ther. 1994, 64, 155–174.
12. Fox, S.B.; Gatter, K.C.; Bicknell, R.; Going, J.J.; Stanton, P.; Cooke, T.G.; Harris, A.L. Relationship of Endothelial Cell Prolif Eration to Tumor Vascularity in Human Breast Cancer. Cancer Res. 1993, 53, 4161–4163.
13. El-Kenawi, A.E.; El-Remessy, A.B. Angiogenesis Inhibitors in Cancer Therapy: Mechanistic Perspective on Classification and Treatment Rationales. Br J Pharmacol. 2013, 170(4), 712–729.
14. Thorpe, P.E. Vascular Targeting Agents as Cancer Therapeutics. Clin Cancer Res. 2004, 10(2), 415–427.
15. Guo, Z.; Jing, X.; Sun, X.; Sun, S.; Yang, Y.; Cao, Y. Tumor Angiogenesis and Anti-Angiogenic Therapy. Chin Med J (Engl). 2024, 137(17), 2043–2051.
16. Liu, Z.L.; Chen, H.H.; Zheng, L.L.; Sun, L.P.; Shi, L. Angiogenic Signaling Pathways and Anti-Angiogenic Therapy for Cancer. Signal Transduct Target Ther. 2023, 8(1), 198.
17. Siemann, D.W. The Unique Characteristics of Tumor Vasculature and Preclinical Evidence for Its Selective Disruption by Tumor-Vascular Disrupting Agents. Cancer Treat Rev. 2011, 37(1), 63–74.
18. Ong, M.S.; Deng, S.; Halim, C.E.; Cai, W.; Tan, T.Z.; Huang, R.Y.; Sethi, G.; Hooi, S.C.; Kumar, A.P.; Yap, C.T. Cytoskeletal Proteins in Cancer and Intracellular Stress: A Therapeutic Perspective. Cancers (Basel). 2020, 12(1), 238.
19. Bremnes, R.M.; Dønnem, T.; Al-Saad, S.; Al-Shibli, K.; Andersen, S.; Sirera, R.; Camps, C.; Marinez, I.; Busund, L.T. The Role of Tumor Stroma in Cancer Progression and Prognosis: Emphasis on Carcinoma-Associated Fibroblasts and Non-Small Cell Lung Cancer. J Thorac Oncol. 2011, 6, 209–217.
20. Murphy, K.J.; Chambers, C.R.; Herrmann, D.; Timpson, P.; Pereira, B.A. Dynamic Stromal Alterations Influence Tumor-Stroma Crosstalk to Promote Pancreatic Cancer and Treatment Resistance. Cancers. 2021, 13, 3481.
21. Kremheller, J.; Vuong, A.T.; Schrefler, B.A.; Wall, W.A. An Approach for Vascular Tumor Growth Based on a Hybrid embedded/homogenized Treatment of the Vasculature Within a Multiphase Porous Medium Model. Int J Numer Method Biomed Eng. 2019, 35(11), e3253.
22. Hanahan, D.; Weinberg, R.A. The Hallmarks of Cancer. Cell. 2000, 100, 57–70.
23. Lugano, R.; Ramachandran, M.; Dimberg, A. Tumor Angiogenesis: Causes, Consequences, Challenges and Opportunities. Cell Mol Life Sci. 2020, 77(9), 1745–1770.
24. Saman, H.; Raza, S.S.; Uddin, S.; Rasul, K. Inducing Angiogenesis, a Key Step in Cancer Vascularization, and Treatment Approaches. Cancers (Basel). 2020, 12(5), 1172.
25. Dudley, A.C.; Griffioen, A.W. Pathological Angiogenesis: Mechanisms and Therapeutic Strategies. Angiogenesis. 2023, 26(3), 313–347.
26. Wilkins, S.E.; Abboud, M.I.; Hancock, R.L.; Schofield, C.J. Targeting Protein-Protein Interactions in the HIF System. ChemMedChem. 2016, 11, 773–786.
27. Jeong, J.-W.; Bae, M.-K.; Ahn, M.-Y.; Kim, S.-H.; Sohn, T.-K.; Bae, M.-H.; Yoo, M.-A.; Song, E.J.; Lee, K.-J.; Kim, K.-W. Regulation and Destabilization of HIF-1alpha by ARD1-Mediated Acetylation. Cell. 2002, 111, 709–720.
28. Huang, L.E.; Gu, J.; Schau, M.; Bunn, H.F. Regulation of Hypoxia-Inducible Factor 1alpha Is Mediated by an O_2-Dependent Degradation Domain via the Ubiquitin-Proteasome Pathway. Proc Natl Acad Sci USA. 1998, 95(14), 7987–7992.
29. Strowitzki, M.; Cummins, E.; Taylor, C. Protein Hydroxylation by Hypoxia-Inducible Factor (HIF) Hydroxylases: Unique or Ubiquitous? Cells. 2019, 8, 384.
30. Koyasu, S.; Kobayashi, M.; Goto, Y.; Hiraoka, M.; Harada, H. Regulatory Mechanisms of Hypoxia-Inducible Factor 1 Activity: Two Decades of Knowledge. Cancer Sci. 2018, 109(3), 560–571

31. Yu, A.Y.; Frid, M.G.; Shimoda, L.A.; Wiener, C.M.; Stenmark, K.; Semenza, G.L. Temporal, Spatial, and Oxygen-Regulated Expression of Hypoxia-Inducible Factor-1 in the Lung. Am J Physiol Lung Cell Mol Physiol. 1998, 275, L818–L826.
32. McKeown, S.R. Defining Normoxia, Physoxia and Hypoxia in Tumours—Implications for Treatment Response. Br J Radiol. 2014, 87, 20130676.
33. Artemov, A.V.; Zhigalova, N.; Zhenilo, S.; Mazur, A.M.; Prokhortchouk, E.B. VHL Inactivation Without Hypoxia Is Sufficient to Achieve Genome Hypermethylation. Sci Rep. 2018, 8, 10667.
34. Iwai, K.; Yamanaka, K.; Kamura, T.; Minato, N.; Conaway, R.C.; Conaway, J.W.; Klausner, R.D.; Pause, A. Identification of the von Hippel-Lindau Tumor-Suppressor Protein as Part of an Active E3 Ubiquitin Ligase Complex. Proc Natl Acad Sci USA. 1999, 96(22), 12436–12441.
35. Amelio, I.; Mancini, M.; Petrova, V.; Cairns, R.A.; Vikhreva, P.; Nicolai, S.; Marini, A.; Antonov, A.A.; le Quesne, J.; Baena Acevedo, J.D.; et al. P53 Mutants Cooperate with HIF-1 in Transcriptional Regulation of Extracellular Matrix Components to Promote Tumor Progression. Proc Natl Acad Sci USA. 2018, 115, E10869–E10878.
36. Zhang, C.; Liu, J.; Wang, J.; Zhang, T.; Xu, D.; Hu, W.; Feng, Z. The Interplay Between Tumor Suppressor p53 and Hypoxia Signaling Pathways in Cancer. Front Cell Dev Biol. 2021, 9, 648808.
37. Mohlin, S.; Hamidian, A.; von Stedingk, K.; Bridges, E.; Wigerup, C.; Bexell, D.; Påhlman, S. PI3K-MTORC2 but Not PI3K MTORC1 Regulates Transcription of HIF2A/EPAS1and Vascularization in Neuroblastoma. Cancer Res. 2015, 75, 4617–4628.
38. Stegeman, H.; Span, P.N.; Peeters, W.J.M.; Verheijen, M.M.G.; Grénman, R.; Meijer, T.W.H.; Kaanders, J.H.A.M.; Bussink, J. Interaction between Hypoxia, AKT and HIF-1 Signaling in HNSCC and NSCLC: Implications for Future Treatment Strategies. Future Sci OA. 2016, 2, FSO84.
39. Shibuya, M. Vascular Endothelial Growth Factor (VEGF) and Its Receptor (VEGFR) Signaling in Angiogenesis: A Crucial Target for Anti- and Pro-Angiogenic Therapies. Genes Cancer. 2011, 2(12), 1097–105.
40. Holmes, D.I.; Zachary, I. The Vascular Endothelial Growth Factor (VEGF) Family: Angiogenic Factors in Health and Disease. Genome Biol. 2005, 6(2), 209.
41. Li, X.; Eriksson, U. Novel VEGF Family Members: VEGF-B, VEGF-C and VEGF-D. Int J Biochem Cell Biol. 2001, 33, 421–426.
42. Liang, L.; Yue, Z.; Du, W.; Li, Y.; Tao, H.; Wang, D.; Wang, R.; Huang, Z.; He, N.; Xie, X.; et al. Molecular Imaging of Inducible VEGFExpression and Tumor Progression in a Breast Cancer Model. Cell Physiol Biochem. 2017, 42, 407–415.
43. Chang, J.; Chaudhuri, O. Beyond Proteases: Basement Membrane Mechanics and Cancer Invasion. J Cell Biol. 2019, 218, 2456–2469.
44. Schaaf, M.B.; Garg, A.D.; Agostinis, P. Defining the Role of the Tumor Vasculature in Antitumor Immunity and Immunotherapy Article. Cell Death Dis. 2018, 9, 115.
45. Duffy, A.M.; Bouchier-Hayes, D.J.; Harmey, J.H. Vascular endothelial growth factor (VEGF) and its role in non-endothelial cells: Autocrine signalling by VEGF. In: Madame Curie Bioscience Database [Internet]. Austin, TX: Landes Bioscience; 2000–2013. Available from: https://www.ncbi.nlm.nih.gov/books/NBK6482/.
46. Matsuda, K.; Ohga, N.; Hida, Y.; Muraki, C.; Tsuchiya, K.; Kurosu, T.; Akino, T.; Shih, S.C.; Totsuka, Y.; Klagsbrun, M.; et al. Isolated Tumor Endothelial Cells Maintain Specific Character during Long-Term Culture. Biochem Biophys Res Commun. 2010, 394, 947–954.
47. Sievert, W.; Tapio, S.; Breuninger, S.; Gaipl, U.; Andratschke, N.; Trott, K.R.; Multhoff, G. Adhesion Molecule Expression and Function of Primary Endothelial Cells in Benign and Malignant Tissues Correlates with Proliferation. PLoS ONE. 2014, 9, e91808.
48. Mehran, R.; Nilsson, M.; Khajavi, M.; Du, Z.; Cascone, T.; Wu, H.K.; Cortes, A.; Xu, L.; Zurita, A.; Schier, R.; et al. Tumor Endothelial Markers Define Novel Subsets of Cancer-Specific Circulating Endothelial Cells Associated with Antitumor Efficacy. Cancer Res. 2014, 74, 2731–2741.
49. Nimlamool, W.; Andrews, R.M.K.; Falk, M.M. Connexin43 Phosphorylation by PKC and MAPK Signals VEGF-Mediated Gap Junction Internalization. Mol Biol Cell. 2015, 26, 2755–2768.
50. Sahni, A.; Francis, C.W. Vascular Endothelial Growth Factor Binds to Fibrinogen and Fibrin and Stimulates Endothelial Cell Proliferation. Blood. 2000, 96(12), 3772–3778.
51. Xiang, D.; Feng, Y.; Wang, J.; Zhang, X.; Shen, J.; Zou, R.; Yuan, Y. Platelet-Derived Growth Factor-BB Promotes Proliferation and Migration of Retinal Microvascular Pericytes by Up-Regulating the Expression of C-X-C Chemokine Receptor Types 4. Exp Ther Med. 2019, 18, 4022–4030.
52. Lindahl, P.; Johansson, B.R.; Levéen, P.; Betsholtz, C. Pericyte Loss and Microaneurysm Formation in PDGF-B-Deficient Mice. Science. 1997, 277, 242–245.

53. Franco, M.; Roswall, P.; Cortez, E.; Hanahan, D.; Pietras, K. Pericytes Promote Endothelial Cell Survival through Induction of Autocrine VEGF-Asignaling and Bcl-w Expression. Blood. 2011, 118, 2906–2917.
54. Libutti, S.K.; Tamarkin, L.; Nilubol, N. Targeting the Invincible Barrier for Drug Delivery in Solid Cancers: Interstitial Fluid Pressure. Oncotarget. 2018, 9, 35723–35725.
55. Padera, T.P.; Stoll, B.R.; Tooredman, J.B.; Capen, D.; di Tomaso, E.; Jain, R.K. Pathology: Cancer Cells Compress Intratumour Vessels. Nature. 2004, 427, 695.
56. Nagy, J.A.; Dvorak, A.M.; Dvorak, H.F. Vascular Hyperpermeability, Angiogenesis, and Stroma Generation. Cold Spring Harb Perspect Med. 2012, 2, a006544.
57. Stylianopoulos, T.; Martin, J.D.; Chauhan, V.P.; Jain, S.R.; Diop-Frimpong, B.; Bardeesy, N.; Smith, B.L.; Ferrone, C.R.; Hornicek, F.J.; Boucher, Y.; et al. Causes, Consequences, and Remedies for Growth-Induced Solid Stress in Murine and Human Tumors. Proc Natl Acad Sci USA. 2012, 109, 15101–15108.
58. Bender, L.H.; Abbate, F.; Walters, I.B. Intratumoral Administration of a Novel Cytotoxic Formulation with Strong Tissue Dispersive Properties Regresses Tumor Growth and Elicits Systemic Adaptive Immunity in in Vivo Models. Int J Mol Sci. 2020, 21, 4493.
59. Sriraman, S.K.; Aryasomayajula, B.; Torchilin, V.P. Barriers to Drug Delivery in Solid Tumors. Tissue Barriers. 2014, 2, e29528.
60. Caswell, D.R.; Swanton, C. The Role of Tumour Heterogeneity and Clonal Cooperativity in Metastasis, Immune Evasion and Clinical Outcome. BMC Med. 2017, 15, 133.
61. Kennedy, K.M.; Scarbrough, P.M.; Ribeiro, A.; Richardson, R.; Yuan, H.; Sonveaux, P.; Landon, C.D.; Chi, J.-T.; Pizzo, S.; Schroeder, T.; et al. Catabolism of Exogenous Lactate Reveals It as a Legitimate Metabolic Substrate in Breast Cancer. PLoS ONE. 2013, 8, e75154.
62. Wang, Y.; Bai, C.; Ruan, Y.; Liu, M.; Chu, Q.; Qiu, L.; Yang, C.; Li, B. Coordinative Metabolism of Glutamine Carbon and Nitrogen in Proliferating Cancer Cells Under Hypoxia. Nat Commun. 2019, 10, 201.
63. Pérez-Escuredo, J.; Dadhich, R.K.; Dhup, S.; Cacace, A.; Van Hée, V.; De Saedeleer, C.J.; Sboarina, M.; Rodriguez, F.; Fontenille, M.-J., Brisson, L.; et al. Lactate Promotes Glutamine Uptake and Metabolism in Oxidative Cancer Cells. Cell Cycle. 2016, 15, 72–83.
64. Rauschner, M.; Lange, L.; Hüsing, T.; Reime, S.; Nolze, A.; Maschek, M.; Thews, O.; Riemann, A. Impact of the Acidic Environment on Gene Expression and Functional Parameters of Tumors In Vitro and In Vivo. J Exp Clin Cancer Res. 2021, 40, 10.
65. Riemann, A.; Schneider, B.; Gündel, D.; Stock, C.; Thews, O.; Gekle, M. Acidic Priming Enhances Metastatic Potential of Cancer Cells. Pflügers Arch Eur J Physiol. 2014, 466, 2127–2138.
66. Wu, H.; Estrella, V.; Beatty, M.; Abrahams, D.; El-Kenawi, A.; Russell, S.; Ibrahim-Hashim, A.; Longo, D.L.; Reshetnyak, Y.K.; Moshnikova, A.; et al. T-Cells Produce Acidic Niches in Lymph Nodes to Suppress Their Own Effector Functions. Nat Commun. 2020, 11, 4113.
67. Halcrow, P.W.; Geiger, J.D.; Chen, X. Overcoming Chemoresistance: Altering pH of Cellular Compartments by Chloroquine and Hydroxychloroquine. Front Cell Dev Biol. 2021, 9, 170.
68. Duswald, T.; Lima, E.A.B.F.; Oden, J.T.; Wohlmuth, B. Bridging Scales: A Hybrid Model to Simulate Vascular Tumor Growth and Treatment Response. ArXiv [Preprint]. 2023 Jun 9: arXiv:2306.05994v1. PMID: 37332572; PMCID: PMC10274951.
69. Welti, J.; Loges, S.; Dimmeler, S.; Carmeliet, P. Recent Molecular Discoveries in Angiogenesis and Antiangiogenic Therapies in Cancer. J Clin Invest. 2013, 123, 3190–3200.
70. Baeriswyl, V.; Christofori, G. The Angiogenic Switch in Carcinogenesis. Semin Cancer Biol. 2009, 19, 329–337.
71. Quail, D.F.; Joyce, J.A. Microenvironmental Regulation of Tumor Progression and Metastasis. Nat Med. 2013, 19(11), 1423––1437.
72. Padera, T.P. et al. Pathology: Cancer Cells Compress Intratumour Vessels. Nature. 2004, 427, 695.
73. Chouaib, S.; Noman, M.Z.; Kosmatopoulos, K.; Curran, M.A. Hypoxic Stress: Obstacles and Opportunities for Innovative Immunotherapy of Cancer. Oncogene. 2017, 36, 439–445.
74. Fukumura, D.; Kloepper, J.; Amoozgar, Z.; Duda, D.G.; Jain, R.K. Enhancing Cancer Immunotherapy Using Antiangiogenics: Opportunities and Challenges. Nat Rev Clin Oncol. 2018, 15(5), 325–340.
75. Reardon, D.A. Update on the Use of Angiogenesis Inhibitors in Adult Patients with Brain Tumors. Clin Adv Hematol Oncol. 2014, 12, 293–303.
76. Winkler, F. et al. Kinetics of Vascular Normalization by VEGFR2 Blockade Governs Brain Tumor Response to Radiation: Role of Oxygenation, Angiopoietin-1, and Matrix Metalloproteinases. Cancer Cell. 2004, 6, 5 53–563.
77. Casazza, A. et al. Impeding Macrophage Entry into Hypoxic Tumor Areas by Sema3A/Nrp1 Signaling Blockade Inhibits Angiogenesis and Restores Antitumor Immunity. Cancer Cell. 2013, 24, 695–709.

78. Westrich, J.A.; Vermeer, D.W.; Colbert, P.L.; Spanos, W.C.; Pyeon, D. The Multifarious Roles of the Chemokine CXCL14 in Cancer Progression and Immune Responses. Mol Carcinog. 2020, 59(7), 794–806.
79. Ferrara, N.; Hillan, K.J.; Novotny, W. Bevacizumab (Avastin), a Humanized Anti-VEGF Monoclonal Antibody for Cancer Therapy. Biochem Biophys Res Commun. 2005, 333(2), 328–335.
80. Goel, S. et al. Normalization of the Vasculature for Treatment of Cancer and Other Diseases. Physiol Rev. 2011, 91, 1071–1121.
81. Stylianopoulos, T.; Jain, R.K. Combining Two Strategies to Improve Perfusion and Drug Delivery in Solid Tumors. Proc Natl Acad Sci USA. 2013, 110, 18632–18637.
82. Weiss, S.A. et al. Immunologic Heterogeneity of Tumor-Infiltrating Lympho Cyte Composition in Primary Melanoma. Hum Pathol. 2016, 57, 116–125.
83. Hatfield, S.M. et al. Immunological Mechanisms of the Antitumor Effects of Supplemental Oxygenation. Sci Transl Med. 2015, 7, 277–230.
84. Huang, Y. et al. Vascular Normalizing Doses of Antiangiogenic Treatment Reprogram the Immunosuppressive Tumor Microenvironment and Enhance Immunotherapy. Proc Natl Acad Sci USA. 2012, 109, 17561–17566.
85. Voron, T. et al. VEGF-A Modulates Expression of Inhibitory Checkpoints on CD8+T Cells in Tumors. J Exp Med. 2015, 212, 139–148.
86. Maes, H. et al. Tumor Vessel Normalization by Chloroquine Independent of Autophagy. Cancer Cell. 2014, 26, 190–206.
87. Starobinets, H. et al. Antitumor Adaptive Immunity Remains Intact Following Inhibition of Autophagy and Antimalarial Treatment. J Clin Invest. 2016, 126, 4417–4429.
88. Potente, M.; Carmeliet, P. The Link between Angiogenesis and Endothelial Metabolism. Annu Rev Physiol. 2017, 79, 43–66.
89. Cantelmo, A.R. et al. Inhibition of the Glycolytic Activator PFKFB3 in Endo Thelium Induces Tumor Vessel Normalization, Impairs Metastasis, and Improves Chemotherapy. Cancer Cell. 2016, 30, 968–985.
90. Stapor, P.; Wang, X.; Goveia, J.; Moens, S.; Carmeliet, P. Angiogenesis Revisited- Role and Therapeutic Potential of Targeting Endothelial Metabolism. J Cell Sci. 127(Pt 20), 4331–4341 (2014).
91. Fasanaro, P. et al. MicroRNA-210 Modulates Endothelial Cell Response to Hypoxia and Inhibits the Receptor Tyrosine Kinase Ligand Ephrin-A3. J Biol Chem. 2008, 283, 15878–15883.
92. Karaa, Z.S. et al. The VEGF IRESes Are Differentially Susceptible to Translation Inhibition by miR-16. RNA. 2009, 15, 249–254.
93. Mao, G. et al. Tumor-Derived microRNA-494 Promotes Angiogenesis in Non-Small Cell Lung Cancer. Angiogenesis. 2015, 18, 373–382.
94. Li, Y. et al. Local Expression of Indoleamine 2,3-Dioxygenase Protects Engraftment of Xenogeneic Skin Substitute. J Invest Dermatol. 2006, 126, 128–136.
95. Holmgaard, R.B.; Zamarin, D.; Munn, D.H.; Wolchok, J.D.; Allison, J.P. Indoleamine 2,3-Dioxygenase Is a Critical Resistance Mechanism in Antitumor T Cell Immunotherapy Targeting CTLA-4. J Exp Med. 2013, 210, 1389–1402.
96. Tian, L. et al. Mutual Regulation of Tumour Vessel Normalization and Immunostimulatory Reprogramming. Nature. 2017, 544, 250–254.
97. Matuszewska, K.; Pereira, M.; Petrik, D.; Lawler, J.; Petrik, J. Normalizing Tumor Vasculature to Reduce Hypoxia, Enhance Perfusion, and Optimize Therapy Uptake. Cancers (Basel). 2021, 13(17), 4444.
98. Gray, L.H.; Conger, A.D.; Ebert, M.; Hornsey, S.; Scott, O.C.A. The Concentration of Oxygen Dissolved in Tissues at the Time of Irradiation as a Factor in Radiotherapy. Br J Radiol. 1953, 26, 638–648.
99. Price, M.; Heilbrun, L.; Kessel, D. Effects of the Oxygenation Level on Formation of Different Reactive Oxygen Species during Photodynamic Therapy. Photochem Photobiol. 2012, 89, 683–686.
100. Nanayakkara, A.K.; Follit, C.A.; Chen, G.; Williams, N.S.; Vogel, P.D.; Wise, J.G. Targeted Inhibitors of P-Glycoprotein Increase Chemotherapeutic-Induced Mortality of Multidrug Resistant Tumor Cells. Sci Rep. 2018, 8, 967.
101. Lv, Y.; Zhao, S.; Han, J.; Zheng, L.; Yang, Z.; Zhao, L. Hypoxia-Inducible Factor-1 Induces Multidrug Resistance Protein in Colon Cancer. OncoTargets Ther. 2015, 8, 1941–1948.
102. Mirzaei, S.A.; Reiisi, S.; Tabari, P.G.; Shekari, A.; Aliakbari, F.; Azadfallah, E.; Elahian, F. Broad Blocking of MDR Efflux Pumps by Acetylshikonin and Acetoxyisovalerylshikonin to Generate Hypersensitive Phenotype of Malignant Carcinoma Cells. Sci Rep. 2018, 8, 3446.
103. Chen, J.; Ding, Z.; Peng, Y.; Pan, F.; Li, J.; Zou, L.; Zhang, Y.; Liang, H. HIF-1 Inhibition Reverses Multidrug Resistance in Colon Cancer Cells via Downregulation of MDR1/P-Glycoprotein. PLoS ONE. 2014, 9, e98882.

104. Thiery, J.P.; Acloque, H.; Huang, R.Y.-J.; Nieto, M.A. Epithelial-Mesenchymal Transitions in Development and Disease. Cell. 2009, 139, 871–890.
105. Saggar, J.K.; Tannock, I.F. Chemotherapy Rescues Hypoxic Tumor Cells and Induces Their Reoxygenation and Repopulation—An Effect That Is Inhibited by the Hypoxia-Activated Prodrug TH-302. Clin Cancer Res. 2015, 21, 2107–2114.
106. Alagoz, T.; Buller, R.E.; Anderson, B.; Terrell, K.L.; Squatrito, R.C.; Niemann, T.H.; Tatman, D.J.; Jebson, P. Evaluation of Hyperbaric Oxygen as a Chemosensitizer in the Treatment of Epithelial Ovarian Cancer in Xenografts in Mice. Cancer. 1995, 75, 2313–2322.
107. Colliez, F.; Gallez, B.; Jordan, B.F. Assessing Tumor Oxygenation for Predicting Outcome in Radiation Oncology: A Review of Studies Correlating Tumor Hypoxic Status and Outcome in the Preclinical and Clinical Settings. Front Oncol. 2017, 7, 10.
108. Ray, S.K.; Mukherjee, S. Innovative Nanomaterials for Targeting Hypoxia to Improve Treatment for Triple-Negative Breast Cancer. Recent Pat Biotechnol. 2024, 18(4), 269–272.
109. Mukherjee, S.; Ray, S.K. Targeting Tumor Hypoxia and Hypoxia-Inducible Factors (HIFs) for the Treatment of Cancer – A Story of Transcription Factors with Novel Approach in Molecular Medicine. Curr Mol Med. 2022, 22(4), 285–286.
110. Yeh, J.J.; Kim, W.Y. Targeting Tumor Hypoxia with Hypoxia-Activated Prodrugs. J Clin Oncol. 2015, 33, 1505–1508.
111. Thews, O.; Vaupel, P. Spatial Oxygenation Profiles in Tumors during Normo- and Hyperbaric Hyperoxia. Strahlenther Und Onkol. 2015, 191, 875–882.
112. Kim, K.J.; Li, B.; Winer, J.; Armanini, M.; Gillett, N.; Phillips, H.S.; Ferrara, N. Inhibition of Vascular Endothelial Growth Factor-Induced Angiogenesis Suppresses Tumour Growth in Vivo. Nature. 1993, 362, 841–844.
113. Van Beijnum, J.R.; Nowak-Sliwinska, P.; Huijbers, E.J.M.; Thijssen, V.L.; Griffioen, A.W. The Great Escape; the Hallmarks of Resistance to Antiangiogenic Therapy. Pharmacol Rev. 2015, 67, 441–461.
114. Jain, R.K. Antiangiogenesis Strategies Revisited: From Starving Tumors to Alleviating Hypoxia. Cancer Cell. 2014, 26, 605–622.
115. Godet, I.; Shin, Y.J.; Ju, J.A.; Ye, I.C.; Wang, G.; Gilkes, D.M. Fate-Mapping Post-Hypoxic Tumor Cells Reveals a ROS-Resistant Phenotype That Promotes Metastasis. Nat Commun. 2019, 10, 4862.
116. Dor, Y.; Porat, R.; Keshet, E. Vascular Endothelial Growth Factor and Vascular Adjustments to Perturbations in Oxygen Homeostasis. Am J Physiol Cell Physiol. 2001, 280, C1367–C1374.
117. Martin, J.D.; Seano, G.; Jain, R.K. Normalizing Function of Tumor Vessels: Progress, Opportunities, and Challenges. Annu Rev Physiol. 2019, 81, 505–534.
118. Perica, K.; Varela, J.C.; Oelke, M.; Schneck, J. Adoptive T Cell Immunotherapy for Cancer. Rambam Maimonides Med J. 2015, 6, e0004.
119. Farkona, S.; Diamandis, E.P.; Blasutig, I.M. Cancer Immunotherapy: The Beginning of the End of Cancer? BMC Med. 2016, 14, 73.
120. Jazirehi, A.R.; Lim, A.; Dinh, T. PD-1 Inhibition and Treatment of Advanced Melanoma-Role of Pembrolizumab. Am J Cancer Res. 2016, 6, 2117–2128.
121. Iafolla, M.A.J.; Juergens, R.A. Updateonprogrammeddeath-1 and Programmed Death-Ligand 1 Inhibition in the Treatment of Advanced or Metastatic Non-Small Cell Lung Cancer. Front Oncol. 2017, 7, 67.
122. Pfirschke, C. et al. Immunogenic Chemotherapy Sensitizes Tumors to Check Point Blockade Therapy. Immunity. 2016, 44, 343–354.
123. Morris, Z.S. et al. In Situ Tumor Vaccination by Combining Local Radiation and Tumor-Specific Antibody or Immunocytokine Treatments. Cancer Res. 2016, 76, 3929–3941.
124. Kroemer, G.; Galluzzi, L.; Kepp, O.; Zitvogel, L. Immunogenic Cell Death in Cancer Therapy. Annu Rev Immunol. 2013, 31, 51–72.
125. Sistigu, A. et al. Cancer Cell-Autonomous Contribution of Type I Interferon Signaling to the Efficacy of Chemotherapy. Nat Med. 2014, 20, 1301–1309.
126. Garg, A.D. et al. Pathogen Response-Like Recruitment and Activation of Neutrophils by Sterile Immunogenic Dying Cells Drives Neutrophil-Mediated Residual Cell Killing. Cell Death Differ. 2017, 24, 832–843.
127. Restifo, N.P.; Smyth, M.J.; Snyder, A. Acquired Resistance to Immunotherapy and Future Challenges. Nat Rev Cancer. 2016, 16, 121–126.
128. Mao, Y. et al. The Value of Tumor Infiltrating Lymphocytes (TILs) for Predicting Response to Neoadjuvant Chemotherapy in Breast Cancer: A Systematic Review and Meta-Analysis. PLoS ONE. 2014, 9, e115103.

11 Novel Strategies for Drug Delivery in Hypoxic Tumor

Kritika Singh
Indian Council of Medical Research, National Institute for Research in Tribal Health, Jabalpur, Madhya Pradesh, India

Saransh Shrivastava
National Yang Ming Chiao Tung University, Hscinchu, Taiwan

Sandeep Kumar
Indian Council of Medical Research, Ansari Nagar, New Delhi, India

Mayank Soni
Rajiv Gandhi Cancer Institute and Research Centre, Rohini, Delhi, India

Shweta Pathak
State Cancer Institute, Netaji Subhash Chandra Bose Medical College, Jabalpur, Madhya Pradesh, India

Tapas Chakma
Indian Council of Medical Research, National Institute for Research in Tribal Health, Jabalpur, Madhya Pradesh, India

Suman Kumar Ray
Department of Biochemistry, Jabalpur, Madhya Pradesh, India

Suyesh Shrivastava
Indian Council of Medical Research, National Institute for Research in Tribal Health, All India Institute of Medical Sciences, Bhopal, India
Academy of Scientific and Innovative Research (AcSIR), Ghaziabad, Uttar Pradesh, India

INTRODUCTION

Hypoxia, characterized by a deficiency in oxygen supply, is a prevalent feature of solid tumors and significantly influences tumor biology, treatment resistance, and patient outcomes. The hypoxic tumor microenvironment presents unique challenges and opportunities for targeted drug delivery systems, particularly in cancer therapy. The development of hypoxia-targeted drug delivery

DOI: 10.1201/9781003477419-11

strategies has gained traction due to the potential to selectively target hypoxic tumor cells while sparing normal tissues, thereby enhancing therapeutic efficacy and minimizing side effects. This synthesis will explore various approaches to hypoxia-targeted drug delivery, including hypoxia-activated prodrugs (HAPs), nanoparticle-based systems, and molecular imaging techniques.

HAPs represent a promising class of therapeutic agents designed to become activated specifically in hypoxic environments. These prodrugs are enzymatically reduced under low oxygen conditions, releasing active cytotoxic agents that can kill hypoxic tumor cells. For instance, TH-302, a HAP, has shown efficacy in targeting hypoxic bone marrow niches in preclinical leukemia models, highlighting the potential of HAPs in treating hematological malignancies [1]. Moreover, the selective activation of HAPs in hypoxic regions allows for a bystander effect, where the released drug can diffuse to adjacent tumor cells, thereby enhancing overall treatment efficacy [2]. Despite the promise of HAPs, clinical trials have yielded mixed results, necessitating further research to optimize their use in combination with other therapies [3].

Nanoparticle-based drug delivery systems have emerged as a versatile platform for targeting hypoxic tumors. These systems can be engineered to respond to the unique biochemical environment of hypoxic tumors, such as elevated levels of reducing agents like glutathione [4]. For example, demonstrated the use of nanoparticle-engineered adipose-derived stem cells to deliver therapeutic agents specifically to hypoxic regions in glioblastoma, showcasing the potential of stem cell-mediated delivery systems in targeting tumor hypoxia [5]. Additionally, the incorporation of hypoxia-responsive elements into nanoparticles can enhance the specificity and efficacy of drug delivery, allowing for controlled release in hypoxic conditions [6]. The combination of HAPs with nanoparticle technology may further improve therapeutic outcomes by enhancing drug solubility, stability, and bioavailability.

Molecular imaging techniques play a crucial role in the development and optimization of hypoxia-targeted therapies. Imaging modalities such as positron emission tomography (PET) using fluoromisonidazole (FMISO) allow for the visualization of hypoxic regions within tumors, enabling personalized treatment planning [7]. The ability to accurately map hypoxic areas can inform the selection of appropriate therapies, including the use of HAPs or other hypoxia-targeted agents. Furthermore, the integration of imaging with therapeutic agents, as seen in theranostic approaches, can facilitate real-time monitoring of treatment response and tumor dynamics [8]. This dual capability of imaging and therapy underscores the importance of hypoxia in guiding clinical decision-making and improving patient outcomes.

The characterization of hypoxia-associated molecular features is essential for the development of effective hypoxia-targeted therapies. Research has identified various biomarkers and signaling pathways associated with hypoxia, such as hypoxia-inducible factors (HIFs), which regulate gene expression in response to low oxygen levels [9]. Targeting HIFs and their downstream signaling pathways has emerged as a strategy to enhance the efficacy of existing therapies and overcome resistance mechanisms [10]. For instance, the inhibition of HIF 1-alpha (HIF-1α) has been shown to sensitize tumors to radiotherapy and chemotherapy, suggesting that HIF-targeted strategies could be integrated into multimodal treatment regimens [11]. However, the complexity of hypoxia-related signaling networks necessitates a comprehensive recognizing of the molecular landscape of individual tumors to tailor therapies effectively.

Despite the advances in hypoxia-targeted drug delivery, several challenges remain. The heterogeneity of tumor hypoxia, characterized by varying degrees of oxygen deprivation within different tumor regions, complicates the development of universally effective therapies [12]. Additionally, the presence of necrotic areas and the dynamic nature of the tumor microenvironment can influence drug distribution and efficacy [13]. Therefore, ongoing research is focused on identifying patient-specific hypoxia profiles and optimizing treatment strategies accordingly. For example, proposed a molecular subtyping system based on hypoxia-related genes to enhance the personalization of targeted therapies in non-small cell lung cancer (NSCLC) [14]. Such approaches aim to improve treatment outcomes by aligning therapeutic interventions with the unique characteristics of each patient's tumor (Figure 11.1).

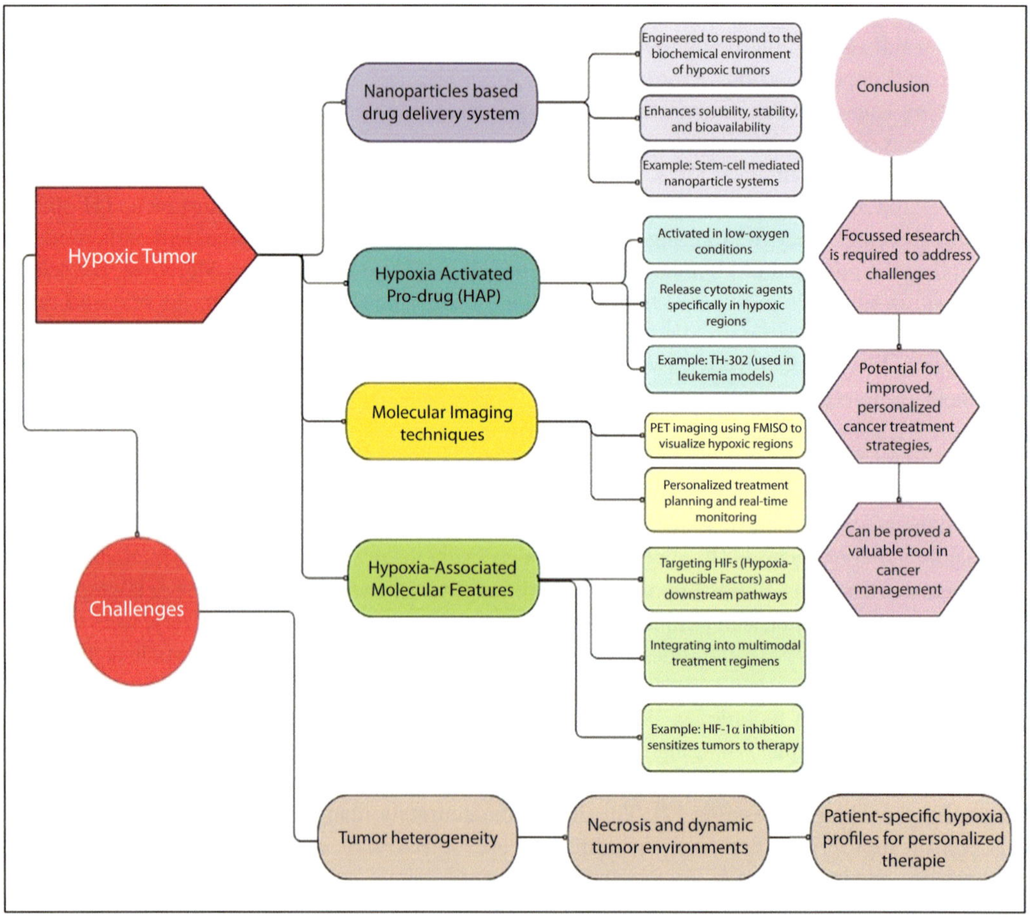

FIGURE 11.1 Targeted drug delivery for hypoxic tumors.

Hypoxia-targeted drug delivery represents a promising avenue for enhancing cancer therapy. The integration of HAPs, nanoparticle-based systems, and advanced molecular imaging techniques offers a multifaceted approach to selectively target hypoxic tumor cells. While significant progress has been made in recognizing the implications of hypoxia in cancer biology, further research is needed to address the challenges associated with tumor heterogeneity and treatment resistance. By leveraging the unique properties of the hypoxic tumor microenvironment, researchers and clinicians can develop more effective and personalized therapeutic strategies that improve patient outcomes in cancer treatment.

NOVEL STRATEGIES AND TARGETED DRUG DELIVERY SYSTEM IN TUMOR HYPOXIA

Many solid tumors exhibit hypoxia, which is a condition of low oxygen tension. Usually, it is linked to aberrant vasculature, which lowers the flow of nutrients and oxygen and makes it more difficult for medications to be delivered. Novel therapeutic approaches are required due to the complex link between hypoxia and tumor growth. By focusing on hypoxia-associated pathways, delivery methods based on nanoparticles can greatly increase the effectiveness of cancer treatments. One typical feature of solid tumors is hypoxia. Low oxygen levels brought on by faulty vascular networks supporting the majority of tumors are the primary cause. A number of prodrug techniques

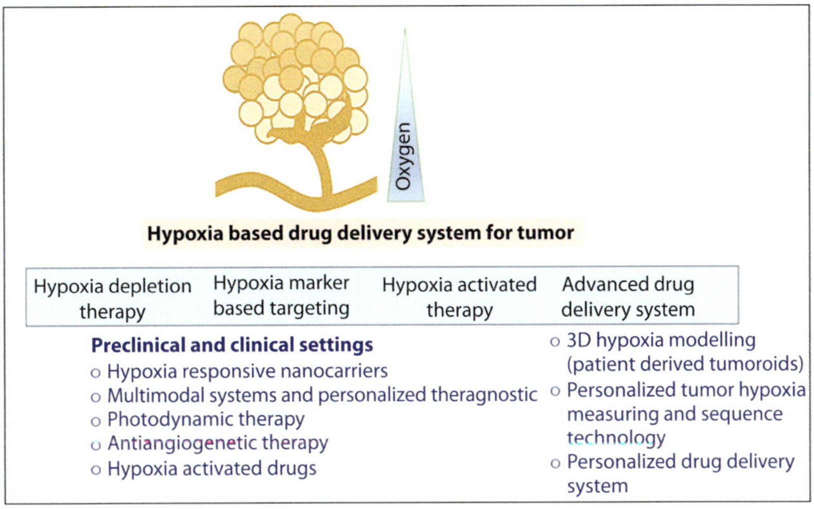

FIGURE 11.2 Hypoxia-based different drug delivery strategy for tumors and personalization.

have been devised to achieve hypoxia-specific delivery of cytotoxic anticancer drugs (Figure 11.2) in an effort to improve the current chemotherapeutic treatment and lessen related adverse effects. As nanotechnology has advanced, new delivery systems that are triggered by the resulting effects of hypoxia have been created. It is currently naïve to build hypoxia-sensitive medication delivery devices, which rely solely on low oxygen levels.

HYPOXIA-ACTIVATED PRODRUGS

HAPs represent a promising therapeutic strategy aimed at selectively targeting hypoxic tumor environments, which are prevalent in many solid tumors. These prodrugs remain inactive under normoxic conditions but are activated in hypoxic regions, thereby minimizing toxicity to normal tissues while maximizing cytotoxic effects on cancer cells. The underlying mechanism involves enzymatic reduction processes that occur in low-oxygen environments, allowing for the release of active cytotoxic agents specifically where they are most needed [15, 16].

The design of HAPs has evolved significantly, with various chemical moieties being employed to enhance their efficacy and selectivity. For instance, the 2-nitroimidazole moiety has been utilized in several prodrug systems, including TH-302 (evofosfamide), which is currently undergoing clinical trials [17, 18]. Additionally, the development of analogues resistant to aerobic metabolism, such as PR-104, has been explored to improve tumor selectivity and reduce off-target effects [19, 20]. The strategic incorporation of bioreductive switches in HAPs allows for a controlled release of cytotoxic agents, which can also diffuse to adjacent tumor cells, thereby inducing a bystander effect that enhances overall therapeutic efficacy [2, 21]. Despite the potential advantages of HAPs, challenges remain in their clinical application. The heterogeneous nature of tumor hypoxia can lead to inconsistent activation of prodrugs, limiting their effectiveness [22]. Furthermore, the lack of patient stratification based on hypoxia levels has been cited as a contributing factor to the limited success of some HAPs in clinical trials [23]. Recent advancements in imaging techniques have been proposed to monitor prodrug activation and distribution within tumors, which could facilitate better patient selection and treatment outcomes [24]. HAPs are a compelling area of research in cancer therapy, leveraging the unique characteristics of tumor hypoxia to deliver targeted treatments (Figure 11.3). Different studies aim to refine their design and application, addressing the challenges of hypoxia heterogeneity and improving patient stratification to enhance clinical efficacy [15, 22].

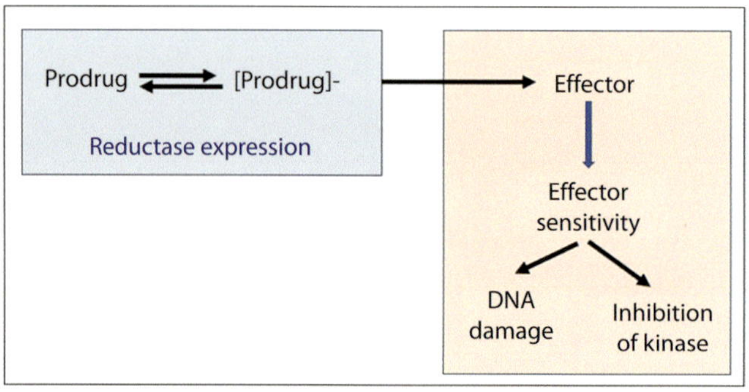

FIGURE 11.3 HAPs are activated in tumors by enzymatic one-electron reduction process to yield a prodrug radical anion. In hypoxia, the radical anion either fragments or is reduced further to produce a cytotoxic effector which have a specific pharmacological role.

The mechanism of action for HAPs involves their selective activation in low-oxygen environments, where they undergo bioreductive conversion to release cytotoxic agents. This selective activation is primarily mediated by various reducing agents that accumulate in hypoxic tumor microenvironments, such as NADH, NADPH, and specific reductases like nitroreductase (NTR) and cytochrome P450 reductase [25–27].

One of the most notable examples of HAPs is TH-302 (evofosfamide), which has been shown to enhance T-cell infiltration and restore sensitivity to immune checkpoint inhibitors in preclinical models of prostate cancer [28, 29]. This prodrug is designed to be inactive under normoxic conditions but becomes cytotoxic in hypoxic regions, thereby targeting the tumor more effectively while sparing normal tissues. Similarly, tirapazamine (TPZ) is another HAP that has been extensively studied for its ability to selectively kill hypoxic tumor cells, demonstrating significant potential in clinical trials [30, 31]. The design of HAPs often involves linking chemotherapeutic agents to moieties that can be selectively reduced in hypoxic conditions. For instance, azobenzene and nitroaromatic groups are commonly used to create stable prodrugs that are activated in the hypoxic tumor microenvironment [32, 33]. These prodrugs can be combined with other therapeutic modalities, such as photothermal therapy, to enhance their efficacy. For example, a recent study developed a HAP conjugated with a photothermal agent, allowing for imaging-guided combination therapy that improves therapeutic outcomes.

Moreover, advancements in nanotechnology have led to the development of hypoxia-responsive nanocarriers that can deliver HAPs more effectively. These nanocarriers can be engineered to respond to the unique biochemical environment of tumors, enhancing the specificity and efficacy of drug delivery [33]. The integration of imaging capabilities with HAPs also allows for real-time tracking of drug delivery and therapeutic response, which is crucial for optimizing treatment strategies [8]. In summary, HAPs leverage the unique metabolic characteristics of tumors, particularly hypoxia, to deliver targeted therapies that can overcome the limitations of traditional cancer treatments. Ongoing research and clinical trials continue to explore the potential of these prodrugs in improving therapeutic outcomes and reducing drug resistance in solid tumors [34–36].

NANOPARTICLE-BASED DRUG DELIVERY SYSTEMS

Nanoparticle-based drug delivery systems have emerged as a promising strategy especially for targeting solid tumors, which are usually resistant to conventional therapies due to their unique tumor microenvironment characterized by low oxygen levels. Nanotechnology-based cancer therapies operate through various approaches, including the use of hypoxia-sensitive materials, engineered bacteria, and advanced nanocarrier designs that enhance drug accumulation in hypoxic regions.

One of the key mechanisms for improving drug delivery to hypoxic tumors is the development of hypoxia-responsive nanoparticles. For instance, Liu et al. demonstrated that azobenzene bonds can serve as effective hypoxia-sensitive moieties, allowing for selective drug release in hypoxic conditions [37, 38]. This approach enables the design of nanocarriers that can respond to the tumor microenvironment, thereby enhancing the therapeutic efficacy of drugs like doxorubicin [39]. Further, Shi and his colleagues demonstrated the effective targeting of hypoxic tumors via utilizing engineered bacteria-driven delivery of drug nanoparticle directly to the site of tumor, and thus improving the therapeutic outcomes of chemotherapy [40].

The size and composition of nanoparticles also play a critical role in their ability to penetrate tumor tissues. Poor vascularization, a characteristic feature of solid hypoxic tumors, poses a barrier for targeted delivery of chemotherapeutic drugs and hence poor outcome of chemotherapy. Therefore, normalization of vasculature in hypoxic tumors could a promising approach for improving the treatment outcome. Several studies have reported that nanoparticles smaller than 20 nm can effectively penetrate deeper into tumor tissues, a crucial step for reaching hypoxic as well as poorly vascularized malignant tissues [41]. Recently, Du et al. have synthesized nanoparticles of lipid derivative conjugates (LGCs) made of anti-angiogenic agents with low molecular weight heparin (LMWH) and gemcitabine (Gem) that improved drug delivery and treatment response via normalizing the tumor vasculature [42]. Moreover, other group has demonstrated the efficacy of gold nanoparticles carrying recombinant human endostatin in normalizing tumor vasculature in H22 xenograft mouse models [43]. Further, combination therapy of h-endostatin nanoparticles with 5-FU resulted in increased 5-FU delivery into the tumor and eventually reduced hypoxia, leaking, improved pericyte coverage and blood perfusion, and overall improvement in therapeutic efficiency.

Photodynamic therapy is a choice of treatment for cancer therapy in clinical settings; however, its efficacy is compromised when it comes to hypoxic tumors. To tackle this barrier, Cui et al. synthesized a semiconducting polymer nanoprodrug (SPNpd) with a well-defined structure for hypoxia-activated synergistic cancer therapy [44]. The SPNpd not only efficiently generated singlet oxygen ($^1O_2$) under NIR photoirradiation but also specifically activated its chemotherapeutic action in hypoxic tumor microenvironment. Furthermore, the use of semiconducting polymeric nanoparticles has been shown to enhance penetration in large solid tumors, thereby addressing the challenges posed by hypoxia. This is complemented by the enhanced permeability and retention (EPR) effect, which allows for passive targeting of nanoparticles to tumor tissues [45]. Another innovative approach involves the use of stimuli-responsive systems that can be activated by external factors such as light or pH changes. For example, developed hypoxia-responsive polyprodrug nanocarriers that release therapeutic agents upon exposure to near-infrared light, thereby amplifying the hypoxic conditions within the tumor and enhancing drug release [46].

Enhanced aerobic/anaerobic glycolysis and increased HIF-mediated proton pumping from tumor cells drive the acidic environment in hypoxic tumors as compared to normal tissue [47]. Therefore, pH gradient in tumor is of great importance to explore as an effective strategy to targeted delivery of pH-sensitive nanoparticles loaded with chemotherapeutic agent(s) especially in case of hypoxic tumors. The pH-dependent nanoparticles could be organic, inorganic, and composite depending upon the material of origin and get charged, swell and release the entrapped anticancer drug on reaching to target site. The most commonly utilized bonds for synthesizing pH-dependent nanoparticles are hydrazone/acyl hydrazone, imine, acetal/ketal, oxime, amide, ester/orthoester, β-thiopropionatent, and borate ester [48].

Recently, Wang et al. (2024) prepared COF-PBA@DOX nanoparticles with reversible charge conversions for the accurate tumor-targeting and enhanced anticancer drug delivery [49]. The group utilized covalent organic frameworks (COFs) and azobenzene (azo) groups for synthesizing nanocarrier and further modified these nanoparticles by pH-sensitive sulfamide-based zwitterionic polymers (PBA). Thus, synthesized pH-dependent nanocarriers were then loaded with the chemotherapeutic drug doxorubicin (DOX). Moreover, Dutta et al. synthesized pH-responsive nanoparticles which released ERK-inhibitor in the hypoxic zone and sensitized free gemcitabine in mutant

K-Ras-addicted pancreatic cancer cells and mouse model [50]. Further, dual approach of using both endogenous (hypoxia) and exogenous (light) stimuli can significantly improve the effectiveness of cancer therapies. To demonstrate the success of this approach, Zhang et al. constructed dual-responsive carriers (DANPCT) that encapsulate the photosensitizer chlorin e6 (Ce6) and HAP TPZ to enable efficient PDT and PDT-boosted hypoxia-activated chemotherapy [51]. These nanoparticles were efficient in inducing transactivator of transcription (TAT) presentation at tumor site in acidic pH condition, a characteristic feature of hypoxic tumors.

Moreover, the integration of macrophage-mediated delivery systems has shown promise in overcoming the limitations of traditional nanoparticle delivery methods. By utilizing macrophages to transport nanoparticles, researchers have been able to bypass the immune system and enhance the accumulation of therapeutic agents in hypoxic tumor regions [52]. This strategy not only improves drug delivery efficiency but also minimizes systemic side effects. In summary, nanoparticle-based drug delivery systems for hypoxic tumors leverage a combination of hypoxia-responsive materials, engineered biological carriers, and advanced nanocarrier designs to enhance drug accumulation and therapeutic efficacy. These innovative approaches are paving the way for more effective treatments for patients with hypoxic tumors, which have historically posed significant challenges in oncology.

MOLECULAR IMAGING TECHNIQUES

Molecular imaging techniques have become increasingly vital in the assessment and treatment of hypoxic tumors, which are characterized by low oxygen levels that often lead to treatment resistance and poor prognosis. Various imaging modalities, including positron emission tomography (PET), single photon emission computed tomography (SPECT), and advanced nanoprobe technologies, have been developed to visualize and quantify hypoxia within tumors.

PET imaging, particularly with radiotracers such as 18F-FMISO and 18F-flortanidazole (HX4), is one of the most established techniques for assessing tumor hypoxia. These tracers accumulate in hypoxic tissues due to their reductive metabolism, allowing for the identification of hypoxic regions that are resistant to therapies such as radiation [45–47]. Studies have demonstrated that the accumulation of these tracers correlates with the levels of HIF-1α, a key regulator of the cellular response to hypoxia [48, 49]. Furthermore, the use of PET imaging can guide treatment planning by identifying hypoxic subvolumes within tumors, enabling dose escalation strategies in radiotherapy [50, 51]. In addition to PET, SPECT imaging has also been utilized to assess tumor hypoxia. Similar to PET, SPECT employs radiotracers that preferentially accumulate in hypoxic regions. The development of novel radiopharmaceuticals for SPECT has expanded the toolkit available for clinicians to evaluate tumor hypoxia, which is crucial for tailoring treatment strategies. Moreover, the integration of imaging modalities, such as combining PET with electron paramagnetic resonance imaging (EPRI), has been proposed to enhance the accuracy of hypoxia assessments by providing quantitative measurements of oxygen levels in tissues [52].

Nanoprobe technologies represent another innovative approach to molecular imaging of hypoxia. For instance, activatable nanoprobes that respond to the unique biochemical environment of hypoxic tumors have been developed. These probes can enter cancer cells and react with specific enzymes, such as NTR, which are upregulated in hypoxic conditions, thereby facilitating real-time imaging of hypoxia at the cellular level [53]. Additionally, advancements in intravital imaging techniques, such as multiphoton microscopy, allow for the visualization of hypoxic tumor cells in vivo, providing insights into their invasive and motility phenotypes [54]. The application of these imaging techniques extends beyond mere visualization; they play a critical role in predicting treatment outcomes. For example, metabolic profiling through hyperpolarized MRI and EPR imaging has been shown to correlate with the efficacy of therapies targeting hypoxic tumors, such as HAPs [55]. Furthermore, the identification of hypoxic regions can inform the selection of patients for specific therapies, enhancing the overall effectiveness of cancer treatment.

Molecular imaging techniques are essential for recognizing and managing hypoxic tumors. The integration of various imaging modalities, including PET, SPECT, and advanced nanoprobe technologies, provides a comprehensive approach to visualize and quantify tumor hypoxia. This not only aids in treatment planning but also enhances the potential for personalized medicine in oncology.

BIOMARKERS AND SIGNALING PATHWAYS IN HYPOXIC TUMORS

The hypoxic tumors as discussed present a unique challenge in cancer biology, as they are characterized by low oxygen levels that significantly influence tumor behavior, including growth, metastasis, and response to therapy. The mechanisms underlying these phenomena are complex and involve various biomarkers and signaling pathways. One of the key players in the hypoxic tumor microenvironment is the HIF, particularly HIF-1α. HIF-1α is a TAT factor that regulates the expression of genes involved in angiogenesis, metabolism, and cell survival under low oxygen conditions. It has been shown that HIF-1α promotes the expression of vascular endothelial growth factor (VEGF), which is crucial for angiogenesis, thereby facilitating tumor growth and metastasis [56, 57]. Additionally, HIF-1α influences the epithelial-mesenchymal transition (EMT), a process that enhances the migratory and invasive properties of cancer cells [58, 59]. For instance, hypoxia-induced EMT is associated with the upregulation of N-cadherin and downregulation of E-cadherin, which are critical markers of this transition. A few basic functions of HIF-1α and its signaling in hypoxic cancer cells are shown in Figure 11.4.

Moreover, hypoxia can alter metabolic pathways within tumors, promoting a shift towards glycolysis, a phenomenon known as the Warburg effect. This metabolic adaptation is largely mediated by HIF-1α, which activates glycolytic genes while inhibiting mitochondrial respiration [60]. This metabolic reprogramming not only supports rapid tumor growth but also contributes to therapeutic resistance, as hypoxic tumors often exhibit reduced sensitivity to radiation and chemotherapy [61]. For example, hypoxia has been linked to increased expression of multidrug resistance proteins in colon cancer, which diminishes the efficacy of standard chemotherapeutic agents [62]. In addition to HIF-1α, other signaling pathways are also implicated in the response of tumors to hypoxia. The hedgehog (Hh) signaling pathway has been shown to play a role in modulating the hypoxic tumor landscape, affecting tumor cell characteristics and the immune microenvironment [63, 64]. Furthermore, the interaction between cancer-associated fibroblasts (CAFs) and hypoxic conditions

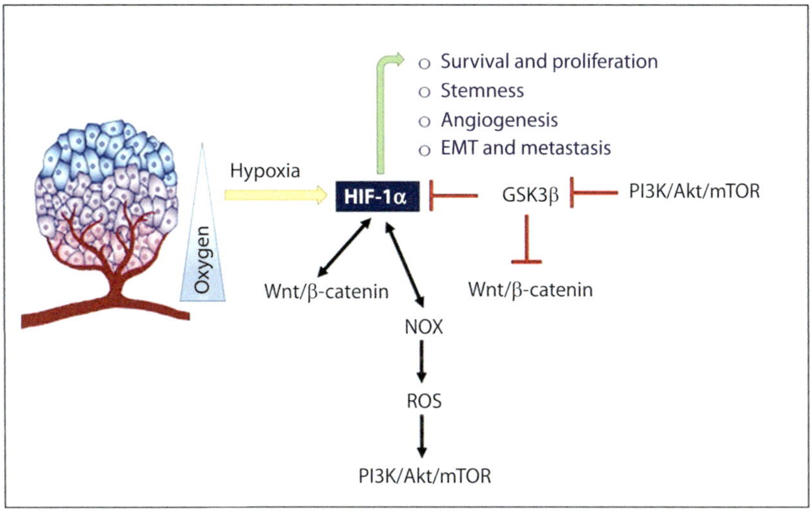

FIGURE 11.4 Basic functions of HIF-1α and its signaling in hypoxic cancer cells.

is critical, as CAFs can be activated by HIF signaling, leading to enhanced tumor progression and immune evasion [65].

Exosomes, which are small extracellular vesicles, also play a significant role in the communication between hypoxic tumor cells and their microenvironment. Hypoxic tumors release exosomes containing various biomolecules, including long non-coding RNAs and microRNAs, which can modulate the behavior of recipient cells and promote tumor growth and metastasis [66, 67]. For instance, hypoxic exosomes have been shown to transfer long non-coding RNA-UCA1, facilitating bladder tumor growth. In summary, the hypoxic tumor microenvironment is characterized by a complex interplay of signaling pathways and biomarkers, primarily driven by HIF-1α. This environment not only promotes tumor growth and metastasis through metabolic reprogramming and EMT but also contributes to therapeutic resistance and immune evasion. Recognizing these mechanisms is crucial for developing targeted therapies that can effectively combat hypoxic tumors.

CHALLENGES IN IMPLEMENTING HYPOXIA-TARGETED DRUG DELIVERY SYSTEMS

Implementing hypoxia-targeted drug delivery systems presents a multitude of challenges that stem from the complex biological and chemical environments of tumors. Hypoxia, characterized by low oxygen levels, is a common feature of solid tumors and significantly complicates therapeutic strategies. The tumor microenvironment is often heterogeneous, leading to variable oxygenation levels that can affect drug efficacy and distribution. This variability poses a significant hurdle for the development of hypoxia-responsive drug delivery systems, as the effectiveness of these systems is contingent upon the precise targeting of hypoxic regions within tumors [9, 33, 68].

One of the primary challenges in hypoxia-targeted drug delivery is the inherent resistance of hypoxic tumor cells to conventional therapies. Hypoxic conditions can lead to the upregulation of various survival pathways, including HIFs, which promote cell survival and resistance to apoptosis [69, 70]. This resistance is aggravated by the fact that hypoxic cells are often located further from blood vessels, resulting in inadequate exposure to systemic therapies. Consequently, the design of drug delivery systems must account for the unique biological behavior of hypoxic cells, necessitating innovative approaches to enhance drug accumulation and retention in these regions.

Moreover, the development of HAPs and redox-responsive nanocarriers has gained traction as a strategy to selectively deliver cytotoxic agents to hypoxic tumor cells [4]. However, the effectiveness of these systems is often limited by the uneven distribution of hypoxia within tumors. Many tumors exhibit areas of varying oxygenation, which can lead to suboptimal activation of prodrugs and insufficient therapeutic response [71]. This heterogeneity necessitates a more nuanced recognizing of tumor biology and the development of advanced delivery systems that can adapt to the dynamic nature of the tumor microenvironment.

Another significant challenge is the biocompatibility and stability of hypoxia-targeted delivery systems. Many nanoparticle-based systems face issues related to stability in the bloodstream and potential toxicity to normal tissues [72, 73]. For instance, the use of nanoparticles that respond to hypoxic conditions must be carefully engineered to ensure that they do not prematurely release their payload in normoxic tissues, which could lead to systemic toxicity. Additionally, the materials used in these systems must be biocompatible and capable of withstanding the harsh conditions often present in the tumor microenvironment, including acidic pH and high interstitial fluid pressure [74].

The complexity of the tumor microenvironment also poses challenges for the monitoring and evaluation of drug delivery systems. Real-time tracking of drug release and distribution within tumors is crucial for assessing the efficacy of hypoxia-targeted therapies [75]. However, current imaging techniques may not provide sufficient resolution or specificity to accurately monitor the behavior of drug delivery systems in vivo. This limitation underscores the need for the development of advanced imaging modalities that can provide real-time feedback on drug distribution and release kinetics in hypoxic regions.

Furthermore, the interplay between hypoxia and the immune microenvironment adds another layer of complexity to hypoxia-targeted drug delivery. Hypoxic conditions can influence the behavior of immune cells, potentially leading to an immunosuppressive environment that hampers the effectiveness of immunotherapies [70]. Recognizing how hypoxia affects immune cell function and how this interaction can be leveraged to enhance therapeutic outcomes is critical for the successful implementation of hypoxia-targeted strategies [70].

In addition to these biological challenges, there are also technical and regulatory hurdles associated with the development of hypoxia-targeted drug delivery systems. The translation of these innovative therapies from the laboratory to clinical practice requires rigorous testing to ensure safety and efficacy [33, 70]. Regulatory pathways for novel drug delivery systems can be complex and may require extensive preclinical and clinical data to demonstrate their benefits over existing therapies. This process can be time-consuming and costly, potentially delaying the availability of effective hypoxia-targeted therapies for patients.

Moreover, the integration of hypoxia-targeted drug delivery systems with existing treatment modalities, such as chemotherapy and radiotherapy, presents additional challenges. Combining these therapies requires a thorough recognizing of the interactions between different treatment modalities and the potential for additive or synergistic effects [33, 68]. Careful consideration must be given to the timing and sequencing of treatments to maximize therapeutic efficacy while minimizing adverse effects.

The economic aspects of developing hypoxia-targeted drug delivery systems also warrant attention. The costs associated with the research, development, and manufacturing of these advanced therapies can be substantial [33, 70]. Ensuring that these therapies are accessible and affordable for patients is a critical consideration that must be addressed by researchers, clinicians, and policymakers alike. Addressing the biological complexities of tumor hypoxia, ensuring the stability and biocompatibility of delivery systems, and navigating the regulatory landscape are all critical factors that must be considered. Furthermore, the integration of these systems with existing therapies and the economic implications of their development are essential components of a comprehensive approach to advancing hypoxia-targeted therapies. Continued research and innovation in this field are necessary to overcome these challenges and realize the full potential of hypoxia-targeted drug delivery systems in clinical oncology.

STRATEGIES FOR SUCCESSFUL IMPLEMENTATION OF HYPOXIA-TARGETED DRUG DELIVERY

The implementation of hypoxia-targeted drug delivery systems in cancer therapy represents a promising frontier in oncology, particularly due to the unique challenges posed by the hypoxic tumor microenvironment. Hypoxia, characterized by reduced oxygen availability, is a common feature in solid tumors and significantly contributes to treatment resistance, tumor progression, and metastasis. Therefore, developing effective strategies to target hypoxic regions within tumors is crucial for enhancing therapeutic efficacy. This response synthesizes various strategies for successfully implementing hypoxia-targeted drug delivery, drawing on recent research and advancements in the field.

One of the primary strategies involves the use of HAPs, which are designed to become cytotoxic only in low-oxygen environments. These prodrugs are activated by reductive processes that occur under hypoxic conditions, allowing for selective targeting of tumor cells while sparing normal tissues. For instance, the prodrug TH-302 has demonstrated efficacy in targeting hypoxic bone marrow niches in leukemia models, highlighting the potential of HAPs in treating hematological malignancies [1]. Moreover, the combination of HAPs with other therapeutic modalities, such as immunotherapy and radiotherapy, has shown promise in enhancing treatment outcomes. Evofosfamide, another HAP, has been evaluated in clinical trials and has demonstrated synergistic effects when combined with other agents in head and neck squamous cell carcinoma [76, 77].

Nanotechnology plays a pivotal role in the development of hypoxia-targeted drug delivery systems. Nanoparticles can be engineered to respond to the hypoxic tumor microenvironment, thereby facilitating the controlled release of therapeutic agents. For example, developed a hypoxia-responsive nano-drug delivery system based on angelica polysaccharide, which effectively released drugs in hypoxic conditions, leading to significant therapeutic effects against liver cancer. Additionally, the use of redox-responsive nanocarriers that incorporate hypoxia-sensitive bonds, such as azo groups, has been explored to enhance drug delivery specificity and efficacy [4]. These nanocarriers can be designed to release their payloads selectively in hypoxic regions, thereby maximizing therapeutic impact while minimizing systemic toxicity.

Another strategy involves the modulation of HIFs, which are critical regulators of cellular responses to hypoxia. Targeting HIF-1α and HIF-2α can disrupt the adaptive responses of tumors to hypoxia, potentially enhancing the effectiveness of conventional therapies [77, 78]. Inhibitors of HIF pathways have been developed and tested in preclinical and clinical settings, although challenges remain in translating these findings into effective clinical strategies. Furthermore, recognizing the molecular subtypes of tumors and their hypoxia-related gene expressions can aid in optimizing targeted therapies, as demonstrated in NSCLC [3, 14].

Molecular imaging techniques are also essential for the successful implementation of hypoxia-targeted therapies. Imaging modalities such as PET using F-18 FMISO can provide real-time insights into tumor hypoxia, allowing for personalized treatment planning [7]. By identifying hypoxic regions within tumors, clinicians can tailor therapeutic approaches to maximize efficacy. The integration of imaging with hypoxia-targeted drug delivery systems can facilitate the monitoring of treatment responses and adjustments in therapeutic strategies based on real-time data [79].

Moreover, the development of theranostic agents that combine therapeutic and diagnostic capabilities is gaining traction in hypoxia-targeted therapies. These agents can provide quantitative monitoring of tumor hypoxia while simultaneously delivering cytotoxic drugs. For instance, the theranostic prodrug NMAC4A-CyNH$_2$ has been designed to respond to hypoxic conditions, enabling targeted drug delivery and real-time tracking of therapeutic efficacy [8]. This dual functionality enhances the precision of cancer treatments and allows for adaptive therapeutic strategies based on tumor responses.

In addition to these strategies, enhancing oxygen delivery to tumors presents another avenue for improving hypoxia-targeted therapies. Techniques such as hyperbaric oxygen therapy and the use of oxygen-generating nanoparticles can potentially alleviate tumor hypoxia, thereby increasing the effectiveness of conventional therapies [9, 78]. By improving oxygenation within tumors, the efficacy of chemotherapeutic agents and radiotherapy can be significantly enhanced, addressing one of the major barriers to successful cancer treatment. Furthermore, the combination of hypoxia-targeted therapies with immunotherapy is an area of active research. Hypoxia can suppress immune responses within tumors, leading to immune evasion and treatment resistance. Strategies aimed at re-oxygenating tumors or modulating the immune microenvironment may enhance the effectiveness of immune checkpoint inhibitors and other immunotherapeutic agents [12, 80]. Recognizing the interactions between hypoxia and immune cell function is critical for developing effective combination therapies that leverage the strengths of both modalities.

CONCLUSION AND FUTURE ASPECT

Several factors that upset the equilibrium of cell survival, proliferation, and differentiation lead to cancer. The significance of tumor hypoxia in oncology and its potential as a therapeutic target have gained more recognition within the last 60 years. It may be possible to pursue novel drug discovery techniques that eventually result in better cancer treatment regimens by using tumor hypoxia to target tumors and release active medications selectively. Since bioreductive methods seem to have the best chance of success right now, special attention has been paid to them. Normal cells are essentially immune to the side effects that could be anticipated in the absence of hypoxia targeting and reductive drug release since the reductive pathways involved in prodrug activation are hypoxia sensitive and negatively associated with available oxygen concentrations. The successful implementation of hypoxia-targeted drug delivery systems in cancer therapy requires a multifaceted approach that integrates various strategies, including the use of HAPs, nanotechnology, molecular imaging, and combination therapies. By addressing the unique challenges posed by the hypoxic tumor microenvironment, these strategies hold the potential to significantly improve treatment outcomes for patients with cancer. Continued research and innovation in this field will be essential for translating these strategies into clinical practice and ultimately enhancing the efficacy of cancer therapies.

It is hoped that this book chapter would serve as a helpful manual for seasoned researchers, enabling them to deepen their knowledge while encouraging investigators who are new to the field to explore the opportunities and problems of hypoxia as a drug discovery technique. In the end, it is anticipated that these initiatives will advance the quickly developing field of personalized cancer medicine and result in new and more efficient therapeutic approaches.

ETHICS AND CONSENT TO PARTICIPATE

Not applicable.

CONSENT FOR PUBLICATION

Not applicable.

AVAILABILITY OF DATA AND MATERIAL

Data of the review are publicly published data. The study does not require ethical approval.

CONFLICT OF INTEREST

The authors declare no conflict of interest.

FUNDING

None.

ACKNOWLEDGMENTS

Declared none.

REFERENCES

1. Benito, J., Ramirez, M., Millward, N., Vélez, J., Harutyunyan, K., Lu, H., … and Konopleva, M. (2016). Hypoxia-activated prodrug TH-302 targets hypoxic bone marrow niches in preclinical leukemia models. Clinical Cancer Research, 22(7), 1687–1698. https://doi.org/10.1158/1078-0432.ccr-14-3378
2. Liew, L., Singleton, D., Wong, W., Cheng, G., Jamieson, S., and Hay, M. (2019). Hypoxia-activated prodrugs of perk inhibitors. Chemistry – An Asian Journal, 14(8), 1238–1248. https://doi.org/10.1002/asia.201801826
3. Ye, Y., Hu, Q., Hu, C., Liang, K., Yuan, Y., Yu, X., … and Han, L. (2019). Characterization of hypoxia-associated molecular features to aid hypoxia-targeted therapy. Nature Metabolism, 1(4), 431–444. https://doi.org/10.1038/s42255-019-0045-8
4. Ma, J., Zhan, Y., Xu, X., Zeng, Y., Liang, J., and Chen, X. (2018). Hypoxia-activated prodrugs and redox-responsive nanocarriers. International Journal of Nanomedicine, 13, 6551–6574. https://doi.org/10.2147/ijn.s173431

5. Jiang, X., Wang, C., Fitch, S., and Yang, F. (2018). Targeting tumor hypoxia using nanoparticle-engineered CXCR4-overexpressing adipose-derived stem cells. Theranostics, 8(5), 1350–1360. https://doi.org/10.7150/thno.22736
6. Xia, Y., Duan, S., Han, C., Jing, C., Xiao, Z., and Li, C. (2022). Hypoxia-responsive nanomaterials for tumor imaging and therapy. Frontiers in Oncology, 12, 1089446. https://doi.org/10.3389/fonc.2022.1089446
7. Rajendran, J. and Krohn, K. (2015). F-18 fluoromisonidazole for imaging tumor hypoxia: imaging the microenvironment for personalized cancer therapy. Seminars in Nuclear Medicine, 45(2), 151–162. https://doi.org/10.1053/j.semnuclmed.2014.10.006
8. Zhao, X., Gao, K., and Shi, Y. (2021). Noncovalent theranostic prodrug for hypoxia-activated drug delivery and real-time tracking. Analytical Chemistry, 93(45), 15080–15087. https://doi.org/10.1021/acs.analchem.1c03153
9. Patel, A. and Sant, S. (2016). Hypoxic tumor microenvironment: opportunities to develop targeted therapies. Biotechnology Advances, 34(5), 803–812. https://doi.org/10.1016/j.biotechadv.2016.04.005
10. Janji, B. and Chouaïb, S. (2022). The promise of targeting hypoxia to improve cancer immunotherapy: mirage or reality?. Frontiers in Immunology, 13. https://doi.org/10.3389/fimmu.2022.880810
11. Salem, A., Asselin, M., Reymen, B., Jackson, A., Lambin, P., West, C., … and Faivre-Finn, C. (2017). Targeting hypoxia to improve non–small cell lung cancer outcome. JNCI Journal of the National Cancer Institute, 110(1), 14–30. https://doi.org/10.1093/jnci/djx160
12. Harris, B., Saleem, S., Cook, N., and Searle, E. (2022). Targeting hypoxia in solid and haematological malignancies. Journal of Experimental and Clinical Cancer Research, 41(1). https://doi.org/10.1186/s13046-022-02522-y
13. Lee, T. (2024). Clinical relevance and therapeutic predictive ability of hypoxia biomarkers in head and neck cancer tumour models. Molecular Oncology, 18(8), 1885–1903. https://doi.org/10.1002/1878-0261.13620
14. Lin, J., Chen, S., Xiao, L., Wang, Z., Lin, Y., and Xu, S. (2022). Identifying molecular subtypes and 6-gene prognostic signature based on hypoxia for optimizing targeted therapies in non-small cell lung cancer. International Journal of General Medicine, 15, 4417–4432.
15. Ikeda, Y., Hisano, H., Nishikawa, Y., and Nagasaki, Y. (2016). Targeting and treatment of tumor hypoxia by newly designed prodrug possessing high permeability in solid tumors. Molecular Pharmaceutics, 13(7), 2283–2289. https://doi.org/10.1021/acs.molpharmaceut.6b00011
16. Cheng, Z., Huang, Y., Shao, P., Wang, L., Zhu, S., Yu, J., … and Lü, W. (2021). Hypoxia-activated albumin-binding exatecan prodrug for cancer therapy. ACS Omega, 7(1), 1082–1089. https://doi.org/10.1021/acsomega.1c05671
17. Karnthaler-Benbakka, C., Groza, D., Koblmüller, B., Terenzi, A., Holste, K., Haider, M., … and Keppler, B. (2016). Targeting a targeted drug: an approach toward hypoxia-activatable tyrosine kinase inhibitor prodrugs. Chemmedchem, 11(21), 2410–2421. https://doi.org/10.1002/cmdc.201600417
18. Hunter, F., Hsu, H., Su, J., Pullen, S., Wilson, W., and Wang, J. (2014). Dual targeting of hypoxia and homologous recombination repair dysfunction in triple-negative breast cancer. Molecular Cancer Therapeutics, 13(11), 2501–2514. https://doi.org/10.1158/1535-7163.mct-14-0476
19. Ashoorzadeh, A., Guise, C., Mowday, A., Mittra, R., Silva, S., Hicks, K., … and Patterson, A. (2021). Restoring tumour selectivity of the bioreductive prodrug PR-104 by developing an analogue resistant to aerobic metabolism by human Aldo-Keto reductase 1C3. Pharmaceuticals, 14(12), 1231. https://doi.org/10.3390/ph14121231
20. Ashoorzadeh, A., Mowday, A., Guise, C., Silva, S., Bull, M., Copp, J., … and Smaill, J. (2022). Interrogation of the structure–activity relationship of a lipophilic nitroaromatic prodrug series designed for cancer gene therapy applications. Pharmaceuticals, 15(2), 185. https://doi.org/10.3390/ph15020185
21. Foehrenbacher, A., Patel, K., Abbattista, M., Guise, C., Secomb, T., Wilson, W., … and Hicks, K. (2013). The role of bystander effects in the antitumor activity of the hypoxia-activated prodrug PR-104. Frontiers in Oncology, 3. https://doi.org/10.3389/fonc.2013.00263
22. Yang, Y., Lu, Y., Abbaraju, P., Azimi, I., Lei, C., Tang, J., … and Liu, C. (2018). Stepwise degradable nanocarriers enabled cascade delivery for synergistic cancer therapy. Advanced Functional Materials, 28(28), 1800706. https://doi.org/10.1002/adfm.201800706
23. Tosun, C., Mallerman, M., Wallabregue, A., Phillips, S., Edwards, C., Conway, S., … and Hammond, E. (2023). Antibody-based imaging of bioreductive prodrug release in hypoxia. ChemRxiv. https://doi.org/10.26434/chemrxiv-2023-9n5s0
24. Bhuniya, S. (2024). Hypoxia-activated theragnostic prodrugs (HATPs): current state and future perspectives. Pharmaceutics, 16(4), 557. https://doi.org/10.3390/pharmaceutics16040557

25. Wang, Y., Shang, W., Niu, M., Hui, H., and Xu, K. (2019). Hypoxia-active nanoparticles used in tumor theranostic. International Journal of Nanomedicine, 14, 3705–3722. https://doi.org/10.2147/ijn.s196959
26. Mistry, I., Thomas, M., Calder, E., Conway, S., and Hammond, E. (2017). Clinical advances of hypoxia-activated prodrugs in combination with radiation therapy. International Journal of Radiation Oncology, Biology, Physics, 98(5), 1183–1196. https://doi.org/10.1016/j.ijrobp.2017.03.024
27. Sharma, A., Arambula, J., Koo, S., Kumar, R., Singh, H., Sessler, J., … and Kim, J. (2019). Hypoxia-targeted drug delivery. Chemical Society Reviews, 48(3), 771–813. https://doi.org/10.1039/c8cs00304a
28. Skwarska, A., Calder, E., Sneddon, D., Bolland, H., Odyniec, M., Mistry, I., … and Hammond, E. (2021). Development and pre-clinical testing of a novel hypoxia-activated KDAC inhibitor. Cell Chemical Biology, 28(9), 1258–1270.e13. https://doi.org/10.1016/j.chembiol.2021.04.004
29. Jayaprakash, P., Ai, M., Liu, A., Budhani, P., Bartkowiak, T., Sheng, J., … and Curran, M. (2018). Targeted hypoxia reduction restores T cell infiltration and sensitizes prostate cancer to immunotherapy. Journal of Clinical Investigation, 128(11), 5137–5149. https://doi.org/10.1172/jci96268
30. Thambi, T., Park, J., and Lee, S. (2016). Hypoxia-responsive nanocarriers for cancer imaging and therapy: Recent approaches and future perspectives. Chemical Communications, 52(55), 8492–8500. https://doi.org/10.1039/c6cc02972h
31. Han, H., Zhang, Y., Dai, X., Zhang, W., Foda, M., Zhang, J., … and Han, H. (2021). Selective thrombosis of tumor for enhanced hypoxia-activated prodrug therapy. Advanced Materials, 33(41). https://doi.org/10.1002/adma.202104504
32. Yang, D., Wen, L., Du, L., Luo, C., Lu, Z., Liu, J., … and Lin, Z. (2022). A hypoxia-activated prodrug conjugated with a bodipy-based photothermal agent for imaging-guided chemo-photothermal combination therapy. ACS Applied Materials and Interfaces, 14(36), 40546–40558. https://doi.org/10.1021/acsami.2c09071
33. Alimoradi, H., Matikonda, S., Gamble, A., Giles, G., and Greish, K (2016). Hypoxia responsive drug delivery systems in tumor therapy. Current Pharmaceutical Design, 22(19), 2808–2820. https://doi.org/10.2174/1381612822666160217130049
34. Zhao, X., Ha, W., Gao, K., and Shi, Y. (2020). Precisely traceable drug delivery of azoreductase-responsive prodrug for colon targeting via multimodal imaging. Analytical Chemistry, 92(13), 9039–9047. https://doi.org/10.1021/acs.analchem.0c01220
35. Lindsay, D., Garvey, C., Mumenthaler, S., and Foo, J. (2016). Leveraging hypoxia-activated prodrugs to prevent drug resistance in solid tumors. PLoS Computational Biology, 12(8), e1005077. https://doi.org/10.1371/journal.pcbi.1005077
36. Graham, K. and Unger, E. (2018). Overcoming tumor hypoxia as a barrier to radiotherapy, chemotherapy and immunotherapy in cancer treatment. International Journal of Nanomedicine, 13, 6049–6058. https://doi.org/10.2147/ijn.s140462
37. Liu, Q., Wang, X., Li, J., Wang, J., Sun, G., Zhang, N., Ren, T., Zhao, L., & Zhong, R. (2021). Development and biological evaluation of AzoBGNU: A novel hypoxia-activated DNA crosslinking prodrug with AGT-inhibitory activity. Biomedicine and Pharmacotherapy, 144, 112338.
38. Zhang, X., Wu, M., Li, J., Lan, S., Zeng, Y., Liu, X., … and Liu, J. (2018). Light-enhanced hypoxia-response of conjugated polymer nanocarrier for successive synergistic photodynamic and chemo-therapy. ACS Applied Materials and Interfaces, 10(26), 21909–21919. https://doi.org/10.1021/acsami.8b06491
39. Zhang, P., Yang, H., Shen, W., Liu, W., Chen, L., and Xiao, C. (2020). Hypoxia-responsive polypeptide nanoparticles loaded with doxorubicin for breast cancer therapy. ACS Biomaterials Science and Engineering, 6(4), 2167–2174. https://doi.org/10.1021/acsbiomaterials.0c00125
40. Shi, H., Chen, L., Liu, Y., Wen, Q., Lin, S., Wen, Q., … and Shao, F. (2023). Bacteria-driven tumor microenvironment-sensitive nanoparticles targeting hypoxic regions enhances the chemotherapy outcome of lung cancer. International Journal of Nanomedicine, 18, 1299–1315. https://doi.org/10.2147/ijn.s396863
41. Wang, X., Wu, M., Li, H., Jiang, J., Zhou, S., Chen, W., … and Jiang, X. (2022). Enhancing penetration ability of semiconducting polymer nanoparticles for sonodynamic therapy of large solid tumor. Advanced Science, 9(6). https://doi.org/10.1002/advs.202104125
42. Du, S., Xiong, H., Xu, C., Lu, Y., & Yao, J. (2019). Attempts to strengthen and simplify the tumor vascular normalization strategy using tumor vessel normalization promoting nanomedicines. Biomaterials Science, 7(3). https://doi.org/10.1039/c8bm01350k
43. Li, W., Zhao, X., Du, B., Li, X., Liu, S., Yang, X. Y., Ding, H., Yang, W., Pan, F., Wu, X., Qin, L., & Pan, Y. (2016). Gold nanoparticle-mediated targeted delivery of recombinant human endostatin normalizes tumour vasculature and improves cancer therapy. Scientific Reports, 6, 30619. https://doi.org/10.1038/srep30619

44. Cui D, Huang J, Zhen X, Li J, Jiang Y, Pu K. A semiconducting polymer nano-prodrug for hypoxia-activated photodynamic cancer therapy. Angewandte Chemie International Edition. 2019;58(18): 5920–5924. https://doi.org/10.1002/anie.201814730. Epub 2019 Mar 26. PMID: 30793456.
45. Singh, R., Nörret, M., House, M., Galabura, Y., Bradshaw, M., Ho, D., … and Iyer, K. (2015). Dose-dependent therapeutic distinction between active and passive targeting revealed using transferrin-coated PGMA nanoparticles. Small, 12(3), 351–359. https://doi.org/10.1002/smll.201502730
46. Dutta, D., Zhou, Q., Mukerabigwi, J., Lu, N., and Ge, Z. (2021). Hypoxia-responsive polyprodrug nanocarriers for near-infrared light-boosted photodynamic chemotherapy. Biomacromolecules, 22(11), 4857–4870. https://doi.org/10.1021/acs.biomac.1c01152
47. Boedtkjer, E., & Pedersen, S. F. (2020). The acidic tumor microenvironment as a driver of cancer. Annual Review of Physiology, 82. https://doi.org/10.1146/annurev-physiol-021119-034627
48. Chu, S., Shi, X., Tian, Y., & Gao, F. (2022). pH-responsive polymer nanomaterials for tumor therapy. Frontiers in Oncology, 12, 855019.
49. Wang, Z., Cheng, Q., Jiang, X., Chu, X., Li, B., Zhang, L., Wu, W., Li, J., Narain, R. (2024). pH/Hypoxia dual-stimuli responsive COF nanocarriers with reversible charge conversions for the accurate tumor-targeting and enhanced anticancer drug delivery. Colloids and Surfaces A: Physicochemical and Engineering Aspects, 703(1), 135277.
50. Dutta, D., Ray, P., De, A., Ghosh, A., Hazra, R.S., Ghosh, P., Banerjee, S., Diaz, F.J., Upadhyay, S.P., Quadir, M., Banerjee, S.K. (2024). pH-responsive targeted nanoparticles release ERK-inhibitor in the hypoxic zone and sensitize free gemcitabine in mutant K-Ras-addicted pancreatic cancer cells and mouse model. PLoS One, 19(4), e0297749.
51. Zhang, Z., Feng, J., Zhang, T., Gao, A., & Sun, C. (2023). Application of tumor pH/hypoxia-responsive nanoparticles for combined photodynamic therapy and hypoxia-activated chemotherapy. Frontiers in Bioengineering and Biotechnology, 11. https://doi.org/10.3389/fbioe.2023.1197404
52. An, L., Wang, Y., Lin, J., Tian, Q., Xie, Y., Hu, J., … and Yang, S. (2019). Macrophages-mediated delivery of small gold nanorods for tumor hypoxia photoacoustic imaging and enhanced photothermal therapy. ACS Applied Materials and Interfaces, 11(17), 15251–15261. https://doi.org/10.1021/acsami.9b00495
53. Nguyen, A. and Kim, H. (2023). Recent developments in PET and SPECT radiotracers as radiopharmaceuticals for hypoxia tumors. Pharmaceutics, 15(7), 1840. https://doi.org/10.3390/pharmaceutics15071840
54. Huizing, F., Hoeben, B., Lok, J., Boerman, O., Heskamp, S., and Bussink, J. (2021). Imaging carbonic anhydrase IX as a method for monitoring hypoxia-related radioresistance in preclinical head and neck cancer models. Physics and Imaging in Radiation Oncology, 19, 145–150. https://doi.org/10.1016/j.phro.2021.08.004
55. Véra, P., Thureau, S., Chaumet-Riffaud, P., Modzelewski, R., Bohn, P., Vermandel, M., … and Dubray, B. (2017). Phase II study of a radiotherapy total dose increase in hypoxic lesions identified by 18F-misonidazole PET/CT in patients with non–small cell lung carcinoma (RTEP5 study). Journal of Nuclear Medicine, 58(7), 1045–1053. https://doi.org/10.2967/jnumed.116.188367
56. Hu, Y., Wu, D., Tian, C., Zhang, W., Wei, Q., and Bian, Y. (2019). Evaluating changes of tumor hypoxia using $^{99}Tc^{m}$-MNLS hypoxic imaging. Iranian Journal of Radiology, 16(4). https://doi.org/10.5812/iranjradiol.86127
57. Muzi, M., Peterson, L., O'Sullivan, J., Fink, J., Rajendran, J., McLaughlin, L., … and Krohn, K. (2015). 18F-fluoromisonidazole quantification of hypoxia in human cancer patients using image-derived blood surrogate tissue reference regions. Journal of Nuclear Medicine, 56(8), 1223–1228. https://doi.org/10.2967/jnumed.115.158717
58. Lyng, H. and Malinen, E. (2017). Hypoxia in cervical cancer: From biology to imaging. Clinical and Translational Imaging, 5(4), 373–388. https://doi.org/10.1007/s40336-017-0238-7
59. Peeters, S., Zegers, C., Biemans, R., Lieuwes, N., Stiphout, R., Yaromina, A., … and Dubois, L. (2015). Th-302 in combination with radiotherapy enhances the therapeutic outcome and is associated with pretreatment [^{18}F]HX4 hypoxia pet imaging. Clinical Cancer Research, 21(13), 2984–2992. https://doi.org/10.1158/1078-0432.ccr-15-0018
60. Kim, H. (2021). *Development of a PET/EPRI combined imaging system for assessing tumor hypoxia.* https://doi.org/10.48550/arxiv.2101.11723
61. Feng, X., Li, Y., Zhang, S., Li, C., and Tian, J. (2022). Quantitative hypoxia mapping using a self-calibrated activatable nanoprobe. Journal of Nanobiotechnology, 20(1). https://doi.org/10.1186/s12951-022-01341-9
62. Wang, Y., Wang, H., Li, J., Entenberg, D., Xue, A., Wang, W., … and Condeelis, J. (2016). Direct visualization of the phenotype of hypoxic tumor cells at single cell resolution in vivo using a new hypoxia probe. Intravital, 5(2), e1187803. https://doi.org/10.1080/21659087.2016.1187803

63. Matsumoto, S., Kishimoto, S., Saito, K., Takakusagi, Y., Munasinghe, J., Devasahayam, N., … and Krishna, M. (2018). Metabolic and physiologic imaging biomarkers of the tumor microenvironment predict treatment outcome with radiation or a hypoxia-activated prodrug in mice. Cancer Research, 78(14), 3783–3792. https://doi.org/10.1158/0008-5472.can-18-0491
64. Petrova, V., Annicchiarico-Petruzzelli, M., Melino, G., and Amelio, I. (2018). The hypoxic tumour microenvironment. Oncogenesis, 7(1). https://doi.org/10.1038/s41389-017-0011-9
65. Rankin, E. and Giaccia, A. (2016). Hypoxic control of metastasis. Science, 352(6282), 175–180. https://doi.org/10.1126/science.aaf4405
66. Lv, W., Liu, Q., An, J., and Song, X. (2019). Scutellarin inhibits hypoxia-induced epithelial-mesenchymal transition in bladder cancer cells. Journal of Cellular Physiology, 234(12), 23169–23175. https://doi.org/10.1002/jcp.28883
67. Terry, S., Buart, S., and Chouaïb, S. (2017). Hypoxic stress-induced tumor and immune plasticity, suppression, and impact on tumor heterogeneity. Frontiers in Immunology, 8, 1625. https://doi.org/10.3389/fimmu.2017.01625
68. Shaikh, D., Zhou, Q., Chen, T., Ibe, J., Raj, J., and Zhou, G. (2012). Camp-dependent protein kinase is essential for hypoxia-mediated epithelial–mesenchymal transition, migration, and invasion in lung cancer cells. Cellular Signalling, 24(12), 2396–2406. https://doi.org/10.1016/j.cellsig.2012.08.007
69. Roy, S., Kumaravel, S., Sharma, A., Duran, C., Bayless, K., and Chakraborty, S. (2020). Hypoxic tumor microenvironment: Implications for cancer therapy. Experimental Biology and Medicine, 245(13), 1073–1086. https://doi.org/10.1177/1535370220934038
70. Lv, Y., Zhao, S., Han, J., Zheng, L., Yang, Z., and Zhao, L. (2015). Hypoxia-inducible factor-1andamp;alpha; induces multidrug resistance protein in colon cancer. Oncotargets and Therapy, 1941. https://doi.org/10.2147/ott.s82835
71. Lama-Sherpa, T., Das, S., Hinshaw, D., Kammerud, S., Song, P., Alsheikh, H., … and Shevde, L. (2021). Quantitative longitudinal imaging reveals that inhibiting hedgehog activity alleviates the hypoxic tumor landscape. Molecular Cancer Research, 20(1), 150–160. https://doi.org/10.1158/1541 7786.mcr-21-0257
72. Liao, C., Zheng, C., and Wang, L. (2020). Down-regulation of FOXR2 inhibits hypoxia-driven ROS-induced migration and invasion of thyroid cancer cells via regulation of the hedgehog pathway. Clinical and Experimental Pharmacology and Physiology, 47(6), 1076–1082. https://doi.org/10.1111/1440-1681.13286
73. Kim, I., Choi, S., Yoo, S., Lee, M., and Kim, I. (2022). Cancer-associated fibroblasts in the hypoxic tumor microenvironment. Cancers, 14(14), 3321. https://doi.org/10.3390/cancers14143321
74. Xue, M., Chen, W., An, X., Wang, R., Chen, H., Pan, J., … and Xu, L. (2017). Hypoxic exosomes facilitate bladder tumor growth and development through transferring long non-coding RNA-UCA1. Molecular Cancer, 16(1). https://doi.org/10.1186/s12943-017-0714-8
75. Sun, X., Zhou, Z., Zhang, Y., Wang, J., Zhao, X., Jin, L., … and Ye, L. (2021). Identification and validation of a hypoxia-related prognostic and immune microenvironment signature in bladder cancer. Cancer Cell International, 21(1). https://doi.org/10.1186/s12935-021-01954-4
76. Smith, P., McKeown, S., and Patterson, L. (2022). Targeting DNA topoisomerase IIα (TOP2A) in the hypoxic tumour microenvironment using unidirectional hypoxia-activated prodrugs (uHAPs). IUBMB Life, 75(1), 40–54. https://doi.org/10.1002/iub.2619
77. Wang, H., Zhao, L., Zhu, L., Wang, Y., Pan, D., Yao, J., … and Guo, Q. (2013). Wogonin reverses hypoxia resistance of human colon cancer HCT116 cells via downregulation of HIF-1α and glycolysis, by inhibiting PI3K/AKT signaling pathway. Molecular Carcinogenesis, 53(S1), E107–E118. https://doi.org/10.1002/mc.22052
78. Jing, X., Yang, F., Shao, C., Wei, K., Xie, M., Shen, H., … and Shu, Y. (2019). Role of hypoxia in cancer therapy by regulating the tumor microenvironment. Molecular Cancer, 18(1). https://doi.org/10.1186/s12943-019-1089-9
79. Zhu, R., He, H., Liu, Y., Cao, D., Jin, Y., Duan, S., … and Yin, L. (2019). Cancer-selective bioreductive chemotherapy mediated by dual hypoxia-responsive nanomedicine upon photodynamic therapy-induced hypoxia aggravation. Biomacromolecules, 20(7), 2649–2656. https://doi.org/10.1021/acs.biomac.9b00428
80. Pullan, J., Dailey, K., Bhallamudi, S., Li, F., Alhalhooly, L., Froberg, J., … and Mallik, S. (2022). Modified bovine milk exosomes for doxorubicin delivery to triple-negative breast cancer cells. ACS Applied Bio Materials, 5(5), 2163–2175. https://doi.org/10.1021/acsabm.2c00015

12 Enhancing Drug Efficacy in Hypoxic Tumor Microenvironments

Nalini Devarajan
Department of Research, Meenakshi Academy of Higher Education and Research, (Deemed to be University), Chennai, Tamil Nadu, India
Faculty of Allied Health Sciences, Meenakshi Academy of Higher Education and Research (Deemed to be University), Chennai, Tamil Nadu, India

Senthil Kumar Ganesan
Laboratory of Functional Genomics, Structural Biology & Bioinformatics Division, CSIR-Indian Institute of Chemical Biology, Salt Lake, Kolkata, India
Academy of Scientific and Innovative Research (AcSIR), Ghaziabad, Uttar Pradesh, India

INTRODUCTION

Cancer remains one of the most formidable challenges in modern medicine, primarily due to its complex, adaptive nature, which demands innovative and multifaceted therapeutic approaches [1]. Among the myriad obstacles to effective cancer treatment, the tumor microenvironment (TME)—and specifically tumor hypoxia—stands out as a critical determinant of therapeutic resistance and disease progression. Hypoxia, characterized by low oxygen levels within tumors, is a hallmark of most solid malignancies [2]. It profoundly influences tumor biology, driving progression, immune evasion, and resistance to conventional treatments, including radiotherapy, chemotherapy, and immunotherapy, the details of which are illustrated in Figure 12.1. Consequently, targeting tumor hypoxia has emerged as a promising strategy to enhance therapeutic outcomes and improve patient prognoses [3–5].

At the cellular level, tumor hypoxia is governed by hypoxia-inducible factors (HIFs), which serve as master regulators of the adaptive response to oxygen deprivation. Dysregulation of HIF signaling is a common feature across diverse cancer types and is closely associated with increased tumor aggressiveness, metastasis, and therapeutic resistance. HIF-mediated processes promote angiogenesis, metabolic reprogramming, and immune modulation, collectively enabling tumor cell survival and fostering a pro-invasive phenotype. Hypoxia-induced metabolic rewiring—marked by increased glucose and amino acid uptake, augmented glycolytic flux, and mitochondrial alterations—further exacerbates therapeutic resistance. Additionally, the acidification of the TME, intracellular alkalinization, and the upregulation of drug efflux transporters under hypoxic conditions amplify chemoresistance, posing significant challenges to conventional cancer therapies [3–5].

Efforts to overcome hypoxia-driven resistance have catalyzed the development of novel therapeutic interventions, such as hypoxia-activated prodrugs (HAPs) and metabolic modifiers.

 DOI: 10.1201/9781003477419-12

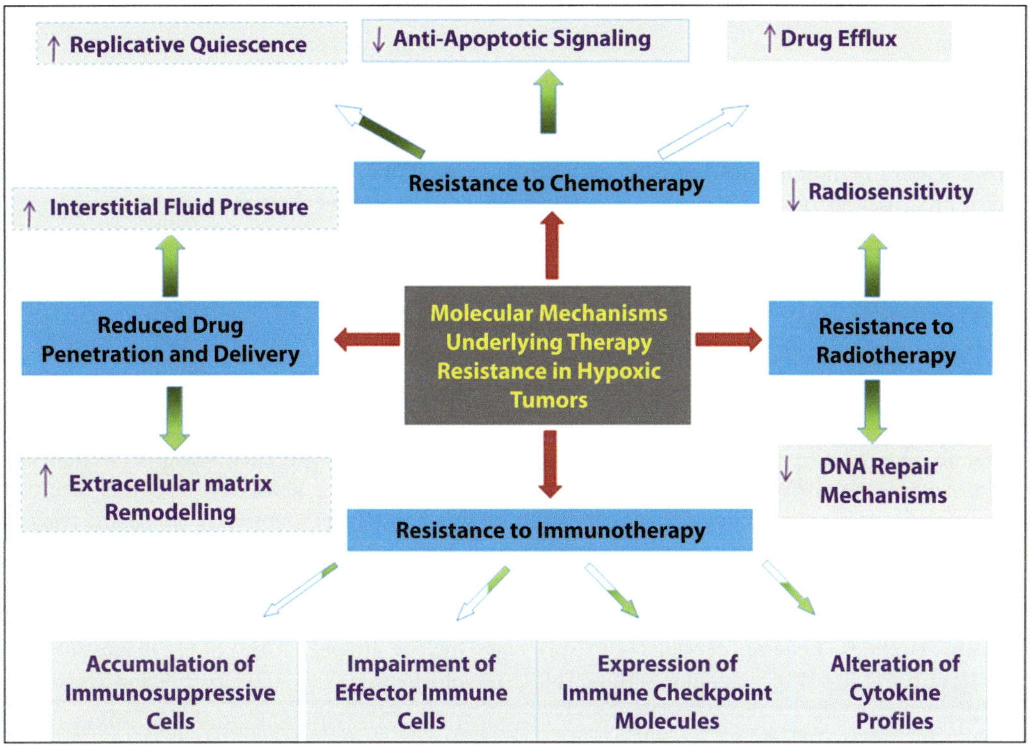

FIGURE 12.1 Molecular mechanisms underlying therapy resistance in hypoxic tumors.

HAPs are bioreductive agents selectively activated in hypoxic tumor regions, providing a targeted mechanism to counter therapeutic resistance. These agents have shown encouraging antitumor efficacy in both preclinical and clinical studies, as standalone treatments and in combination with standard therapies. Metabolic modifiers, on the other hand, aim to reverse hypoxia-induced metabolic alterations, sensitizing tumor cells to conventional therapies. The use of nanoparticle (NP)-based delivery systems has further enhanced the precision and efficacy of these approaches, enabling selective targeting of hypoxic tumor areas while minimizing systemic toxicity.

Understanding the intricate interplay between hypoxia and tumor progression necessitates the development of advanced experimental models. While traditional two-dimensional (2D) in vitro models have been instrumental in elucidating hypoxia-driven molecular mechanisms, three-dimensional (3D) cell culture models provide a more physiologically relevant framework. These 3D systems better recapitulate the structural and functional complexity of the TME, enabling the study of hypoxia-driven immunosuppressive pathways and immune cell infiltration dynamics. Such models serve as robust platforms for evaluating the efficacy of novel hypoxia-targeted therapies and combinatorial treatment regimens.

Despite substantial progress, significant gaps persist in the understanding and clinical application of hypoxia-targeted strategies. The heterogeneity of the TME and the limited translation of preclinical findings to clinical success remain formidable challenges. However, emerging approaches, including advanced NP-based drug delivery platforms, combinatorial therapies, and next-generation HIF inhibitors, hold immense promise. These strategies aim to mitigate hypoxia-mediated resistance, enhance therapeutic precision, and ultimately improve patient survival, underscoring the critical need for integrative, multimodal approaches in cancer treatment.

This chapter provides a comprehensive exploration of the pivotal role of hypoxia in cancer biology, with a particular focus on its impact on therapeutic resistance and the potential of hypoxia-targeted interventions. By unraveling the molecular and metabolic intricacies of hypoxia-driven pathways and highlighting cutting-edge therapeutic innovations, this work aspires to advance the field of precision oncology, paving the way for transformative cancer treatments and better patient outcomes.

STRATEGIES TO OVERCOME HYPOXIA-MEDIATED THERAPY RESISTANCE IN CANCER

Hypoxia-Activated Prodrugs (HAPs)

HAPs, also known as bioreductive agents, represent a sophisticated approach to cancer treatment, capitalizing on the distinct hypoxic microenvironment of tumors [6]. These drugs remain inactive under normal oxygen levels but are enzymatically reduced in oxygen-deprived conditions, releasing potent cytotoxic agents that selectively target hypoxic tumor cells while minimizing damage to healthy tissues [7]. Over the past few decades, significant advancements have been made in developing various classes of HAPs, including quinones, nitroaromatics, aliphatic N-oxides, and heteroaromatic N-oxides. Leading candidates in this class include tirapazamine [8–11], banoxantrone (AQ4N) [12], PR-104 [13], apaziquone (EO9) [14, 15], evofosfamide (TH-302) [16–20], and SN30000 [21, 22].

Since the 1980s, HAPs have undergone systematic evaluation, progressing from preclinical studies to clinical trials. While these agents have demonstrated notable anticancer efficacy, several challenges have hindered their clinical application. A primary hurdle lies in the development of advanced screening techniques to identify the most effective drug candidates for tumors with hypoxic profiles. In this regard, non-invasive imaging technologies such as PET/CT have shown considerable promise, enabling precise visualization of HAP distribution and real-time monitoring of therapeutic responses [19].

Another critical aspect of optimizing HAP therapy involves identifying biomarkers to predict patient-specific drug sensitivity. The activation of HAPs depends on specific enzymes that catalyze the bioreduction process. Detecting and quantifying these enzymes in tumor tissues could provide valuable insights into individual responsiveness, thereby facilitating more targeted and effective treatment strategies.

Additionally, the transient nature of hypoxic regions within tumors presents a significant challenge. Evidence suggests that hypoxic tumor cells typically survive for only two to three days before undergoing necrosis, underscoring the need for a deeper understanding of the dynamic hypoxic TME. This necessitates a shift in therapeutic focus, integrating hypoxia-targeted strategies with approaches that address the broader tumor architecture and metabolic adaptability. To fully unlock the potential of HAPs, future research must address these limitations by refining patient selection processes, developing more robust biomarkers, and improving our understanding of hypoxia's complex role in tumor biology. By overcoming these barriers, HAPs could pave the way for a new era of precision oncology, offering targeted solutions for one of cancer's most elusive hallmarks.

Targeting Hypoxia-Inducible Factors (HIFs)

Targeting tumor hypoxia through the inhibition of the HIF pathway represents a compelling avenue in cancer therapy [23]. However, as HIF is an intracellular transcription factor with few accessible active sites, direct inhibition poses significant challenges. Initial efforts focused on compounds indirectly impeding HIF activity by reducing its mRNA expression, translation, degradation, or transcriptional activity. Examples such as PX-478 and digoxin demonstrated potential by inhibiting hypoxia-inducible factor 1-alpha (HIF-1α) protein expression through the disruption of heat shock protein 90 (Hsp90) activity. Despite promising results in preclinical models involving cancer cell lines and mice, these compounds lacked specificity and exhibited excessive toxicity, preventing their progression to clinical trials [23].

In recent years, new HIF-1α inhibitors have emerged. Chetomin, for instance, disrupts the DNA-binding ability of the HIF complex by interfering with the HIF-1/Hsp90 interaction. It has shown antitumor efficacy in human myeloma cell lines, patient samples, and prostate cancer models [24, 25]. Similarly, acriflavine, a small molecule, inhibits the interaction between HIF-1α and its binding partner p300, reducing the activation of specific HIF target genes. This has led to increased cell death in glioma cells and improved survival outcomes in both *in vitro* and *in vivo* studies [26]. Additionally, natural plant-derived compounds, or phytocompounds, such as baicalein and oroxylin, have demonstrated potential in reducing HIF activity and enhancing cytotoxicity through diverse mechanisms [27]. However, the observed cytotoxic effects of these compounds require further investigation to establish whether they are solely attributable to HIF inhibition. A key challenge with existing HIF-1 inhibitors remains their limited specificity. Most function indirectly, leading to significant off-target effects, including DNA intercalation, which interferes with DNA replication and the cell cycle.

In contrast, targeting HIF-2 has been more successful [28]. Unlike HIF-1 inhibitors, which were identified through compound screening, HIF-2 inhibitors were discovered using structural biology approaches. Two prominent HIF-2 inhibitors, PT2385 (and its second-generation derivative PT2977) and PT2399 (belzutifan), selectively bind to HIF-2α, preventing its dimerization with HIF-1β. These inhibitors have shown remarkable antitumor effects in both *in vitro* and *in vivo* models, particularly in clear cell renal cell carcinoma (ccRCC), where HIF-2 is a critical oncogenic driver. Phase I clinical trials of PT2385 and PT2399 demonstrated good antitumor activity and safety profiles, while a Phase II trial revealed substantial efficacy in treating ccRCC and other tumors associated with von Hippel-Lindau (VHL) disease, leading to Food and Drug Administration (FDA) approval of belzutifan. Despite these advancements, resistance mechanisms, such as mutations in HIF-2 preventing inhibitor binding and alternative escape pathways involving p53, have been reported. Not all patients respond equally to HIF-2 inhibition, highlighting the need for predictive biomarkers to stratify responsive patient populations [28, 29].

The discovery of HIF inhibitors offers significant potential for enhancing combination therapies. For example, HIF-1 inhibitors are being evaluated in combination with chemotherapy, radiotherapy, and immunotherapy. However, the indirect nature of current HIF-1 inhibitors complicates the attribution of therapeutic benefits solely to HIF-1 inhibition. Developing more specific inhibitors could enable more effective combinations with anti-PD-1 immunotherapies, potentially reducing PD-L1 expression in tumor cells. Additionally, there is growing interest in combining HIF-2 inhibitors with immunotherapeutic agents. Unlike other cancer types, ccRCC's PD-L1 expression is primarily regulated by HIF-2α. Preclinical studies in pancreatic ductal adenocarcinoma (PDAC) have shown that stromal HIF-2 activity can reduce the efficacy of anti-CTLA-4 and anti-PD-1 therapies, underscoring the potential of combining HIF-2 inhibition with immune checkpoint inhibitors. This approach is currently being evaluated in clinical trials, such as the combination of PT2385 with nivolumab (an anti-PD-L1 antibody) in advanced ccRCC [30].

Despite these advancements, targeting HIF in cancer remains challenging. Complete inhibition of HIF activity could cause unintended toxicity in tissues reliant on HIF for normal physiological functions. While a specific HIF-2 inhibitor has been developed, HIF-1 inhibitors predominantly function through indirect mechanisms, necessitating further research to develop more precise inhibitors.

A promising strategy to overcome these challenges lies in understanding the transcriptional specificity of HIF. Although many HIF coactivators have been identified, the mechanisms by which they collaborate to facilitate the HIF response remain unclear. Future studies should focus on delineating how HIF and its coactivators initiate transcriptional activity at individual target genes. Detailed structural investigations into the interactions between HIF isoforms and their activators could provide deeper mechanistic insights and identify new drug targets. This approach may pave the way for designing novel inhibitors that specifically disrupt these interactions, enhancing the therapeutic potential of HIF-targeting strategies while minimizing off-target effects.

Targeting Tumor Metabolism

Hypoxia serves as a selective pressure, compelling cancer cells to undergo metabolic rewiring to adapt to oxygen deprivation [31]. Central to this adaptive mechanism is the HIF-1α, a transcription factor that regulates a myriad of genes linked to cell proliferation, epithelial-to-mesenchymal transition (EMT), metastasis, drug efflux, stem cell-like properties, and metabolic reprogramming. This metabolic shift, often termed the "hypoxic signature," includes the following:

Enhanced Glycolysis: Elevated glucose uptake and fermentation to lactate provide adenosine triphosphate (ATP) and biosynthetic intermediates necessary for survival and proliferation.

Altered pH Dynamics: Acidification of the extracellular environment (decreased extracellular pH, pHe) and intracellular alkalization (increased intracellular pH, pHi) neutralize weakly basic chemotherapeutic agents and promote their sequestration in lysosomes, rendering them ineffective.

Reduced Oxidative Phosphorylation (OXPHOS): A diminished tricarboxylic acid (TCA) cycle and mitochondrial respiration reduce reliance on oxygen-dependent ATP production.

Increased Mitophagy: Enhanced mitochondrial turnover ensures sustained ATP production and metabolic flexibility.

Antioxidant Defense: Elevated synthesis of glutathione (GSH) and other antioxidant metabolites, coupled with sub-lethal mitochondrial reactive oxygen species (mtROS), primes cells to withstand oxidative damage induced by chemotherapeutic agents.

Hypoxic tumors leverage these metabolic adaptations to withstand chemotherapy-induced stress [31]. For instance, the glycolytic shift not only sustains energy demands but also drives biosynthesis essential for tumor progression. Simultaneously, altered pH dynamics impair the cytotoxicity of chemotherapeutic agents, while antioxidant defenses mitigate oxidative damage. Collectively, these mechanisms establish a robust chemoresistant phenotype.

Given the central role of HIF-1α in mediating hypoxia-induced chemoresistance, its inhibition represents an attractive therapeutic strategy. However, HIF-1α inhibitors often exhibit significant toxicity, as HIF-1α is indispensable for physiological processes such as ischemia-reperfusion response in non-cancerous tissues. An alternative approach involves targeting HIF-1α-regulated metabolic pathways to reprogram cancer cell metabolism toward a normoxic state. This strategy holds promise for enhancing chemotherapeutic efficacy and mitigating resistance.

The distinct metabolic profile of hypoxic cancer cells—characterized by high anaerobic glycolysis and reduced mitochondrial metabolism—provides a quantitative therapeutic window. Precision medicine strategies can leverage this difference to selectively target cancer cells while sparing normal tissues. Key approaches include the following:

1. *Metabolic Modifiers*: Agents targeting glycolysis, lactate production, or antioxidant defenses have shown potential in preclinical and clinical settings. While off-target effects remain a concern, the unique metabolic landscape of hypoxic tumors may enable selective targeting.
2. *Nanotechnology-Driven Drug Delivery*: NPs and liposomes can enhance the tumor-specific delivery of metabolic modifiers, improving therapeutic efficacy while minimizing systemic toxicity.
3. *Endogenous Metabolites*: Molecules such as pyruvate and melatonin exhibit chemosensitizing properties, modulating metabolic pathways with reduced toxicity compared to conventional drugs.

The integration of metabolic insights into cancer therapeutics offers a promising avenue for overcoming chemoresistance. By tailoring interventions to exploit the metabolic vulnerabilities of hypoxic tumors, precision medicine can revolutionize the treatment of aggressive and refractory cancers. Future research should focus on refining these strategies, balancing efficacy with safety, and leveraging advancements in nanotechnology to maximize therapeutic outcomes.

Through a nuanced understanding of hypoxia-induced metabolic rewiring, the development of innovative chemosensitizing strategies could transform the landscape of cancer treatment, offering hope for patients with otherwise intractable tumors.

ADVANCEMENTS IN DRUG DELIVERY SYSTEMS TO OVERCOME HYPOXIA MEDIATED

DRUG RESISTANCE

Recent advancements in drug delivery systems, including hypoxia-responsive nanocarriers, oxygen releasing therapeutics, and hypoxia-targeted molecular inhibitors, show promising results to overcome hypoxia-induced therapy resistance. By integrating these strategies with existing treatments, researchers are redefining the potential of precision medicine in managing hypoxic tumors and improving therapeutic outcomes.

Nanotechnology in Targeting Hypoxic Tumors

NPs smaller than 50 nm exhibit an extraordinary ability to penetrate cells efficiently, interact with biological systems both at the cellular surface and intracellular levels, and serve as transformative agents in cancer therapies. Nanomedicines have emerged as a promising avenue to address challenges in pharmaceutical delivery, including poor water solubility, limited bioavailability, and systemic toxicity. Despite substantial progress, only a handful of nanoformulations have successfully reached the market, such as Abraxane® (albumin-bound paclitaxel), Onivyde®, DaunoXome® (liposomal daunorubicin), Doxil®, and Myocet® (liposomal doxorubicin (DOX)). These examples underscore the potential of nanomedicines in enhancing therapeutic outcomes while highlighting the need for further advancements [32, 33].

Lipoidal Nanoparticles

Lipoidal NPs have emerged as effective tools for drug delivery due to their non-toxic nature, ease of production, and high biocompatibility. These features position them as safer alternatives to traditional nanocarriers [34]. Gliomas, a highly invasive and aggressive form of malignant brain tumor, present significant challenges to effective treatment. Hypoxia-responsive lipid-polymer NPs have been developed to tackle these issues in therapies such as photodynamic therapy (PDT), photothermal therapy, chemotherapy, and fluorescence-guided surgery [35]. For instance, NPs co-loaded with DOX, indocyanine green (ICG), glioma-targeting peptide angiopep-2, and poly(nitroimidazole) (P-(Nis)25) exploit hypoxia-responsive mechanisms for improved outcomes. Upon 808 nm laser irradiation, ICG generates a localized hypoxic environment, while DOX suppresses glioma growth [34].

Innovative formulations, such as O_2 self-sufficient liposomes (LipoMB/CaO_2), integrate calcium oxide (CaO_2) and methylene blue (MB) to generate oxygen and induce lipid peroxidation upon brief irradiation. This reduces tumor hypoxia, inhibits growth, and minimizes metastasis with minimal side effects. To ensure controlled drug delivery, lipid NPs have been engineered to release free radicals only under near-infrared (NIR) light, exhibiting a photothermal effect at 44°C. Similarly, perfluorocarbon (PFC) nanodroplets loaded with photosensitizers have been designed to overcome oxygen shortages in TMEs, significantly improving PDT efficiency [36].

Another breakthrough involves liposomal carriers like LEAF-4L6715, encapsulating trans-crocetin (TC) to enhance oxygenation in vascular tissues. This approach has demonstrated superior reoxygenation properties in vitro and extended drug half-life in vivo, with clinical trials underway to evaluate its efficacy in preoperative hypo-fractionated radiotherapy for soft tissue sarcomas [37].

Polymeric Nanoparticles

Polymeric NPs offer distinct advantages, including protection of drugs from degradation, controlled drug release, and enhanced bioavailability. Commonly used polymers include poly(ε-caprolactone) (PCL), poly lactic-co-glycolic acid (PLGA), polylactic acid (PLA), and polyethylene glycol (PEG), which can be tailored into reservoir-based (nanocapsules) or matrix-based (nanospheres) structures [38].

To address the limitations of catalase (CAT) in alleviating tumor hypoxia, researchers have encapsulated CAT within PLGA NPs. This strategy overcomes challenges such as short half-life, protease degradation, and immunogenicity by enabling the NPs to release CAT in response to hydrogen peroxide (H_2O_2). The resultant oxygen generation alleviates hypoxia and enhances therapeutic effectiveness. Additionally, platinum-based drugs have been co-encapsulated within these formulations to synergize oxygen therapy and chemotherapy [36].

Hypoxia-induced immunosuppression in TMEs poses significant barriers to natural killer (NK) cell-based therapies. To counteract this, manganese dioxide (MnO_2) NPs coated with PLGA have been designed to degrade tumor-derived H_2O_2, generating oxygen and improving NK cell cytotoxicity. These NPs also downregulate HIF-1α, thereby reducing the immunosuppressive nature of the microenvironment [39].

In leukemia treatment, PEG-, poly-L-lysine (PLL)-, and PLGA-based NPs functionalized with transferrin and loaded with daunorubicin have demonstrated increased drug sensitivity under hypoxic conditions. These transferrin-functionalized NPs represent a promising approach for hypoxia-targeted leukemia therapy [40].

Metal Nanoparticles

Metallic nanoparticles (MNPs) offer exceptional versatility in drug delivery due to their tunable surfaces and capacity for functionalization with ligands and antibodies. To address oxygen delivery challenges, PFC-loaded hollow Bi_2Se_3 NPs have been developed to release oxygen under NIR light, enhancing radiation therapy by overcoming hypoxia-induced radioresistance.

Additionally, TaO_x NPs conjugated with PFC nanodroplets and stabilized with PEG have been shown to enhance oxygen delivery and radiation energy concentration, amplifying the destruction of tumor cells [41]. Gold nanoparticles (GNPs) have also garnered significant attention for their roles in photothermal cancer therapy and radiotherapy. GNPs with silica cores and gold shells have exhibited enhanced antitumor effects when combined with radiotherapy, offering a promising strategy to mitigate hypoxia-induced resistance.

The landscape of NP-based therapies for hypoxia-targeted cancer treatment continues to evolve, offering transformative solutions to the limitations of conventional therapies. With ongoing advancements in nanotechnology, these innovative approaches hold great promise for improving therapeutic outcomes, enabling precision medicine, and offering new hope to cancer patients worldwide. The future of nanomedicine lies in its ability to integrate cutting-edge research with clinical applications, paving the way for more effective and personalized cancer treatments.

ADVANCEMENTS IN PRECLINICAL MODELS FOR HYPOXIA RESEARCH

To investigate hypoxia in preclinical settings, researchers utilize advanced models that replicate the intricate cellular, molecular, and tissue-level dynamics of hypoxic microenvironments. Two major categories—3D tumor models and organ-on-chip systems, as well as animal models—offer invaluable platforms for exploring hypoxia-related mechanisms and therapeutic strategies [42].

Spheroid and Organoid Models: Insights into Hypoxic Tumor

Microenvironments

Spheroid models have emerged as a pivotal tool for mimicking the hypoxic TME [43]. These cohesive clusters of tumor cells simulate tumor-like niches, with their utility highly influenced by factors like spheroid size (200–500 μm) and culture conditions. The size of spheroids plays a critical role in establishing hypoxia within their core. For instance, glioblastoma spheroid models integrating U87, U251, and SNB19 cell lines have been used to investigate cellular adaptation to 1% oxygen tension and their phenotypic reversion upon normoxia. This model effectively addressed how hypoxia modulates glioblastoma proliferation, migration, and angiogenesis, although questions remain regarding the duration of hypoxic exposure required to render pathological changes irreversible [44].

Spheroids also offer a unique platform for studying tumor-initiating cells (TICs) under hypoxia. One study demonstrated that spheroids enhance the clonogenic capacity of TIC cultures, highlighting hypoxia's role in fostering tumorigenic potential. This approach requires fewer cells and yields in vivo-like results, making it a cost-effective and efficient model for hypoxic TME studies [45].

Organoids, an advanced 3D model, take TME recreation further by capturing tissue-specific architecture and heterogeneity. Patient-derived organoids bridge the gap between traditional in vitro and in vivo models, offering realistic spatial arrangements of stem cell niches. For example, organoid-derived xenografts have replicated single-cell phenotypes from original tumors. Similarly, cerebral organoids have been employed to study the effects of hypoxic injury on neuroprogenitor cells, effectively mirroring in vivo conditions by simulating oxygen deprivation [46].

Despite their potential, organoids face challenges, such as limited oxygen diffusion and cell death during extended cultures. Additionally, engineering cellular complexity in a controlled manner remains a hurdle. Nevertheless, organoid platforms continue to provide critical insights into hypoxia-driven pathologies, aiding the development of targeted therapeutic strategies.

Scaffold-Based Models

Biotech companies and academic researchers are striving to create advanced 3D scaffolds that mimic TME oxygenation profiles, enabling improved drug development strategies. A notable example is the *Cell-Mate 3D®* scaffold, developed by Brit Life Sciences, which incorporates hyaluronic acid and chitosan to replicate hypoxic TME features. Though proprietary, this model underscores the value of 3D systems that replicate oxygen gradients to enhance therapeutic design [47].

A bone marrow-derived scaffold demonstrated the ability to generate oxygen and drug gradients by altering scaffold height, revealing steeper gradients than conventional 2D or 3D platforms. This innovation facilitated studying the interplay between oxygen gradients and drug resistance. Similarly, a gelatin-based oxygen-controllable platform addressed oxygen gradient challenges by using a laccase-mediated cross-linking reaction during fabrication. This hydrogel can adapt to oxygen conditions in real time, making it suitable for *in vitro* drug screening or injectable therapeutic testing [48].

These scaffold-based models pave the way for advanced therapies, offering a deeper understanding of how oxygen dynamics influence cancer progression and drug efficacy.

Microfluidic Models

Microfluidic 3D platforms have significantly advanced hypoxia studies in solid tumors by incorporating fluid-flow dynamics through innovative microchannel designs [49]. Song et al. developed a microfluidic model to systematically investigate specific TME molecular factors and their pathological effects, which are challenging to assess in complex in vivo systems. Their model utilized microvascular networks within a microfluidic chip to study the extravasation potential of breast cancer cell lines (MCF10A, MCF-7, and MDA-MB-231) under varying oxygen conditions, including normoxia (21% oxygen) and hypoxia (1–3% oxygen). This platform highlighted the critical role of HIF-1α signaling in hypoxia-mediated TME dynamics and successfully recreated hallmark tumor features, such as morphological changes and cell viability shifts [42].

Unlike earlier 2D models, which struggled with visualization and failed to elucidate factors like CXCR4-mediated cancer cell adhesion, this 3D system demonstrated key TME characteristics, including E-cadherin loss and vimentin upregulation. However, it could not fully explain the mechanisms driving these changes under hypoxia or establish a direct link between elevated HIF-1α levels and TME invasiveness, indicating areas for further refinement.

CONCLUSION

Cancer remains a significant challenge in modern medicine due to its complex, adaptive nature. The TME is a critical determinant of therapeutic resistance and disease progression. Hypoxia, characterized by low oxygen levels within tumors, is a hallmark of most solid malignancies. Targeting tumor hypoxia has emerged as a promising strategy to enhance therapeutic outcomes and improve patient prognoses. HIFs govern the adaptive response to oxygen deprivation, and dysregulation of HIF signaling is closely associated with increased tumor aggressiveness, metastasis, and therapeutic resistance.

Efforts to overcome hypoxia-driven resistance have catalyzed the development of novel therapeutic interventions, such as HAPs and metabolic modifiers. HAPs are bioreductive agents selectively activated in hypoxic tumor regions, providing a targeted mechanism to counter therapeutic resistance. Metabolic modifiers aim to reverse hypoxia-induced metabolic alterations, sensitizing tumor cells to conventional therapies. The use of NP-based delivery systems has further enhanced the precision and efficacy of these approaches, enabling selective targeting of hypoxic tumor areas while minimizing systemic toxicity. Table 12.1 summarizes the different approaches to overcome hypoxia-induced drug resistance.

TABLE 12.1
Approaches to Overcome Hypoxia-Induced Drug Resistance

Strategy	Mechanism of Action	Examples	Advantages	Challenges and Future Directions
Hypoxia-activated prodrugs (HAPs)	Prodrugs remain inactive under normal oxygen levels but are activated in hypoxic tumor regions, releasing cytotoxic agents.	Tirapazamine, evofosfamide	• Specifically targets hypoxic cells, reducing harm to healthy tissues. • Can be combined with chemotherapy and radiotherapy for improved effectiveness.	• Requires better penetration into deeply hypoxic tumor regions. • Further optimization of stability and activation mechanisms is needed.
Inhibition of hypoxia-inducible factors (HIFs)	Direct inhibition of HIF proteins or interference with regulatory pathways to suppress tumor adaptation to hypoxia.	PT2385, acriflavine	• Reduces tumor survival mechanisms such as angiogenesis and metabolic reprogramming. • Potential application in multiple cancer types.	• Off-target effects may cause toxicity. • Tumors may develop alternative pathways to bypass inhibition.
Metabolic targeting in hypoxic tumors	Disrupting metabolic adaptations such as increased glycolysis, lactate production, and alternative nutrient utilization.	2-Deoxyglucose, 3-AZD3965, CB-839	• Exploits the metabolic vulnerabilities of hypoxic tumors. • Can enhance conventional cancer treatments.	• Metabolic differences among tumor types may affect response. • Potential side effects due to systemic metabolic disruption.
Nanotechnology-based drug delivery	Utilizing nanoparticles to deliver drugs selectively to hypoxic tumor regions or enhance drug retention.	Hypoxia-sensitive nanoparticles, reactive oxygen species (ROS)-generating nanoparticles, theranostic nanocarriers	• Improves drug accumulation in hypoxic areas. • Minimizes toxicity to normal cells. • Supports combination therapies.	• Ensuring controlled and efficient drug release remains a challenge. • Large-scale clinical translation requires further development.
Liposomal and polymer-based drug carriers	Encapsulation of drugs in liposomes or polymer-based systems for targeted release in hypoxic conditions.	PEGylated liposomes, PLGA-based polymers	• Enhances drug bioavailability and retention at tumor sites. • Enables selective drug activation in hypoxic environments.	• Optimizing tumor penetration for effective drug delivery. • Stability and immune system interactions require further refinement.
Oxygen-releasing therapeutics	Introducing oxygen-releasing agents to alleviate hypoxia and restore drug sensitivity.	Calcium and magnesium peroxides, perfluorocarbon-based oxygen carriers	• Directly addresses hypoxia-mediated drug resistance. • Improves effectiveness of chemo/radiotherapy.	• Achieving sustained and controlled oxygen release. • Risk of oxidative stress and associated toxicities.
Preclinical models for hypoxia research	Developing advanced laboratory models to simulate hypoxic tumor environments for better therapeutic testing.	3D tumor spheroids and bioprinted models, hypoxia-adapted animal models, tumor-on-chip systems	• Replicates actual tumor behavior compared to traditional 2D cultures. • Allows better evaluation of drug responses under hypoxic conditions.	• Differences between model systems and human tumors need to be addressed. • Expanding accessibility for widespread research applications.
Clinical applications and personalized therapies	Integrating hypoxia-targeted approaches into precision medicine to improve treatment outcomes.	Hypoxia-specific imaging techniques	• Enables tailored treatment plans for better patient response. • Optimizes therapy selection based on tumor oxygen status.	• Need for reliable and widely accepted hypoxia biomarkers. • High costs and regulatory challenges in clinical trials.

Understanding the intricate interplay between hypoxia and tumor progression necessitates the development of advanced experimental models. 3D cell culture models provide a more physiologically relevant framework for evaluating the efficacy of novel hypoxia-targeted therapies and combinatorial treatment regimens. However, significant gaps persist in the understanding and clinical application of hypoxia-targeted strategies. Emerging approaches, including advanced NP-based drug delivery platforms, combinatorial therapies, and next-generation HIF inhibitors, hold immense promise. By overcoming these barriers, HAPs could pave the way for a new era of precision oncology, offering targeted solutions for one of cancer's most elusive hallmarks.

REFERENCES

1. Anand U, Dey A, Chandel AKS, Sanyal R, Mishra A, Pandey DK, De Falco V, Upadhyay A, Kandimalla R, Chaudhary A, Dhanjal JK, Dewanjee S, Vallamkondu J, Pérez de la Lastra JM. Cancer chemotherapy and beyond: Current status, drug candidates, associated risks and progress in targeted therapeutics. Genes Dis. 2022;10(4):1367–401. doi: 10.1016/j.gendis.2022.02.007.
2. Chen Z, Han F, Du Y, et al. Hypoxic microenvironment in cancer: Molecular mechanisms and therapeutic interventions. Sig Transduct Target Ther. 2023;8:70. doi: 10.1038/s41392-023-01332-8.
3. Shi R, Liao C, Zhang Q. Hypoxia-driven effects in cancer: Characterization, mechanisms, and therapeutic implications. Cells. 2021;10(3):678. doi: 10.3390/cells10030678.
4. Ciepła J, Smolarczyk R. Tumor hypoxia unveiled: Insights into microenvironment, detection tools and emerging therapies. Clin Exp Med. 2024;24:235. doi: 10.1007/s10238-024-01501-1.
5. Teicher BA. Hypoxia and drug resistance. Cancer Metastasis Rev. 1994;13(2):139–68. doi: 10.1007/BF00689633.
6. Baran N, Konopleva M. Molecular pathways: Hypoxia-activated prodrugs in cancer therapy. Clin Cancer Res. 2017;23(10):2382–90. doi: 10.1158/1078-0432.CCR-16-0895.
7. Li Y, Zhao L, Li XF. Targeting hypoxia: Hypoxia-activated prodrugs in cancer therapy. Front Oncol. 2021;11:700407. doi: 10.3389/fonc.2021.700407.
8. Elwell JH, Siim BG, Evans JW, Brown JM. Adaptation of human tumor cells to tirapazamine under aerobic conditions: Implications of increased antioxidant enzyme activity to mechanism of aerobic cytotoxicity. Biochem Pharmacol. 1997;54(2):249–57. doi: 10.1016/s0006-2952(97)00171-8.
9. Birincioglu M, Jaruga P, Chowdhury G, Rodriguez H, Dizdaroglu M, Gates KS. DNA base damage by the antitumor agent 3-amino-1,2,4-benzotriazine 1,4- dioxide (tirapazamine). J Am Chem Soc. 2003;125(38):11607–15. doi: 10.1021/ja0352146.
10. Hong B, Lui VW, Hui EP, Ng MH, Cheng SH, Sung FL, Tsang CM, Tsao SW, Chan AT. Hypoxia-targeting by tirapazamine (TPZ) induces preferential growth inhibition of nasopharyngeal carcinoma cells with Chk1/2 activation. Invest New Drugs. 2011;29(3):401–10. doi: 10.1007/s10637-009-9356-z.
11. Brown JM. Exploiting tumour hypoxia and overcoming mutant p53 with tirapazamine. Br J Cancer. 1998;77(Suppl 4):12–14. doi: 10.1038/bjc.1998.430.
12. Albertella MR, Loadman PM, Jones PH, Phillips RM, Rampling R, Burnet N, Alcock C, Anthoney A, Vjaters E, Dunk CR, Harris PA, Wong A, Lalani AS, Twelves CJ. Hypoxia-selective targeting by the bioreductive prodrug AQ4N in patients with solid tumors: Results of a phase I study. Clin Cancer Res. 2008;14(4):1096–104. doi: 10.1158/1078-0432.CCR-07-4020.
13. Singleton RS, Guise CP, Ferry DM, Pullen SM, Dorie MJ, Brown JM, Patterson AV, Wilson WR. DNA cross-links in human tumor cells exposed to the prodrug PR-104A: Relationships to hypoxia, bioreductive metabolism, and cytotoxicity. Cancer Res. 2009;69(9):3884–91. doi: 10.1158/0008-5472.CAN-08-4023.
14. Bando T, Kasahara K, Shibata K, Numata Y, Heki U, Shirasaki H, Iwasa K, Fujimura M, Matsuda T. Cytotoxicity of a novel indoloquinone eo9 in hypoxic non-small-cell lung-cancer cell-lines. Int J Oncol. 1995;7(4):789–93. doi: 10.3892/ijo.7.4.789.
15. Robertson N, Haigh A, Adams GE, Stratford IJ. Factors affecting sensitivity to EO9 in rodent & human tumour cells in vitro: DT-diaphorase activity & hypoxia. Eur J Cancer. 1994;30A(7):1013–19. doi: 10.1016/0959-8049(94)90134-1.
16. Nytko KJ, Grgic I, Bender S, Ott J, Guckenberger M, Riesterer O, Pruschy M. The hypoxia-activated prodrug evofosfamide in combination with multiple regimens of radiotherapy. Oncotarget. 2017;8(14):23702–12. doi: 10.18632/oncotarget.15784.

17. Liapis V, Zinonos I, Labrinidis A, Hay S, Ponomarev V, Panagopoulos V, Zysk A, DeNichilo M, Ingman W, Atkins GJ, Findlay DM, Zannettino AC. Evdokiou anticancer efficacy of the hypoxia-activated prodrug evofosfamide (TH-302) in osteolytic breast cancer murine models. Cancer Med. 2016;5(3):534–45. doi: 10.1002/cam4.599.
18. Zhang L, Marrano P, Wu B, Kumar S, Thorner P, Baruchel S. Combined antitumor therapy with metronomic topotecan and hypoxia-activated prodrug, evofosfamide, in neuroblastoma and rhabdomyosarcoma preclinical models. Clin Cancer Res. 2016;22(11):2697–708. doi: 10.1158/1078-0432.CCR-15-1853.
19. Sun JD, Liu Q, Ahluwalia D, Ferraro DJ, Wang Y, Jung D, Matteucci MD, Hart CP. Comparison of hypoxia-activated prodrug evofosfamide (TH-302) and ifosfamide in preclinical non-small cell lung cancer models. Cancer Biol Ther. 2016;17(4):371–80. doi: 10.1080/15384047.2016.1139268.
20. Stokes AM, Hart CP, Quarles CC. hypoxia imaging with PET correlates with antitumor activity of the hypoxia-activated prodrug evofosfamide (TH-302) in rodent glioma models. Tomography. 2016; 2(3):229–37. doi: 10.18383/j.tom.2016.00259.
21. Hicks KO, Siim BG, Jaiswal JK, Pruijn FB, Fraser AM, Patel R, Hogg A, Liyanage HD, Dorie MJ, Brown JM, Denny WA, Hay MP, Wilson WR. Pharmacokinetic/pharmacodynamic modeling identifies SN30000 and SN29751 as tirapazamine analogues with improved tissue penetration and hypoxic cell killing in tumors. Clin Cancer Res. 2010;16(20):4946–57. doi: 10.1158/1078-0432.CCR-10-1439.
22. Mao X, McManaway S, Jaiswal JK, Hong CR, Wilson WR, Hicks KO. Schedule- dependent potentiation of chemotherapy drugs by the hypoxia- activated prodrug SN30000. Cancer Biol Ther. 2019;20(9): 1258–69. doi: 10.1080/15384047.2019.1617570.
23. Xu R, Wang F, Yang H, Wang Z. Action sites and clinical application of HIF-1α inhibitors. Molecules. 2022;27(11):3426. doi: 10.3390/molecules27113426.
24. Viziteu E, Grandmougin C, Goldschmidt H, Seckinger A, Hose D, Klein B, Moreaux J. Chetomin, targeting HIF-1α/p300 complex, exhibits antitumour activity in multiple myeloma. Br J Cancer. 2016;114(5):519–23. doi: 10.1038/bjc.2016.20.
25. Fernandez EV, Reece KM, Ley AM, Troutman SM, Sissung TM, Price DK, Chau CH, Figg WD. Dual targeting of the androgen receptor and hypoxia- inducible factor 1α pathways synergistically inhibits castration-resistant prostate cancer cells. Mol Pharmacol. 2015;87(6):1006–12. doi: 10.1124/mol.114.097477.
26. Ma S, Wang F, Dong J, Wang N, Tao S, Du J, Hu S. Inhibition of hypoxia- inducible factor 1 by acriflavine renders glioblastoma sensitive for photodynamic therapy. J Photochem Photobiol B. 2022;234:112537. doi: 10.1016/j.jphotobiol.2022.112537.
27. Wang P, Zhu P, Liu R, Meng Q, Li S. Baicalin promotes extracellular matrix synthesis in chondrocytes via the activation of hypoxia-inducible factor-1α. Exp Ther Med. 2020;20(6):226. doi: 10.3892/etm.2020.9356.
28. Toledo RA, Jimenez C, Armaiz-Pena G, Arenillas C, Capdevila J, Dahia PLM. Hypoxia-inducible factor 2 alpha (HIF2α) inhibitors: Targeting genetically driven tumor hypoxia. Endocr Rev. 2023;44(2): 312–22. doi: 10.1210/endrev/bnac025.
29. Courtney KD, Infante JR, Lam ET, Figlin RA, Rini BI, Brugarolas J, Zojwalla NJ, Lowe AM, Wang K, Wallace EM, Josey JA, Choueiri TK. Phase I dose-escalation trial of PT2385, a first-in-class hypoxia-inducible factor-2α antagonist in patients with previously treated advanced clear cell renal cell carcinoma. J Clin Oncol. 2018;36(9):867–74. doi: 10.1200/JCO.2017.74.2627.
30. Garcia Garcia CJ, Huang Y, Fuentes NR, Turner MC, Monberg ME, Lin D, Nguyen ND, Fujimoto TN, Zhao J, Lee JJ, Bernard V, Yu M, Delahoussaye AM, Jimenez Sacarello I, Caggiano EG, Phan JL, Deorukhkar A, Molkentine JM, Saur D, Maitra A, Taniguchi CM. Stromal HIF2 regulates immune suppression in the pancreatic cancer microenvironment. Gastroenterology. 2022;162(7):2018–31. doi: 10.1053/j.gastro.2022.02.024.
31. Belisario DC, Kopecka J, Pasino M, Akman M, De Smaele E, Donadelli M, Riganti C. Hypoxia dictates metabolic rewiring of tumors: Implications for chemoresistance. Cells. 2020;9(12):2598. doi: 10.3390/cells9122598.
32. Yao Y, Zhou Y, Liu L, Xu Y, Chen Q, Wang Y, Wu S, Deng Y, Zhang J, Shao A. Nanoparticle-based drug delivery in cancer therapy and its role in overcoming drug resistance. Front Mol Biosci. 2020;7:193. doi: 10.3389/fmolb.2020.00193.
33. Wu Z, Chen J, Wang B, Wen Q, Fu S. Nanoparticle-Based drug delivery strategies for targeted therapy to hypoxic solid tumors. Chem Eng J. 2024;502:158081. doi: 10.1016/j.cej.2024.158081
34. Graván P, Aguilera-Garrido A, Marchal JA, Navarro-Marchal SA, Galisteo- González F. Lipid-core nanoparticles: Classification, preparation methods, routes of administration and recent advances in cancer treatment. Adv Colloid Interface Sci. 2023;314:102871. doi: 10.1016/j.cis.2023.102871.

35. Xu H, Han Y, Zhao G, Zhang L, Zhao Z, Wang Z, Zhao L, Hua L, Naveena K, Lu J, et al. Hypoxia-responsive lipid–polymer nanoparticle-combined imaging-guided surgery and multitherapy strategies for glioma. ACS Appl Mater Interfaces. 2020;12:52319–28.
36. Li X, Wu Y, Zhang R, Bai W, Ye T, Wang S. Oxygen-based nanocarriers to modulate tumor hypoxia for ameliorated anti-tumor therapy: Fabrications, properties, and future directions. Front Mol Biosci. 2021;8:683519. doi: 10.3389/fmolb.2021.683519.
37. Europe I de Cancérologie S. Study of Preoperative Radiation Therapy with Concomitant Liposomal Transcrocetin (L-TC) in Soft Tissue Sarcomas. https://clinicaltrials.gov/study/NCT06476704?cond=Hypoxia, cancer&page=23&rank=221
38. Zhou Q, Mohammed F, Wang Y, Wang J, Lu N, Li J, Ge Z. Hypoxia-responsive block copolymer poly-prodrugs for complementary photodynamic-chemotherapy. J Control Release. 2021;339:130–42. doi: 10.1016/j.jconrel.2021.09.023.
39. Murphy DA, Cheng H, Yang T, Yan X, Adjei IM. Reversing hypoxia with PLGA-encapsulated manganese dioxide nanoparticles improves natural killer cell response to tumor spheroids. Mol. Pharm. 2021;18:2935–46.
40. Liu P, Zhang H, Wu X, Guo L, Wang F, Xia G, Chen B, Yin H, Wang Y, Li X. Tf-PEG-PLL-PLGA nanoparticles enhanced chemosensitivity for hypoxia-responsive tumor cells. Onco Targets Ther. 2016;9:5049–59.
41. Song G, Ji C, Liang C, Song X, Yi X, Dong Z, Yang K, Liu Z. TaOx decorated perfluorocarbon nanodroplets as oxygen reservoirs to overcome tumor hypoxia and enhance cancer radiotherapy. Biomaterials. 2017;112:257–63.
42. Bhattacharya S, Calar K, de la Puente P. Mimicking tumor hypoxia and tumor-immune interactions employing three-dimensional in vitro models. J Exp Clin Cancer Res. 2020;39(1):75. doi: 10.1186/s13046-020-01583-1.
43. Riffle S, Hegde RS. Modeling tumor cell adaptations to hypoxia in multicellular tumor spheroids. J Exp Clin Cancer Res. 2017;36(1):102. doi: 10.1186/s13046-017-0570-9.
44. Alves SR, Calori IR, Bi H, Tedesco AC. Characterization of glioblastoma spheroid models for drug screening and phototherapy assays. Open Nano. 2023;9:100116. doi: 10.1016/j.onano.2022.100116.
45. Arora S, Singh S, Mittal A, Desai N, Khatri DK, Gugulothu D, Lather V, Pandita D, Vora LK. Spheroids in cancer research: Recent advances and opportunities. J Drug Deliv Sci Technol. 2024;100:106033. doi: 10.1016/j.jddst.2024.106033.
46. Gaston-Breton R, Maïza Letrou A, Hamoudi R, Stonestreet BS, Mabondzo A. Brain organoids for hypoxic-ischemic studies: From bench to bedside. Cell Mol Life Sci. 2023;80(11):318. doi: 10.1007/s00018-023-04951-0.
47. Abuwatfa WH, Pitt WG, Husseini GA Scaffold-based 3D cell culture models in cancer research. J Biomed Sci. 2024; 31:7. doi: 10.1186/s12929-024-00994-y.
48. Zhao Y, Wu Q, Zhao C, Zhou H, Wu L. Progress of structural scaffold biomaterials for bone tissue defect repair: A cutting-edge review. Compos Struct. 2024;349–350:118542. doi: 10.1016/j.compstruct.2024.118542.
49. Shahpouri M, Adili-Aghdam MA, Mahmudi H, Jaymand M, Amoozgar Z, Akbari M, Hamblin MR, Jahanban-Esfahlan R. Prospects for hypoxia-based drug delivery platforms for the elimination of advanced metastatic tumors: From 3D modeling to clinical concepts. J Control Release. 2023;353:1002–22. doi: 10.1016/j.jconrel.2022.12.009.

13 Biomarkers and Diagnosis in the Context of Hypoxic Tumors

Neha Masarkar and Sukhes Mukherjee
Department of Biochemistry, All India Institute of Medical Sciences, Bhopal, Madhya Pradesh, India

INTRODUCTION

Hypoxia is a common feature of solid tumors; the rapid proliferation of tumors outgrows their surrounding vasculature, resulting in a drop of normal oxygen levels of 2–9% to hypoxic levels of less than 2%. Regions with low oxygen levels are generally termed hypoxic regions [Jing et al., 2019]. The lack of improved outcomes from hypoxia targeting could be partially attributed to poor patient selection for hypoxia-targeted therapies. Therefore, considerable efforts have been devoted to identifying markers for tumor hypoxia. These hypoxic markers could be used to identify patients most likely to benefit from a hypoxia-sensitizing treatment regimen [Le and Courter, 2008]. Biomarkers are biological molecules produced by the body or a tumor in a person with cancer. Biomarkers are vital in healthcare as they provide valuable insights into disease diagnosis, prognosis, treatment response, and personalized medicine [Das et al., 2023]. They serve as objective indicators, enabling early detection and intervention, leading to improved patient outcomes and reduced costs [Walsh et al., 2014]. Diagnostic biomarkers are used to confirm the presence of cancer or to identify a subtype of cancer. The usefulness of these biomarkers is that proper diagnosis can lead to proper treatment and, therefore, the best chances of survival. Some screening biomarkers are also used as diagnostic biomarkers [Sarhadi and Armengol, 2022]. The diverse types of biomarkers used to detect hypoxia are hypoxia-inducible factor-1α (HIF-1α), vascular endothelial growth factor (VEGF), glucose transporter 1 (GLUT 1), PDK1, carbonic anhydrase (CA) IX (CAIX), pimonidazole, etc. Whereas HIF-1α expression is rapidly induced in acute hypoxia, prolonged hypoxia is most likely required in order to induce detectable CAIX and GLUT-1 expression. VEGF is a proangiogenic cytokine that promotes the proliferation and migration of endothelial cells (ECs) and increases vessel permeability. As VEGF expression is induced by the HIF-1, VEGF could serve as an indirect hypoxia marker [Rühle et al., 2022]. The PDK1 protein is also induced under hypoxia, and it is known to play a role in maintaining adenosine triphosphate (ATP) production, which can be used as a marker to detect hypoxia. Pimonidazole is a hypoxia-specific marker. It is administered intravenously prior to biopsy and undergoes reduction in hypoxic cells to form adducts that bind irreversibly to macromolecules [Bernstein et al., 2014]. These Biomarkers also guide treatment decisions by predicting disease outcomes and facilitating individualized treatment plans. Detecting hypoxic tumors using biomarkers involves various invasive and noninvasive techniques. Several of these modalities, either individually or in combination with other imaging techniques, provide functional and physiological information of tumor hypoxia that can significantly improve the course of treatment [Walsh et al., 2014].

TUMOR HYPOXIA

In intensively proliferating and expanding tumor tissue, oxygen demand is surpassed by oxygen supply, and the distance between cells and the existing vasculature increases, hampering oxygen diffusion and creating an even more hypoxic milieu [Muz et al., 2015]. Hypoxia is a common and important feature of solid tumors [Kamilla, 2024]. It is generally accepted that the oxygen level in

DOI: 10.1201/9781003477419-13

hypoxic tumor tissues is poorer than the oxygenation of the respective normal tissues, and on average it is between 1% and 2% O_2 and below [Muz et al., 2015]. Tissue is generally classified as hypoxic if the oxygen tension falls below 10 mmHg, compared to 40–60 mmHg in most normal tissue [Li, 2021]. This has detrimental effects on cells, as they require oxygen for their function. In tumors, hypoxia arises due to a mismatch between oxygen delivery and consumption [Kamilla, 2024]. Hypoxia is closely associated with tumor progression, increased aggressiveness, and enhanced metastatic potential, resistance to radiotherapy or chemotherapy, and lower overall survival of various tumor types [Li, 2021]. Solid tumor hypoxia is typically classified into two subtypes: acute or chronic hypoxia. These two subtypes can lead to completely different hypoxia-related responses, which may directly affect tumor development and response to treatment [Yan Zhuang, 2023]. The lack of improved outcomes from hypoxia Targeting could be partially attributed to poor patient selection for hypoxia-targeted therapies. The detection and assessment of tumor hypoxia now plays a critical role in both the validation and development of hypoxia modification therapies for their eventual adoption into routine clinical practice. Recent clinical trial data appear to demonstrate how patients identified by their hypoxic tumor status have beneficial treatment responses to hypoxia-modified therapies compared with standard therapies, while high-risk patients with hypoxic tumors receiving the control therapies performed poorly. However, despite current research into hypoxia-modification therapies, measurement of tumor hypoxia within lesions is not performed routinely and, consequently, has hindered the development of these therapies [Walsh et al., 2014]. Therefore, considerable efforts have been devoted to identifying clinical markers for hypoxia. These hypoxic markers could be used to identify patients most likely to benefit from hypoxia-sensitizing treatment regimens [Le and Courter, 2008]. Biomarkers enabling the detection and monitoring of tumor hypoxia could be highly advantageous in aiding the translation of novel normalization strategies to clinical application, alone or in combination with other treatment modalities, such as immunotherapy [Abou Khouzam et al., 2021].

Characteristics of Tumor Hypoxia

Most solid tumors are just like normal tissues in that they need a regular supply of oxygen and nutrients to be able to exist, as well as processes for the elimination of the waste products of cellular metabolism. Solid tumors meet these requirements by utilizing the host organ's blood supply, eventually developing their own functional vascular supply through angiogenesis [Horsman and Vaupel, 2016]. Compared to the well-organized blood supply of normal tissues, in tumors, the system is primitive and chaotic. The tumor vascular supply shows abnormal vascular density, contour irregularities, enlarged vessels, vessels with blind ends, and transiently blocked vessels. In addition, there is a loss of hierarchy, a lack of regulatory control mechanisms, and the vessel walls can be structurally defective, causing increased vascular permeability. These factors result in the development of diffusion-limited chronic hypoxia and perfusion-limited acute hypoxia [Sørensen and Horsman, 2020] (Figure 13.1).

Pathophysiology of Hypoxia

Hypoxia is a pathophysiological property that is defined as a state of depressed oxygen tension. Hypoxia can be present in tissues, including tumors, causing the impairment of cellular or organ functions once critical oxygen levels are breached. The proteomic and genomic transformations of tumor cells in response to hypoxia lead to permanent alterations in their cellular composition that are regulated predominantly by HIFs. HIF-1 functions as a master regulator of the cellular and systemic homeostatic response to hypoxia by activating transcription of many genes, including those involved in energy metabolism, angiogenesis, apoptosis, and other genes whose protein products increase oxygen delivery or facilitate metabolic adaptation to hypoxia. HIFs (HIF-1 and HIF-2) are heterodimers consisting of α and β subunits. Both subunits are members of the basic helix-loop-helix Per-Arnt-Sim (bHLH-PAS) transcription factor family [Zimna et al., 2015]. PAS

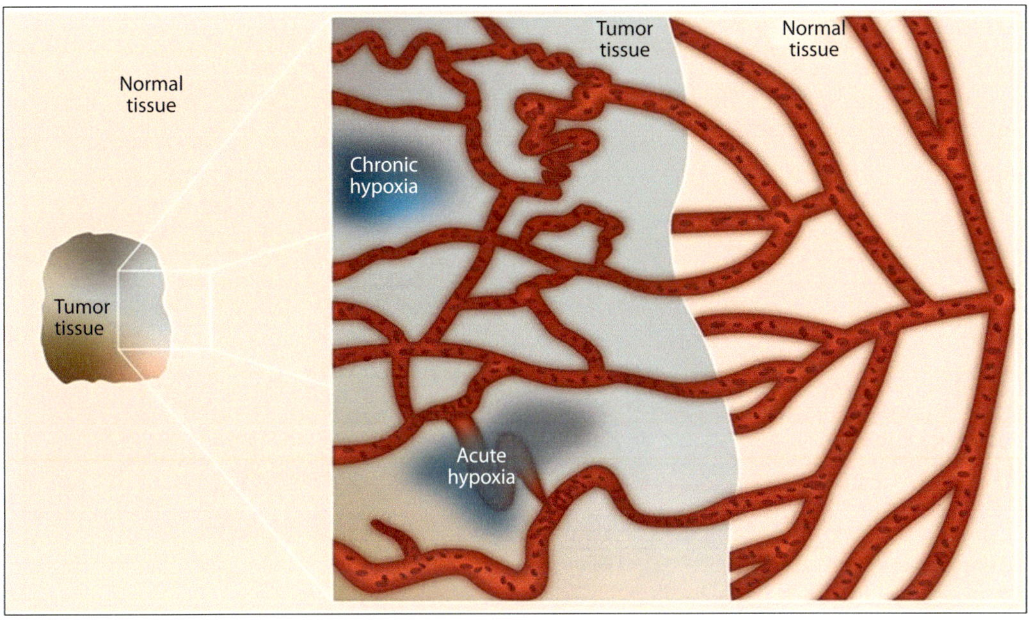

FIGURE 13.1 Schematic illustration of the vascular networks in tumors and associated normal tissues.

and bHLH motifs are required for heterodimerization between the HIF-1α and HIF-1β subunits. HIF-1α plays an integrative role in the cellular response to hypoxia. HIF-1α contains two transactivation domains known as the N-terminal activation domain (N-TAD) and the C-terminal activation domain (C-TAD). C-TAD regulates HIF-1α transcriptional activation under hypoxia, while N-TAD modulates the stability of HIF-1α [Walsh et al., 2014]. Moreover, HIF-1β is a constitutively expressed subunit, while HIF-1α, after translation, is degraded via a ubiquitination-driven proteasomal process under normoxic conditions. On the other hand, HIF-α is stabilized under hypoxic conditions [Della Rocca et al., 2022].

Under normoxic conditions, amino-acid-specific hydroxylations deactivate HIF-1α activity. Prolyl hydroxylase domain protein (PHD) hydroxylates pro line residues on HIF-1α in an oxygen-dependent fashion, enabling von Hippel-Lindau (VHL) tumor suppressor protein to bind HIF-1α for subsequent ubiquitylation and targeted degradation by 26S proteasome (Fig. 13.2). HIF-1α can also undergo hydroxylation by factor inhibiting HIF-1, which inhibits the recruitment of HIF-1α coactivators and the expression of downstream HIF-1α target genes. However, when intracellular levels of oxygen decrease, the rate of HIF-1α hydroxylation by PHD and FIH-1 also decreases. Consequently, VHL fails to bind to HIF-1α, leading to an accumulation of HIF-1α in the cell. This enables HIF-1α to interact with CREB-binding protein/E1A-binding protein p300 (CBP/p300), a transcriptional co-factor, followed by heterodimerization with HIF-1β. The heterodimer readily binds to the HIF-responsive element (HRE) of DNA, leading to the transcriptional activation and up-regulation of multiple HIF-1α target genes. Other factors affecting HIF-1α activation will be discussed in a subsequent section [Walsh et al., 2014] (Figure 13.2).

Through the onset of hypoxia, HIF-1α initiates multiple hypoxia-derived molecular processes that drive tumor growth, proliferation, and metastatic potential. Growth and survival mechanisms such as angiogenesis via VEGF, pH regulation via CA-IX, metabolism via GLUT-1, and oxygen management are upregulated in response to hypoxia. Transcription factors that control cell proliferation, cell survival via nuclear factor kappa-light-chain-enhancer of activated B cells (NF-kB), and apoptosis via signal transducer and activator of transcription 3 (STAT3, p53) are also up-regulated in hypoxic tumor cells. The up-regulation of these proteins directly influences the

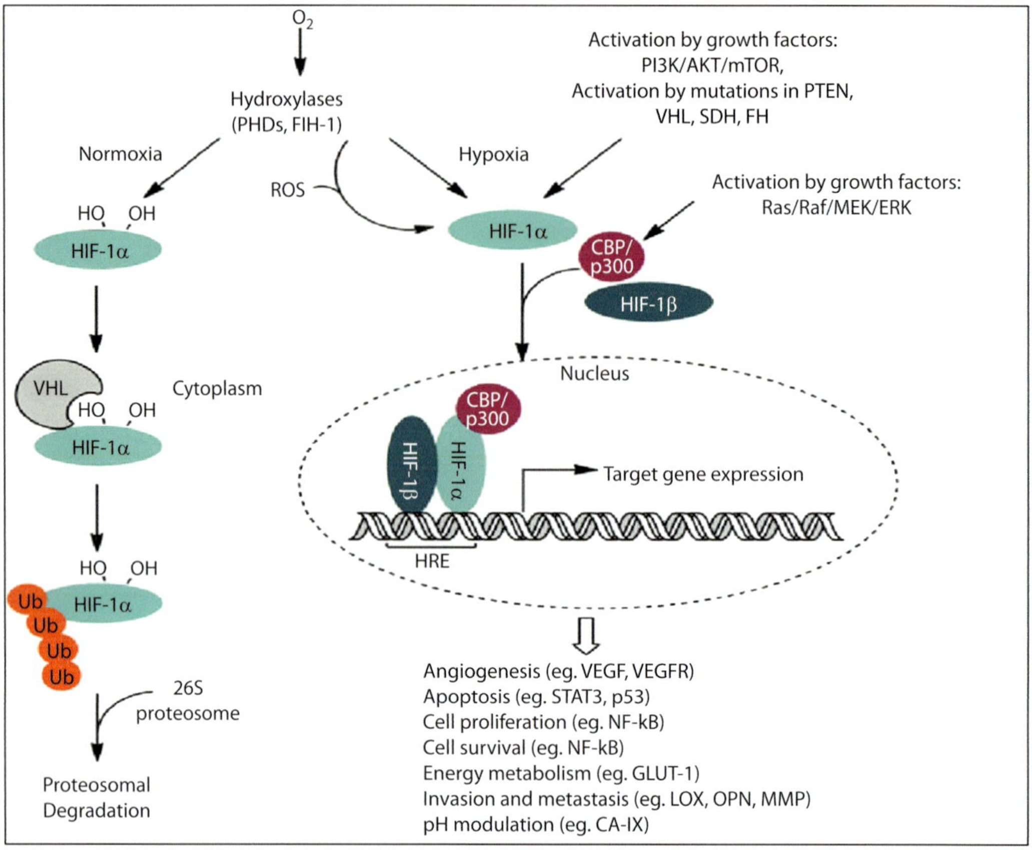

FIGURE 13.2 Regulation of HIF-1α and protein signaling under normoxic and hypoxic conditions.

malignancy of hypoxic tumors, including a propensity for the development of metastatic disease by propagating cells that have lost their apoptotic potential through decreased p53 expression, increased mutant p53 or bcl-2 protein expression, increased angiogenesis, and overall increases in proteinase activity.

BIOMARKERS

A biomarker is an objective indication of a medical state that can be measured with accuracy and reproducibility and used to identify a disease or indicate treatment response [Yang and West, 2019]. Clinical applications of biomarkers are extensive. They can be used as tools for cancer risk assessment, screening, and early detection of cancer, accurate diagnosis, patient prognosis, prediction of response to therapy, and cancer surveillance and monitoring response. Therefore, they can help to optimize decision-making in clinical practice. Moreover, precision oncology is needed for newly developed targeted therapies, as they are functional only in patients with specific cancer genetic mutations, and biomarkers are the tools used for the identification of these subsets of patients [Sarhadi and Armengol, 2022]. According to the National Cancer Institute, Cancer biomarkers are a wide variety of endogenous molecules, including DNA, transcription factors, cell surface receptors, metabolites, and secreted proteins produced by the tumor tissue or by other tissues in response to the presence of the cancer. Cancer biomarkers can also be processes, such as apoptosis, angiogenesis, or proliferation. These molecules can be found in blood, other body fluids, or tissues, and their amounts or structure modifications may indicate the tumor state, progression characteristics, and response to therapies [Silva, 2015].

USE OF BIOMARKERS TO DETECT HYPOXIC TUMORS

Hypoxia is one of such conditions where the human system is deprived of an adequate oxygen supply and requires immediate treatment. Hypoxia markers have been proven to be beneficial in the timely management of cancer [Cui et al., 2017]. They are either produced by the cancer cells or by noncancerous cells in response to cancer. The usefulness of these biomarkers is that proper diagnosis can lead to proper treatment and, therefore, the best chances of survival [Sarhadi and Armengol, 2022]. Biomarkers can be detected in the circulation (whole blood, serum, or plasma) or excretions or secretions (stool, urine, sputum, or nipple discharge), and thus easily assessed non-invasively and serially, or can be tissue-derived, and require either biopsy or special imaging for evaluation [Henry and Hayes, 2012]. Many studies have suggested that direct measurements of pO_2 in tumors or indirect staining for tumor hypoxia markers (e.g. HIF-1α-related markers) in situ can predict outcome following radiation therapy or surgery [Boström et al., 2016]. Indirect tumor hypoxia may be measured with immunohistochemistry using antibodies against intrinsic hypoxia biomarkers, such as HIF-1α, CAIX, and GLUT-1. Whereas HIF-1α expression is rapidly induced in acute hypoxia, prolonged hypoxia is most likely required in order to induce detectable CAIX and GLUT-1 expression. More advanced analyses include measurement of systemically administered extrinsic hypoxia markers, 2-nitroimidazoles, such as pimonidazole, which undergo detectable structural changes under hypoxic conditions. Radiolabeled 2-nitroimidazoles may also be detected with positron emission tomography (PET) [Boström et al., 2016].

DIFFERENT TYPES OF BIOMARKERS TO DETECT HYPOXIC TUMORS

HIF-1α

HIF-1 is a transcription factor that responds to changes in oxygen levels and enables organisms to adapt to low-oxygen environments. HIF-1 is composed of two different subunits: one α-subunit that is regulated by oxygen levels, and one β-subunit that is expressed continuously regardless of oxygen levels [Maciejewska, 2023]. HIF-1 plays a pivotal role in tumor biology, particularly in hypoxic environments. Over the past few decades, a number of HIF-1 inhibitors have been identified as potential therapeutic agents for various cancers [Bui et al., 2022]. Activating HIF-1α expression in human cancer has ties to both hypoxic and normoxic signaling pathways. Activation of the phosphoinositide 3 kinase (PI3K)/Akt/mammalian target of rapamycin apoptosis pathway leads to increased gene expression of HIF-1α. In addition, mutated variants of phosphatase and tensin homolog (PTEN), VHL, succinate dehydrogenase, or fumarate hydratase are also known to increase HIF-1α transcription. Various growth factors, such as insulin-like growth factor and epidermal growth factor, stabilize the protein under normoxic conditions. Lastly, the formation of mitochondrial ROS can stimulate the accumulation of HIF-1α. Mechanistically, ROS may oxidize iron in the active site of PHD, blocking its ability to hydroxylate HIF-1α [Walsh et al., 2014].

CA IX

CA IX is a membrane-associated glycoprotein, belonging to the family of α-CAs that catalyze the reversible hydration of carbon dioxide to bicarbonate ions and protons. Sixteen isoforms of CA have been identified in humans: five are cytosolic (CA I, II, III, VII and XIII), five are membrane-bound (CA IV, IX, XII, XIV and XV), two reside in the mitochondria (CA VA and VB) and one is secreted in milk and saliva (CA VI). Moreover, three non-catalytic isoforms have been described and designated CA-related proteins (CARP VIII, X, and XI). The over-expression of CA IX in cancer tissues is strongly regulated by hypoxia, through the HIF-1 mediated transcription. Indeed, the ability of the enzyme to neutralize intracellular pH, by facilitating bicarbonate transport across the plasma membrane, confers to cancer cells a survival advantage when they are exposed to hypoxic and acidic microenvironments. Moreover, by intensifying the extracellular acidosis, CA IX facilitates the activation of proteases that degrade the extracellular matrix, stimulating migration and invasion of the surrounding tissues [Ambrosio et al., 2016].

GLUT-1

GLUT-1 is a membrane protein facilitating the translocation of glucose across cell membranes. Due to the intensification of glycolysis under hypoxic conditions [Walsh et al., 2014]. It is ubiquitously expressed in normal tissue, and it is expressed at higher levels in a number of tumors. Hypoxia induces a reduction of mitochondrial ATP production and increases cellular glycolytic ATP production (Pasteur Effect), leading to an increase in glucose transport and consumption (Warburg effect). The latter has been considered beneficial for the survival of tumor cells, conferring a growth advantage in a relatively hypoxic tumor environment [Abbondati et al., 2013]. Indirect tumor hypoxia may be measured with immunohistochemistry using antibodies against intrinsic hypoxia biomarkers, such as HIF-1α and GLUT-1. Whereas HIF-1α expression is rapidly induced in acute hypoxia, prolonged hypoxia is most likely required in order to induce detectable GLUT-1 expression [Boström et al., 2016]. This transporter is up-regulated to satisfy the elevated glucose consumption of hypoxic cells. Multiple types of tumors display high levels of this protein, and its over-expression is associated with hypoxia in tumors of the head and neck and cervix. Poor treatment outcomes are related to the expression of this protein in cancer [Walsh et al., 2014]. More advanced analyses include measurement of systemically administered extrinsic hypoxia markers [Boström et al., 2016].

VEGF

VEGF is a frequently studied angiogenic factor in cancer and is considered to have an important role in the progression of cancer [Liang et al., 2015]. VEGF, also known as vascular permeability factor (VPF), is an adimer glycoprotein that binds to the VEGF receptor (VEGFR) on the surface of the cells. VEGFA is produced by most cells in the body but is upregulated in hypoxia. In tumors, VEGF is produced by hypoxic tumor cells, ECs, and infiltrating myeloid cells, termed tumor-associated macrophages (TAMs) [Claesson-Welsh, 2013]. Hypoxia is the principal regulator of VEGF expression, as it is a direct transcriptional target of both HIF-1α and HIF-2α [Krock et al., 2011]. The most potent hypoxia proangiogenic factors VEGF-A. VEGF-A, -B, -C, -D, and PGF are secreted and act on ECs by binding VEGFR (VEGF receptor)-1 and -2. This activates pathways that promote EC proliferation and survival, such as the ERK (extracellular regulated kinase) and PI3K (phosphatidylinositol 3-kinase)/AKT (protein kinase B) pathways. EC migration, like Rho GTPases and ECM degradation for invasion and sprouting *via* expression of MT-MMP (membrane type matrix metalloproteinase), MMP-2, MMP-9, and urokinase plasminogen activator. In addition, VEGF-A plays a key role in vascular permeability that is required for normal tissue homeostasis. Vascular hyperpermeability, due to the increased interstitial pressure in the tumor, enhances extravasation of tumor cells into the blood circulation and their metastasis. Indeed, while physiological angiogenesis gives rise to functional vessels, those arising in tumors are abnormal in structure and function, leading to inadequate tumor perfusion [Abou Khouzam et al., 2021].

PDK1

HIF-1α-induced PDK1 plays a pivotal role in regulating mitochondrial activity. PDK1 acts as a gatekeeping mitochondrial enzyme that downregulates PDH activity, decreases the oxidation of pyruvate in mitochondria, and increases the conversion of pyruvate to lactate in the cytosol [Ognibene et al., 2017]. Moreover, through screening hypoxia-related long non-coding RNAs (lncRNAs) in PDK1-positive tissue, we find that lncRNA is responsible for glycolysis and BCSC maintenance. Furthermore, knockdown decreases PDK1 expression in hypoxia, and ablation of *PDK1* counteracts mediated glycolysis and self-renewal ability *in vitro* and *in vivo*. Accordingly, PDK1 expression exhibits strong correlations in primary breast carcinomas. Let-7 releases HIF-1α, leading to an increase in PDK1 expression. Lastly, aspirin markedly attenuates glycolysis and cancer stem-like characteristics by suppressing PDK1. Thus, these novel findings demonstrate that the glycolysis gatekeeper PDK1 has a critical role in BCSC reprogramming and provides a potential therapeutic strategy for breast malignancy [Peng et al., 2018].

Pimonidazole

Due to the critical role of hypoxia in tumorigenesis, a marker that effectively identifies hypoxic areas in a tumor could provide a better understanding of how a solid tumor develops, and serve as a prognostic marker to discriminate between indolent and aggressive disease as well. One of these markers is pimonidazole, a 2-nitroimidazole-based compound that is reductively activated at oxygen levels below 1.3% and binds covalently to macromolecules [Rios-Colon et al., 2022]. Pimonidazole was originally developed as a radiosensitizer to be more effective than misonidazole (MISO), but it failed to demonstrate efficiency in follow-up clinical trials. Pimonidazole is now used as an exogenous marker for hypoxia [Walsh et al., 2014]. We have effectively utilized this hypoxic marker to identify areas of low oxygen that can harbor more aggressive cells in tumor sphere models [Rios-Colon et al., 2022].

DETECTION METHODS

Early detection and monitoring of hypoxia are crucial for timely intervention and treatment. Understanding hypoxia within a particular type of cancer can provide information regarding the relationship between hypoxia, cancer aggressiveness, and altered therapeutic responses [Perez et al., 2023]. Biomarkers, which are measurable indicators of biological status or conditions, are valuable tools for detecting hypoxia. A biomarker detects or confirms the presence of a disease or condition of interest, or identifies an individual with a subtype of the disease. Detecting hypoxic tumors using biomarkers involves various invasive and noninvasive techniques, such as polarographic needle electrodes, immunohistochemical staining, radionuclide imaging (PET, magnetic resonance imaging (MRI), and optical imaging (bioluminescence and fluorescence), each leveraging specific types of biomarkers indicative of hypoxia in the tumor microenvironment. Here are some of the key detection methods.

NONINVASIVE DETECTION

Understanding the relationship between noninvasive detection methods of hypoxia and particular types of cancer can provide new information regarding cancer aggressiveness and therapeutic responses. Several noninvasive clinically relevant imaging modalities can detect hypoxic areas within the tumor microenvironment. Additional advantages of imaging include the possibility of visualizing the entirety of the involved tissue. The most relevant techniques available to image hypoxia can be broadly categorized as molecular, i.e., positron imaging tomography (PET), functional, i.e., MRI and optical imaging [Perez et al., 2023].

Positron Emission Tomography (PET)

PET imaging was developed in the early 1960s. It is based on administering targeted drugs labeled with radioactive isotopes that are referred to as tracers [Perez et al., 2023]. Starting with

TABLE 13.1
Different PET Imaging Techniques of Tumor Hypoxia

PET Tracers	Cancers Studied
PET—18F-FMISO	• Breast • Head and neck • Lung
PET—18F-FAZA	• Glioma • Lymphoma • Lung • Head and neck • Cervical • Rectal
PET—FETNIM	• Esophageal • Head and neck • Cervical
PET—18F-RP-170	• Glioma • Lung
PET—18F-EF5	• Head and neck • Cervical
PET—18F-HX4	• Lung • Head and neck • Esophageal • Pancreatic
PET—Cu-ATSM	• Head and neck • Lung • Cervical • Rectal • Glioma • Prostate

the 2-nitroimidazole family of compounds in the early 1980s, a great number of PET tracers have been developed for the identification of hypoxia in living tissues and solid tumors (Table 13.1). Each has its own set of advantages and practical uses in PET imaging [Lopci et al., 2014].

Among these PET Tracers, 18F-fluromisonidazole (18F-FMISO) is the most widely used PET tracer derivative for detecting hypoxia. This tracer is successfully used to detect hypoxia in breast cancer, head and neck tumors, and lung cancer, and it is also used to stratify patients for radiotherapy. 18F-FMISO uptake is associated with tumor grade and expression of biomarkers of hypoxia, including CA-IX, HIF-1α, and VEGF [Perez et al., 2023]. 18F FMISO-PET relies on the entrapment of nitroimidazole compounds in hypoxic cells upon binding intracellular macromolecules, which allows for 3D visualization of intra-tumoral hypoxia [Abou Khouzam et al., 2021]. Thus, quantitative information for evaluating tumor aggressiveness, making treatment decisions, and tracking therapy response is provided by PET imaging with hypoxia biomarkers.

MAGNETIC RESONANCE IMAGING (MRI)

MRI techniques are also powerful tools in detecting and analyzing hypoxic conditions in solid tumors. Unlike PET, MRI does not use ionizing radiation. It uses a strong external magnetic field provided by a superconducting magnet and radiofrequency radiation to generate tomographic images in any plane [Smith and McCarthy, 1992]. The hydrogen atom is the most useful MRI source, as it is the most abundant element in the body. It is also the element with the highest gyromagnetic ratio, which is given as the ratio of its magnetic dipole moment to its angular momentum; this offers an advantage in MRI. However, when a subject is placed within a strong magnetic field, the nuclei tend to align in the direction of the field, producing a net magnetization, along the axis, parallel to the scanner bore [Vassiliou et al., 2018]. The contrast between different tissues is based upon multiple factors that can be explained in terms of the magnetic properties of matter [Smith and McCarthy, 1992]. MRI can detect hypoxia in a number of ways, including:

Dynamic Contrast-Enhanced (DCA) MRI

This technique can reflect a range of hypoxia levels in tumors. DCE-MRI employs the use of several contrast agents (CAs), the most common of which are gadolinium (Gd) based [Perez et al., 2023]. In this method a paramagnetic CA is injected intravenously, and the CA uptake in organs or tumors is studied by recording multiple images within a few minutes. The uptake of CA in tumor tissue depends on several microenvironmental parameters, including blood perfusion, vessel wall permeability, cell density, extracellular volume fraction, and extracellular matrix density [Gaustad et al., 2020]. DCE MRI can be used combination with other methods such as BOLD MRI, and MRSI.

Magnetic Resonance Spectroscopic Imaging (MRSI)

MRSI is an advanced MRI technique that combines both MRI and spectroscopy. MRSI detects changes in metabolites like lactate and choline, which are often elevated in hypoxic conditions. This technique uses compounds such as perfluorocarbons or hexamethyldisiloxane (HMDSO) that have oxygen-dependent relaxivity. After injecting these compounds into the tumor, oxygen tensions can be determined from changes in relaxivity [Kakkad et al., 2019].

Blood Oxygenation Level Dependent MRI (BOLD MRI)

BOLD MRI imaging, contrast rests on the balance between paramagnetic deoxyhemoglobin and diamagnetic oxyhemoglobin, and the effect of the latter on MR signals. Although BOLD MRI does not require injection of an exogenous CA, its signal can be influenced by factors other than hypoxia, including blood flow, CO_2 tension, hematocrit, pH, and biphosphoglycerate [Le and Courter, 2008).

OPTICAL IMAGING

Optical imaging is fast and easy to perform, and is relatively inexpensive compared to the other molecular imaging modalities. Optical imaging uses visible light and the special properties of photons to obtain detailed images of organs and tissues, as well as smaller structures, including cells and molecules. Some of the optical imaging methods to evaluate hypoxia, such as those used in histology, require tumor specimens to detect targeted HIFs, such as HIF-1 or VEGF. These endogenous biomarkers are frequently used to test the validity of other biomarkers of hypoxia [Daimiel, 2019]. There are two categories of optical imaging methods that produce light from two different sources.

Fluorescence Imaging

Fluorescence imaging relies on illumination of fluorescently labeled proteins or other intracellular molecules with a defined wavelength of light, ideally near the peak of the fluorophor excitation spectrum, and detection of light emitted at a longer wavelength [Ettinger and Wittmann, 2014]. Fluorescence imaging for detecting hypoxia involves using hypoxia-sensing fluorescent probes that allow the detection and imaging of hypoxia with high sensitivity and spatiotemporal resolution [Wallabregue et al., 2023]. Fluorescence imaging is typically done using a fluorescence microscope, which can excite the fluorescent probes and capture the emitted light.

Bioluminescence Imaging

Bioluminescence imaging is a highly sensitive imaging technique characterized by low background noise. Unlike fluorescence, bioluminescence does not require light observation in order to emit light at a longer wavelength [Badr and Tannous, 2011]. This imaging utilizes the light produced by a chemical reaction between luciferase and its substrate (luciferin) [Miyabara et al., 2023]. Luciferases encompass a wide range of enzymes that produce bioluminescence in living organisms. Although there are a lot of luminous species in the natural world, they are typically found in lower organisms like coelenterates, annelids, mollusks, bacteria, and crustaceans [Badr and Tannous, 2011]. Bioluminescence imaging has been useful for many applications, including monitoring HIF activity, imaging of tumor growth kinetics, detection of metastasis, evaluation of effects of genetic alterations on cancer progression, and testing of tumor response to various therapies [Viola et al., 2008].

INVASIVE DETECTION

Invasive methods to detect hypoxia involve directly accessing tissues or blood to measure parameters indicative of low oxygen levels. These techniques provide high accuracy and direct measurement of oxygen levels or related biochemical markers. This technique involves inserting an electrode into a tumor or metastatic lymph node and measuring oxygen from several points. Measurements are only taken in a point-based manner [Perez et al., 2023]. Direct O_2 measurements have been made in solid tumors of cancer patients using Oxygen polarographic electrodes, fiber-optic devices, and immunohistochemical detection. These methods are crucial in clinical settings for the precise detection and management of hypoxia.

Oxygen Polarographic Electrodes

Oxygen polarographic electrodes were developed in 1956 by Leland Clark. The polarographic electrode is a direct method for measuring tissue oxygen concentration based on the electrochemical reduction of oxygen molecules [Walsh et al., 2014]. This method plays an important role in the study of oxygen dynamics due to its high sensitivity and ability to provide real-time quantitative measurements (Figure 13.3).

Oxygen polarographic electrode is a sensor that measures oxygen tension in blood using a platinum cathode and silver/silver chloride anode in a buffered electrolyte solution. The sensor is separated from blood by a gas-permeable membrane. Oxygen tension in blood equilibrates with the electrolyte solution, forming silver chloride and reducing oxygen, which combines with water to form hydroxide ions. The sensor's current is proportional to oxygen tension in the electrolyte solution and the blood sample. The sensor requires a small voltage and is temperature-dependent, typically kept at 37°C to maintain pO_2. The oxygen polarographic electrode detection method offers several advantages, including direct measurement of oxygen levels in biological samples, which is crucial for understanding cellular respiration, tissue metabolism, and the impact of hypoxia on various physiological processes.

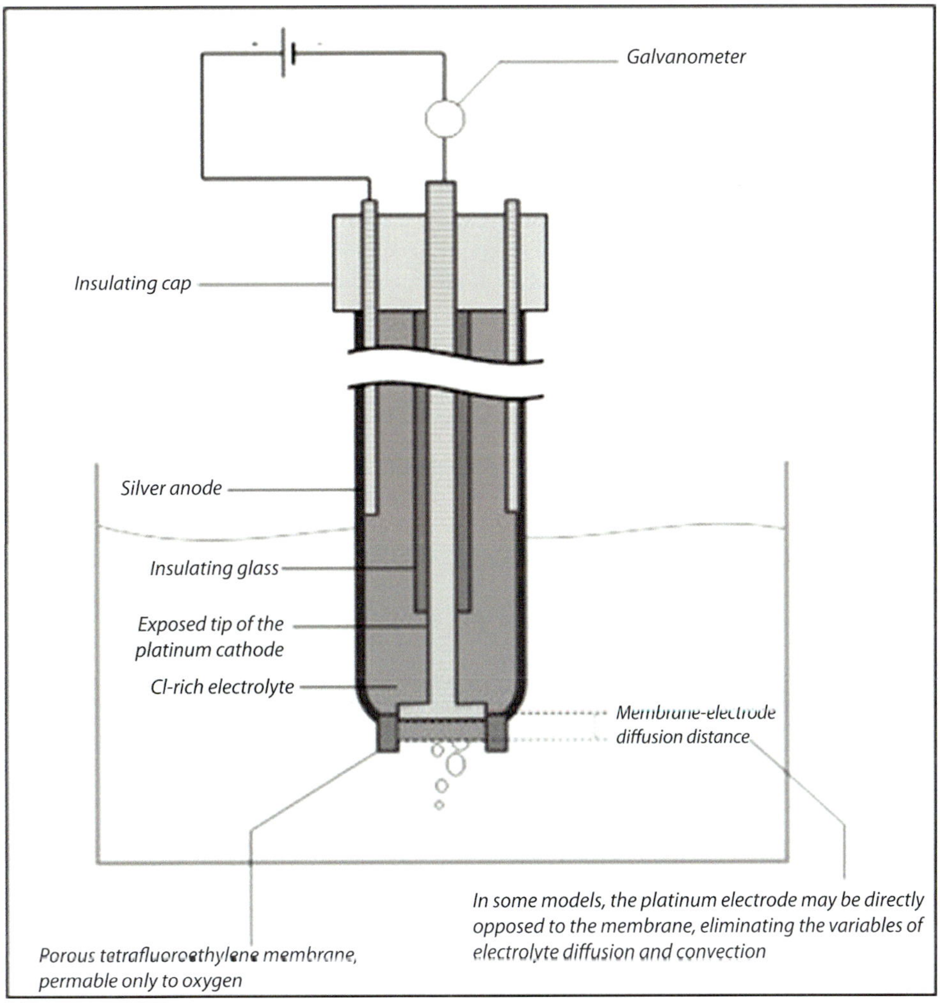

FIGURE 13.3 Diagram of oxygen polarographic electrode.

Fiber-Optic Sensor

Another way to assess tumor oxygenation is to use fiber-optic oxygen-sensing devices. In this system, photodiodes stimulate a fluorophore embedded in a silicon rubber polymer at the end of the probe tip. The lifespan of the fluorescent pulses is inversely proportional to the oxygen tension in the probe tip [Gallez, 2022]. This rapidly equilibrates with PO_2 in the surrounding medium, so a continuous readout of tissue PO_2 can be obtained. Prototypes used a laser to generate the stimulatory pulses, but the commercial fiber-optic devices use chaper, blue light-emitting diodes [Griffiths and Robinson, 1999] (Figure 13.4).

Immunohistochemical Detection

Immunohistochemical detection of hypoxia is a technique that can identify and label specific cellular proteins in hypoxic tissue and cells. It is routinely used both diagnostically and in research to label and identify specific cellular proteins of interest. This method employs antibodies that specifically bind to the target antigen. During this process, antibodies are designed against the GLUT-1, VEGF, CA IX, and HIF-1α [Young and Möller, 2010]. After using primary antibodies to attach

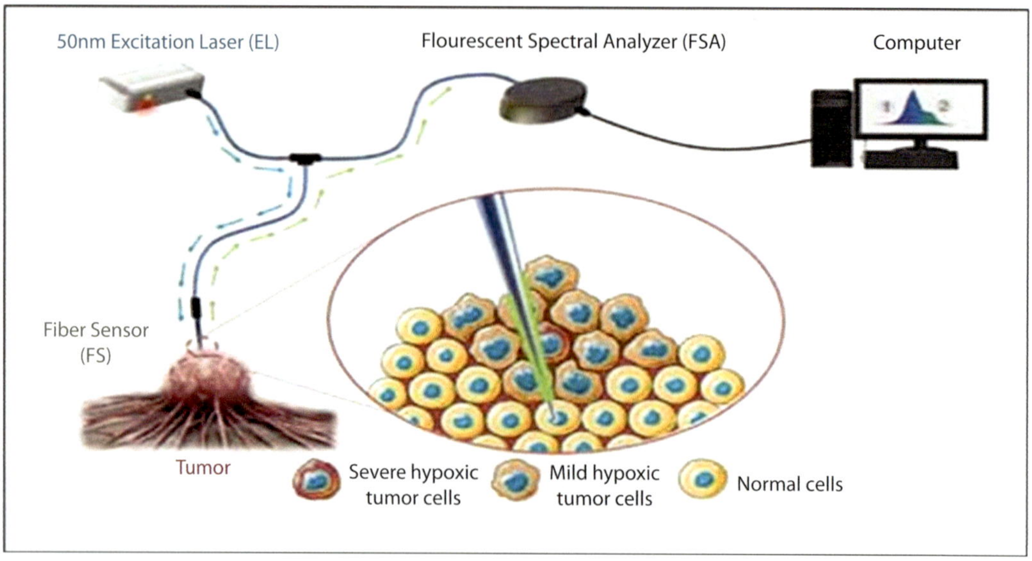

FIGURE 13.4 Diagram of the fiber optical sensor.

to particular protein targets in tissue sections, a secondary antibody is connected to a recognition molecule. The results are visualized under a microscope. The results are typically in the form of an alteration in color or fluorescence, indicating the target protein's existence and location [Das et al., 2023].

CONCLUSION

Tumor hypoxia denotes regions within solid tumors where the oxygen partial pressure is approximately below 10 mmHg. An exact threshold for tumor hypoxia is difficult to define because oxygenation varies over time and between different tissues. In tumors, hypoxia arises due to a mismatch between oxygen delivery and consumption. Hypoxia promotes tumor progression, aggressiveness, and metastatic potential. A common characteristic of hypoxic cancer cells is that they exhibit a greater degree of resistance to radiation- and chemotherapy than their well-oxygenated counterparts. Consequently, hypoxia is known to contribute to treatment failure and thereby to cancer recurrence. Detecting hypoxia promptly and accurately is essential for effective clinical management. Biomarkers play a pivotal role in this detection by providing measurable indicators of hypoxic conditions in the body. Biomarkers have the ability to estimate the likely outcome of radiation and chemotherapy. Biomarkers are either produced by the cancer cells or by noncancerous cells in response to cancer. These biomarkers can be classified into several categories, including HIFs, VEGF, GLUT-1, PDK1, CAIX, and pimonidazole. Their levels provide insights into the extent of hypoxic stress and aid in the diagnosis and management of various hypoxia-related conditions. Detecting hypoxic tumors using biomarkers involves various invasive and noninvasive techniques, including polarographic needle electrodes, immunohistochemical staining, radionuclide imaging (PET, MRI, and optical imaging (bioluminescence and fluorescence). With the help of these techniques, hypoxia status may be continuously monitored, which is helpful for evaluating the efficacy of treatments and the course of the illness. As we move into the era of precision medicine, this type of biomarker will evolve considerably. Such biomarkers may be used not only to identify people with a disease, but to redefine the classification of the disease. For example, the detection of cancer is moving rapidly toward a molecular and imaging-based classification rather than a largely organ-based classification scheme.

REFERENCES

Abbondati, E., Del-Pozo, J., Hoather, T. M., Constantino-Casas, F., & Dobson, J. M. (2013). An immunohistochemical study of the expression of the hypoxia markers GLUT-1 and Ca-IX in Canine sarcomas. Veterinary Pathology, 50(6), 1063–1069. https://doi.org/10.1177/0300985813486810

Abou Khouzam, R., Brodaczewska, K., Filipiak, A., Zeinelabdin, N. A., Buart, S., Szczylik, C., Kieda, C., & Chouaib, S. (2021). Tumor hypoxia regulates immune escape/invasion: influence on angiogenesis and potential impact of hypoxic biomarkers on cancer therapies. Frontiers in Immunology, 11, 613114. https://doi.org/10.3389/fimmu.2020.613114

Ambrosio, M. R., Di Serio, C., Danza, G., Rocca, B. J., Ginori, A., Prudovsky, I., Marchionni, N., Del Vecchio, M. T., & Tarantini, F. (2016). Carbonic anhydrase IX is a marker of hypoxia and correlates with higher Gleason scores and ISUP grading in prostate cancer. Diagnostic Pathology, 11(1), 45. https://doi.org/10.1186/s13000-016-0495-1

Badr, C. E., & Tannous, B. A. (2011). Bioluminescence imaging: progress and applications. Trends in Biotechnology, 29(12), 624–633. https://doi.org/10.1016/j.tibtech.2011.06.010

Bernstein, J. M., Homer, J. J., & West, C. M. (2014). Dynamic contrast-enhanced magnetic resonance imaging biomarkers in head and neck cancer: potential to guide treatment? A systematic review. Oral Oncology, 50(10), 963–970. https://doi.org/10.1016/j.oraloncology.2014.07.011

Boström, P. J., Thoms, J., Sykes, J., Ahmed, O., Evans, A., van Rhijn, B. W., Mirtti, T., Stakhovskyi, O., Laato, M., Margel, D., Pintilie, M., Kuk, C., Milosevic, M., Zlotta, A. R., & Bristow, R. G. (2016). Hypoxia marker GLUT-1 (glucose transporter 1) is an independent prognostic factor for survival in bladder cancer patients treated with radical cystectomy. Bladder Cancer (Amsterdam, Netherlands), 2(1), 101–109. https://doi.org/10.3233/BLC-150033

Bui, B. P., Nguyen, P. L., Lee, K., & Cho, J. (2022). Hypoxia-inducible factor-1: a novel therapeutic target for the management of cancer, drug resistance, and cancer-related pain. Cancers, 14(24), 6054. https://doi.org/10.3390/cancers14246054

Cui, W., Wu, F., & Ma, L. (2017). Hypoxia associated biomarkers in lung cancer – an update. European Review for Medical and Pharmacological Sciences, 21(3Suppl), 43–46.

Daimiel I. (2019). Insights into hypoxia: non-invasive assessment through imaging modalities and its application in breast cancer. Journal of Breast Cancer, 22(2), 155–171. https://doi.org/10.4048/jbc.2019.22.e26

Das, S., Dey, M. K., Devireddy, R., & Gartia, M. R. (2023). Biomarkers in cancer detection, diagnosis, and prognosis. Sensors (Basel, Switzerland), 24(1), 37. https://doi.org/10.3390/s24010037

Della Rocca, Y., Fonticoli, L., Rajan, T. S., Trubiani, O., Caputi, S., Diomede, F., Pizzicannella, J., & Marconi, G. D. (2022). Hypoxia: molecular pathophysiological mechanisms in human diseases. Journal of Physiology and Biochemistry, 78(4), 739–752. https://doi.org/10.1007/s13105-022-00912-6

Ettinger, A., & Wittmann, T. (2014). Fluorescence live cell imaging. Methods in Cell Biology, 123, 77–94. https://doi.org/10.1016/B978-0-12-420138-5.00005-7

Gallez B. (2022). The role of imaging biomarkers to guide pharmacological interventions targeting tumor hypoxia. Frontiers in Pharmacology, 13, 853568. https://doi.org/10.3389/fphar.2022.853568

Gaustad, J. V., Hauge, A., Wegner, C. S., Simonsen, T. G., Lund, K. V., Hansem, L. M. K., & Rofstad, E. K. (2020). DCE-MRI of tumor hypoxia and hypoxia-associated aggressiveness. Cancers, 12(7), 1979. https://doi.org/10.3390/cancers12071979

Griffiths, J. R., & Robinson, S. P. (1999). The oxylite: a fibre-optic oxygen sensor. The British Journal of Radiology, 72(859), 627–630. https://doi.org/10.1259/bjr.72.859.10624317

Henry, N. L., & Hayes, D. F. (2012). Cancer biomarkers. Molecular Oncology, 6(2), 140–146. https://doi.org/10.1016/j.molonc.2012.01.010

Horsman, M. R., & Vaupel, P. (2016). Pathophysiological basis for the formation of the tumor microenvironment. Frontiers in Oncology, 6, 66.

Jing, X., Yang, F., Shao, C., Wei, K., Xie, M., Shen, H., & Shu, Y. (2019). Role of hypoxia in cancer therapy by regulating the tumor microenvironment. Molecular Cancer, 18(1), 157. https://doi.org/10.1186/s12943-019-1089-9

Kakkad, S., Krishnamachary, B., Jacob, D., Pacheco-Torres, J., Goggins, E., Bharti, S. K., Penet, M. F., & Bhujwalla, Z. M. (2019). Molecular and functional imaging insights into the role of hypoxia in cancer aggression. Cancer Metastasis Reviews, 38(1–2), 51–64. https://doi.org/10.1007/s10555-019-09788-3

Krock, B. L., Skuli, N., & Simon, M. C. (2011). Hypoxia-induced angiogenesis: good and evil. Genes & Cancer, 2(12), 1117–1133.

Le, Q. T., & Courter, D. (2008). Clinical biomarkers for hypoxia targeting. Cancer Metastasis Reviews, 27(3), 351–362. https://doi.org/10.1007/s10555-008-9144-9

Liang, B., He, Q., Zhong, L., Wang, S., Pan, Z., Wang, T., & Zhao, Y. (2015). Circulating VEGF as a biomarker for diagnosis of ovarian cancer: a systematic review and a meta-analysis. OncoTargets and Therapy, 8, 1075–1082. https://doi.org/10.2147/OTT.S83616

Lopci, E., Grassi, I., Chiti, A., Nanni, C., Cicoria, G., Toschi, L., Fonti, C., Lodi, F., Mattioli, S., & Fanti, S. (2014). PET radiopharmaceuticals for imaging of tumor hypoxia: a review of the evidence. American Journal of Nuclear Medicine and Molecular Imaging, 4(4), 365–384.

Miyabara, H., Hirano, R., Watanabe, S., Soriano, J. C. C., Watanabe, H., Kuchimaru, T., Kitada, N., Kadonosono, T., Maki, S. A., Kondoh, G., & Kizaka-Kondoh, S. (2023). In vivo optical imaging of tumor stromal cells with hypoxia-inducible factor activity. Cancer Science, 114(10), 3935–3945. https://doi.org/10.1111/cas.15907

Muz, B., de la Puente, P., Azab, F., & Azab, A. K. (2015). The role of hypoxia in cancer progression, angiogenesis, metastasis, and resistance to therapy. Hypoxia (Auckland, N.Z.), 3, 83–92. https://doi.org/10.2147/HP.S93413

Ognibene, M., Cangelosi, D., Morini, M., Segalerba, D., Bosco, M. C., Sementa, A. R., Eva, A., & Varesio, L. (2017). Immunohistochemical analysis of PDK1, PHD3 and HIF-1α expression defines the hypoxic status of neuroblastoma tumors. PLoS ONE, 12(11), e0187206. https://doi.org/10.1371/journal.pone.0187206

Peng, F., Wang, J. H., Fan, W. J., Meng, Y. T., Li, M. M., Li, T. T., Cui, B., Wang, H. F., Zhao, Y., An, F., Guo, T., Liu, X. F., Zhang, L., Lv, L., Lv, D. K., Xu, L. Z., Xie, J. J., Lin, W. X., Lam, E. W., Xu, J., … Liu, Q. (2018). Glycolysis gatekeeper PDK1 reprograms breast cancer stem cells under hypoxia. Oncogene, 37(8), 1062–1074. https://doi.org/10.1038/onc.2017.368

Perez, R. C., Kim, D., Maxwell, A. W. P., & Camacho, J. C. (2023). Functional imaging of hypoxia: PET and MRI. Cancers, 15(13), 3336. https://doi.org/10.3390/cancers15133336

Rios-Colon, L., Kim, S., Su, Y., Kumar, D., & Deep, G. (2022). Immunofluorescence-based method to assess cancer biomarker in the hypoxic region of the tumor. Methods in Molecular Biology (Clifton, N.J.), 2413, 37–43. https://doi.org/10.1007/978-1-0716-1896-7_5

Rühle, A., Grosu, A. L., Wiedenmann, N., Ruf, J., Bieber, B., Stoian, R., Thomsen, A. R., Gkika, E., Vaupel, P., Baltas, D., Weber, W. A., Mix, M., & Nicolay, N. H. (2022). The value of plasma hypoxia markers for predicting imaging-based hypoxia in patients with head-and-neck cancers undergoing definitive chemoradiation. Clinical and Translational Radiation Oncology, 33, 120–127. https://doi.org/10.1016/j.ctro.2022.02.008

Sarhadi, V. K., & Armengol, G. (2022). Molecular biomarkers in cancer. Biomolecules, 12(8), 1021. https://doi.org/10.3390/biom12081021

Silva M. L. (2015). Cancer serum biomarkers based on aberrant post-translational modifications of glycoproteins: clinical value and discovery strategies. Biochimica et biophysica acta, 1856(2), 165–177. https://doi.org/10.1016/j.bbcan.2015.07.002

Smith, R. C., & McCarthy, S. (1992). Physics of magnetic resonance. The Journal of Reproductive Medicine, 37(1), 19–26.

Sørensen, B. S., & Horsman, M. R. (2020). Tumor hypoxia: impact on radiation therapy and molecular pathways. Frontiers in Oncology, 10, 562. https://doi.org/10.3389/fonc.2020.00562

Vassiliou, V. S., Cameron, D., Prasad, S. K., & Gatehouse, P. D. (2018). Magnetic resonance imaging: physics basics for the cardiologist. JRSM Cardiovascular Disease, 7, 2048004018772237. https://doi.org/10.1177/2048004018772237

Viola, R. J., Provenzale, J. M., Li, F., Li, C. Y., Yuan, H., Tashjian, J., & Dewhirst, M. W. (2008). In vivo bioluminescence imaging monitoring of hypoxia-inducible factor 1alpha, a promoter that protects cells, in response to chemotherapy. AJR. American Journal of Roentgenology, 191(6), 1779–1784. https://doi.org/10.2214/AJR.07.4060

Wallabregue, A. L. D., Bolland, H., Faulkner, S., Hammond, E. M., & Conway, S. J. (2023). Two color imaging of different hypoxia levels in cancer cells. Journal of the American Chemical Society, 145(4), 2572–2583. https://doi.org/10.1021/jacs.2c12493

Walsh, J. C., Lebedev, A., Aten, E., Madsen, K., Marciano, L., & Kolb, H. C. (2014). The clinical importance of assessing tumor hypoxia: relationship of tumor hypoxia to prognosis and therapeutic opportunities. Antioxidants & Redox Signaling, 21(10), 1516–1554. https://doi.org/10.1089/ars.2013.5378

Yang, L., & West, C. M. (2019). Hypoxia gene expression signatures as predictive biomarkers for personalising radiotherapy. The British Journal of Radiology, 92(1093), 20180036. https://doi.org/10.1259/bjr.20180036

Young, R. J., & Möller, A. (2010). Immunohistochemical detection of tumour hypoxia. Methods in Molecular Biology (Clifton, N.J.), 611, 151–159. https://doi.org/10.1007/978-1-60327-345-9_12

14 Precision Medicine Approaches in Hypoxic Cancers

Suman Kumar Ray and Sukhes Mukherjee
Department of Biochemistry, All India Institute of Medical Sciences, Bhopal, Madhya Pradesh, India

INTRODUCTION

Precision medicine entails adapting the course of treatment based on the tumor's unique sensitivities [1]. Therefore, molecular genetics, circulating molecular diagnostics, and histochemical molecular diagnostics are all commonly available for malignancies. The development of treatments is influenced by the availability of genetic indicators of tumor resistance and prognosis [2]. In breast cancer, for instance, HER2/neu receptor status reveals which individuals had a good prognosis before Herceptin treatment but are now in the clear [3]. In its absence, HER2/neu enhances survival signaling pathways and tumor growth. It would have been extremely challenging, if not impossible, to conduct a successful Herceptin randomized clinical adjuvant trial without that molecular marker, since many cancers do not express the receptor [4]. The improvement in survival rates with even the most effective molecularly targeted treatments has been minimal and, in most cases, has necessitated meta-analyses to confirm the benefit. Hypoxia was one of the first and, to this day, one of the most influential factors in determining how well a treatment worked. However, developing reliable methods to assess hypoxia *in vivo*, especially during treatment, continues to be a challenge [5]. The reason being, hypoxia is a dynamic condition that might change drastically throughout the course of treatment. However, other randomized trials have demonstrated positive therapeutic outcomes without the capacity to specifically target patients with hypoxic tumors. Being able to identify diagnostic and prognostic markers is, hence, crucial for customized medicine to be successful [6].

The rate of cancer incidence and prevalence is rising alarmingly, but therapy advancements have been sluggish, and the advantages of treatment are not seen for weeks or months. Pathological examination, disease symptoms, and drug histories have traditionally formed the basis of medical care [7]. Thanks to developments in diagnostics and early detection markers, it is now possible to catch some cancers before they cause any noticeable symptoms. Biochemical, epigenetic, genetic, imaging, metabolomic, and proteomic markers are all part of this set. With the capability of multiplexing, technologies can be utilized to identify these markers in clinical samples. The use of many markers in a single sample improves the accuracy and timeliness of cancer diagnoses by increasing the sensitivity and specificity of the test [8]. Because the existence and stage of cancer may be determined from the profiles of markers outlined above, this information is very important because it allows for the construction of individual-specific treatment regimens. The clinical gold standard for diagnosis is pathology; however, molecular diagnostics that incorporate

DOI: 10.1201/9781003477419-14

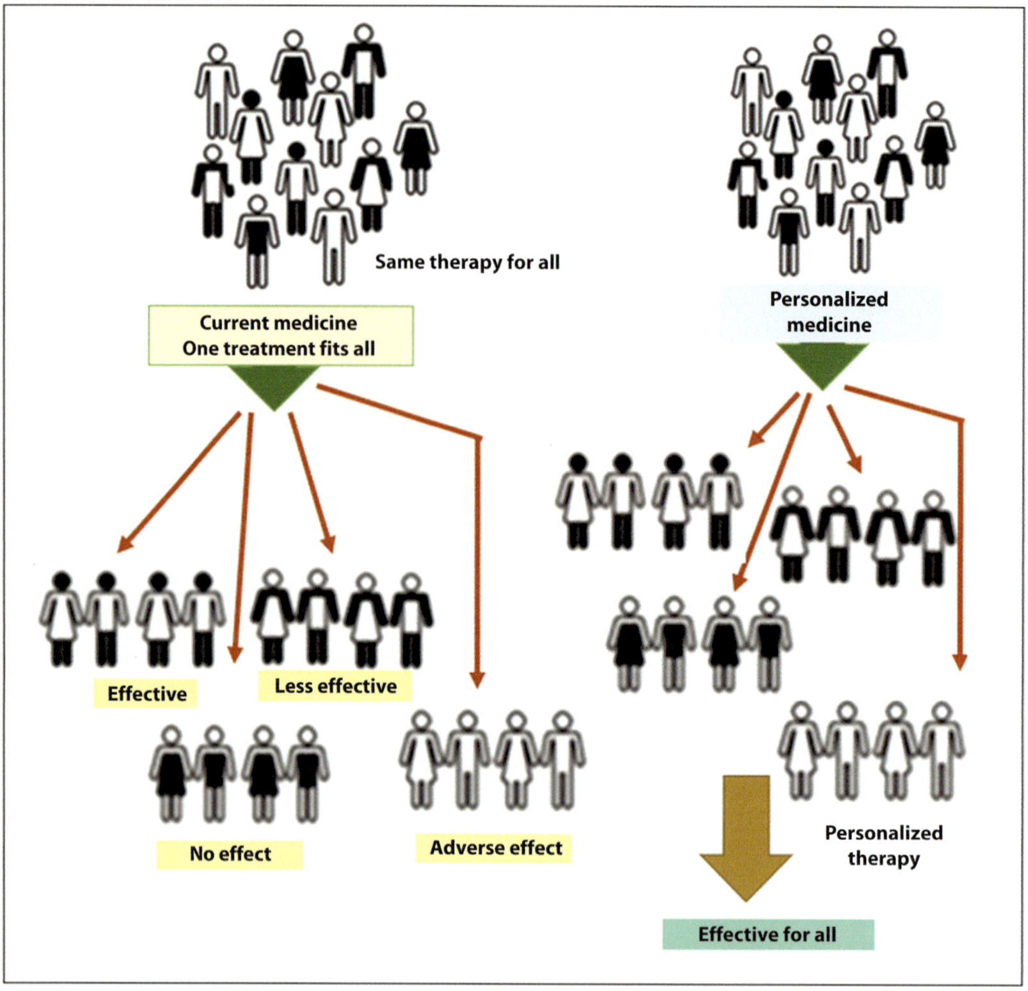

FIGURE 14.1 Basic diagram showing the effectiveness of personalized medicine and current medicine approaches with a one-treatment-fits-all model.

extra data may differ from pathology [9]. We reviewed that hypoxia is probably the single most important factor influencing the efficacy of cancer treatments and discussed and assessed various clinical approaches for monitoring hypoxia in precision oncology [10]. In Figure 14.1, we have shown the effectiveness and therapeutic approaches of personalized medicine and the one treatment fits all model.

REVOLUTION OF TUMOR TREATMENT: FROM TUMOR SITE TO MOLECULAR ALTERATIONS

Recent years have seen a dramatic shift in cancer patient therapy, including cancer hypoxia, as a number of molecular changes have been discovered to cause cancer initiation and progression [11]. The traditional progression of this biomarker-based strategy has been from laboratory work to clinical confirmation. Consequently, biomarkers, rather than the specific tumor's anatomic location of origin, are increasingly being considered treatment decision determinants [12]. This shift allowed for the effective treatment of patient populations with a single targeted medication whose cancers had a common molecular characteristic. Endocrine therapy for luminal breast cancer was the initial application of molecular-based medicine to cancer patients [13].

A turning point in cancer research was reached with the discovery of pharmacologically alterable molecular changes [14]. Results in breast, lung, and melanoma were the most significant [14]. Mutations in human epidermal growth factor receptor 2 (ERBB2) or phosphatidylinositol 4,5-bisphosphate 3-kinase catalytic subunit alpha isoform (PIK3CA) have revolutionized the treatment strategy for luminal breast cancer patients, in addition to the identification of hormonal receptors as potential therapeutic agents in breast cancer [15]. Another significant class of individuals who unquestionably gain from anti-HER2 inhibition in all therapeutic contexts has been identified thanks to the identification of HER2 amplification as a driver [16]. People who were found to have non-small-cell lung cancer (NSCLC) also experienced a significant change. Advancements in illness outcomes have been influenced by the discovery of mutations in the epidermal growth factor receptor (EGFR) [17] and the echinoderm microtubule-associated protein-like 4-anaplastic lymphoma kinase (EML4-ALK) translocation [18]. In addition, individuals with advanced melanoma have shown markedly better clinical outcomes after BRAF-V600E mutant detection and therapy with B-Raf proto-oncogene, serine/threonine kinase (BRAF) and mitogen-activated protein kinase kinase (MEK) inhibitors [19]. These are only a handful of the many ways in which precision medicine is changing the face of everyday clinical practice. Many solid tumors, including so-called orphan diseases like extrahepatic cholangiocarcinoma, have been greatly affected by the genetic revolution in recent years [20].

Regardless of the location of the hypoxic tumor, treatment decisions could be guided by identifying specific molecular features, such as microsatellite instability in all solid tumors, somatic or germline mutations (e.g., breast cancer gene (BRCA1 and BRCA2) (BRCA), BRAF, or ERBB2), or gene fusions (e.g., fibroblast growth factor receptor (FGFR) and neurotrophic tropomyosin receptor kinase (NTRK)) [21]. Ultimately, determining which patient groups are likely to benefit or not from this sort of therapy by discovering certain biomarkers predictive of response or resistance is crucial for the effective application of these molecular-based medicines [22]. It can be challenging to determine which driver is most important to target when multiple molecular changes are apparent; in such circumstances, proteomic analysis may be useful [23]. Metabolomic research is another vital area to investigate for ways to enhance precision medicine [24] in tumor hypoxia. Not only is it important for finding targetable biomarkers, but it can also help us understand the processes of inter-patient variability in response to medication therapy by revealing pharmacological phenotypes [25]. There are chances to develop new therapeutic methods [24] that can be aided by metabolomics' ability to assess medication resistance and disease relapse [26, 27] (Figure 14.2).

Different types of solid tumors with a common driver molecular alteration are chosen and treated with a specific inhibitor in basket trials, whereas patients with the same type of solid tumors are treated according to their molecular features in umbrella trials [28].

WHY PERSONALIZED MEDICINE IS NEEDED IN THE CASE OF HYPOXIC TUMOR

While all cells have the same DNA, genes that code for specific organs (and their cells) act differently. While many cancer hypoxic tumors may have the same DNA, the way genes are expressed varies

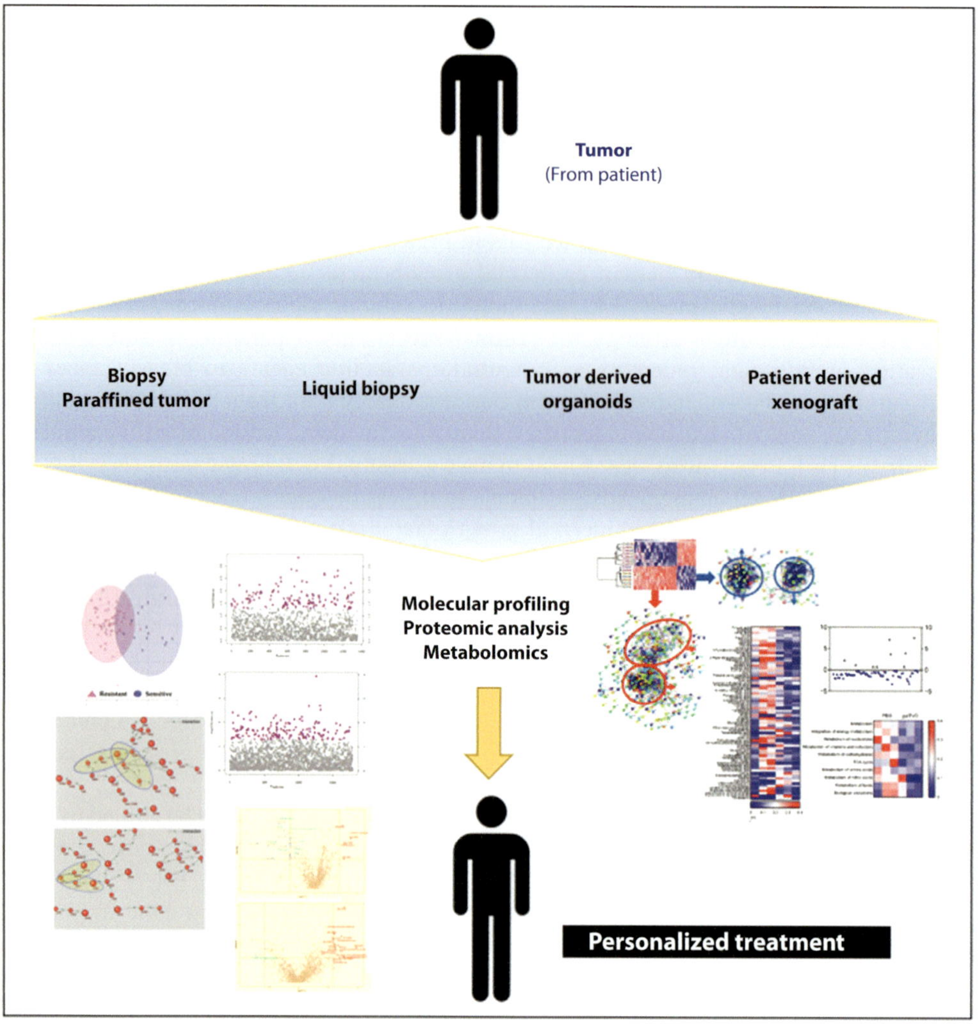

FIGURE 14.2 Personalized treatment and modern approaches in tumor hypoxia.

greatly throughout tumor types. Modern technology has made it possible to compare normal profiling to cancer-related profiles by analyzing hundreds of genes simultaneously using gene-expression microarray [29]. Conventional medical practice has been dominated for decades by population-level findings from cohort-based epidemiological studies that fail to take individual genetic diversity into consideration [30]. A patient's medical history and genetic composition are considered in the development of a treatment plan in contemporary personalized medicine. Care in conventional customized medicine has always focused on the individual's genetic makeup, socioeconomic status, environmental factors, and way of life [31]. The foundation of contemporary personalized medicine is targeted treatment. Access to data regarding the altered route and cancer-causing components is crucial for targeted therapy. Patients with breast cancer who are female and have elevated HER-2 expression levels are candidates for the drug Herceptin [32]. Chronic myeloid leukemias are treated with Gleevec, an inhibitor of tyrosine kinase [33]. The hyperactivation of abl-driven protein signaling is caused by the reciprocal translocation that happens in these patients between chromosomes 9 and 20 [34]. Prevention and treatment strategies, along with the most recent information about the cancer type, inform the development of individualized health care plans [35] (Table 14.1). In

TABLE 14.1
Prevention and Treatment Strategies of the Most Common Cancers, Along With Recent Information and Development of Individualized Health Care Plans

Type of Cancer	Description of the Modern Approaches
Breast Cancer	• Preventative measures like mammograms and BRCA1 and BRCA2 mutation screenings are common among the population. • Customized treatment approaches are not foolproof due to individual variances in genetic predisposition and environmental susceptibility. • Research suggests modifying behavior in high-risk individuals as a first line of defense, identifying and closely monitoring those who are genetically susceptible, and treating early-stage cancer cases noninvasively as a second line of defense. • Molecular characterization of breast cancer allows for the development and implementation of tailored preventive methods for personalized health care. • Tamoxifen treatment is affected by CYP2D6 genotyping, which highlights the importance of individualized medicine in patient care. • Aromatase inhibitors should not be given to women who are either past menopause or in the early stages of menopause. • Two existing diagnostic technologies that rely on expression profiling show promise in personalized therapy: MammPrint and Oncotype DX. • Future "omics" research may contribute valuable information in the personalized treatment of breast cancer.
Colon Cancer	• Colon cancer can be identified using biomarkers and genetics, and can be treated with surgery, radiation, and chemotherapy. • Coloscopy has improved cancer detection timing, allowing for earlier detection of polyps. • A correlation analysis of hypermethylation, mutations, and microsatellite instability in tumors from specific patients is being completed. • Early detection and treatment can lead to better outcomes for patients. Many patients can survive for at least five years if the disease is caught and treated early. • However, stage IV cancer is typically not treatable. The five-year survival rate decreases with increasing cancer stage, and late recurrences are known to occur in colon cancer and other tumors. • Specific treatments are ineffective in colorectal cancer, as tumors harboring KRAS mutations become insensitive to cetuximab or panitumumab. • Pharmacogenomics of colon cancer has been explored, with studies showing a relationship between illness prediction and variation in genes involved in oxaliplatin metabolism.
Lung Cancer	• Small-cell lung cancer (SCLC) and non-small-cell lung cancer (NSCLC) are the two most common forms of lung cancer, accounting for 20% of all cases. • Treatment primarily involves surgery and chemotherapy, with therapeutic targets such as EGFR, K-ras, ALK, MET, CBL, and COX2 being explored. • Recent studies have shown that crizotinib can be used to treat non-small-cell lung cancer. • The anaplastic lymphoma kinase (ALK) inhibitor crizotinib has shown promising activity in treating lung cancer. • Erlotinib and EGFR mutant lung cancer have also shown significant clinical benefits. • The severity and progression of the disease are assessed considering histological data and the patient's medical history. • Genetic variants in EGFR and ERCC1 are associated with medication response in small-cell lung cancer patients, and ABCC1 polymorphism is connected with lung cancer susceptibility in chemotherapy patients in the Chinese population.

(Continued)

TABLE 14.1 *(Continued)*

Prevention and Treatment Strategies of the Most Common Cancers, Along With Recent Information and Development of Individualized Health Care Plans

Type of Cancer	Description of the Modern Approaches
Prostate Cancer	• Prostate cancer is the second-leading killer of men, particularly in the elderly. • Detection methods include digital rectal exams and PSA tests. Treatment for localized, biochemically recurrent, and later-stage prostate cancer is challenging due to its long development time. • Common therapies include radiation therapy, surgery, hormonal therapy, and chemotherapy. • Age-related changes, including metastatic illness, can influence the risk-benefit ratio. • The Comprehensive Geriatric Assessment is a new tool for predicting treatment response and determining patient survival. • SRD5A1 and SRD5A2 variants have been shown to predict biochemical recurrence after radical prostatectomy. • BCL2 polymorphisms in prostate cancer patients are more likely to have a poor prognosis.
Myeloid Neoplasia	• Myeloid neoplasia is a condition influenced by genetic and epigenetic changes, affecting cellular proliferation and hematopoietic differentiation. • Treatment involves various medications. • Customized genomics is being explored by combining pathology and genetic data. • Lymphoid leukemias, similar to lymphomas, start in lymphocytes but primarily affect the blood and bone marrow. • They fall under the category of hematological neoplasms. • Patients with chronic phase myeloid leukemia have CYP3A5 polymorphisms affecting their imatinib trough concentration and clinical response.
Lymphoma and Leukemia	• Lymphoma is a cancer that can spread to other organs, including the digestive tract, bones, brain, and skin. • It is characterized by solid lymphoid tumors and can metastasize to other organs. • Researchers are working on improving clinical prognostic models, utilizing high-throughput technology, and developing anti-idiotype vaccines to stratify lymphoma subtypes. • Chemotherapy, radiation, and bone marrow transplantation are the main treatments. The PML-RARA fusion gene and all-trans retinoic acid (ATRA) have been successful treatments for various cancers. • However, genetic-based treatments like crizotinib and erlotinib have shown minimal effectiveness in various cancer types. • Researchers are working to improve the effectiveness of apoptosis-based treatments.

addition, we have included breast, colon, lung, prostate, myeloid neoplasia, leukemia, and lymphoma below because it is impossible to cover every type of cancer in a single article.

ROLE OF HYPOXIA IN TUMOR RESISTANCE TO THERAPY AND PRECISION MEDICINE

One of the earliest findings in cancer treatment was the effect of reduced oxygen on tumor resistance [36]. For instance, when comparing proliferating cells exposed to radiation at less than 2.5 mmHg to those exposed to radiation at more than 10 mmHg, a dose-modifying factor ranging from 2.5 to 3.0 is observed. Therefore, in order to destroy hypoxic cells at 60 Gy (60 times 2.5 or 3), which is typically curative for euoxic tumors, >150 Gy would be required. According to the calculations, this has a significant impact, turning a treatment that was previously effective with a surviving fraction of 10^9 or 10^{10} into one that is ineffective with more than 1% of cells still alive [37].

Most chemotherapeutic medicines need oxygen to drive DNA oxidation processes; thus, this would have a similar impact on most regimens. However, some chemotherapeutic agents are hypoxia-only cytotoxic, so including them in a regimen for hypoxic tumors would be beneficial [38]. Hypoxia is linked to metabolic pathways that allow tumor resistance. Inflammation due to hypoxia or reoxygenation injury, for instance, might trigger the synthesis of growth factors and receptors for these factors. If the tumor was determined to be euoxic, signaling through HIF-1, which is seen as a potential therapeutic target, would be diminished or eliminated [39]. Similarly, hypoxia reperfusion damage gives tumors ways to resist treatment and grow malignantly by selecting for survival signaling proteins like p53 [40, 41]. Thus, resolving hypoxia could potentially target numerous signaling pathways linked to treatment resistance.

ROLE OF HYPOXIC TUMORS ON LOCAL CONTROL AND SURVIVAL

Much research has examined the impact of hypoxic tumors on regional management and prognosis [42] (Figure 14.3).

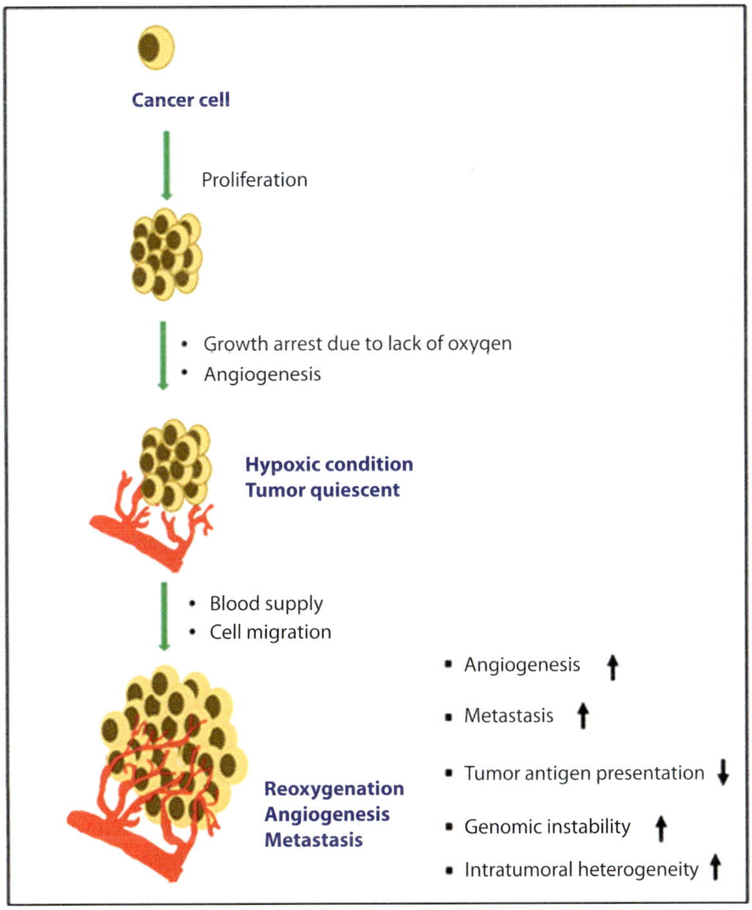

FIGURE 14.3 Cancer cell to metastasis-role of hypoxia, reoxygenation, blood supply, angiogenesis, and cellular migration.

In a nutshell, clinical evidence has consistently shown that hypoxia affects outcomes [43]. When measuring hypoxia, the Eppendorf electrode is considered the "gold standard" technique. We now have experimental and clinical evidence of the function of oxygen in patient outcomes, thanks to its usage, despite some well-established limitations. The criteria for identifying a hypoxic tumor have varied across publications. A portion of the measurements has been selected from the lowest oxygen bin, which is less than 2.5 mmHg. Median pO_2 and other criteria have been employed by others. Evidence from research on a variety of tumor types—including breast cancer [43], head and neck cancer [44], sarcomas [45], uterine cervix [46], and prostate cancer [47, 48]—indicates strikingly different outcomes when comparing hypoxic and non-hypoxic tumors. Crucially, almost 50% of the tumors are determined to be hypoxic for the majority of cancer types, including lung malignancies [49]. Therefore, on any particular therapy day, not all tumors in patients will be hypoxic. The most reliable human data on this topic comes from 18 positron emission tomography (PET) imaging investigations using F-misonidazole (MISO) [49, 50]. However, every study agrees that measuring the level of hypoxia is necessary because it cannot be anticipated with any degree of certainty.

There are alternative, less complicated methods for determining the level of hypoxia. Delivering 18 F-MISO or a comparable chemical that binds to DNA in hypoxic cells is a prominent technique among others [51]. There may be more useful labeling methods that have not yet been tested on humans, such as immunohistochemistry or oxidative tests [52]. Histochemical analysis of HIF-1 and its downstream components is another method. The function of HIF-1 and the validity of its correlation with hypoxia remain debatable. The levels of downstream signaling proteins, like Glut-1, VEGF, Ca9, and NDRG1, tend to scale with hypoxia level [53–56], even though HIF-1 staining is typically not microanatomically associated with hypoxia regions, and these regions do not always overlap with tumor immunopathology. Biopsy specimens must be flash-frozen immediately due to the fleeting nature of hypoxia and the sensitivity of these proteins.

THE CONTRIBUTION OF "OMICS" TO PERSONALIZED MEDICINE IN HYPOXIC CANCER

Precision oncology, traditionally reactive, now involves a comprehensive review of a patient's family history and genetic makeup before recommending treatment. Understanding the relationship between genomic alterations and cancer is crucial for identifying cancer risk factors [57, 58]. The goal of cancer genomics is to improve personalized medicine by discovering new genetic changes linked to specific tumors through DNA sequencing and analysis of cancer cells from patients. To aid in the development of better methods for cancer diagnosis, treatment, and prevention, it is necessary to compile a complete inventory of the important genetic alterations in the main categories and subtypes of cancer. Genomic abnormalities cause cancer, and more and more information regarding different kinds of tumors supports the idea that every tumor has its unique genetic alterations.

More effective treatment techniques are being developed as a result of our growing understanding of the genetic alterations and gene expression profiles found in cancer cells [59]. These strategies are being customized to match the unique genetic profile of each patient's cancer. Projects such as the Cancer Genome Atlas (TCGA) at the National Institutes of Health (NIH) seek to fill gaps in our knowledge about cancer genomes, the value of tumor samples for genomic studies, and the potential of cancer genomics to inform individualized medical care. Personalized therapy benefits not just from genomic information but also from proteomic information. As part of the Human Proteome Project, researchers compared the protein and peptide profiles of cancer patients with those of clinically healthy individuals [60]. Through the analysis of all 21,000 genes in the human genome, the Human Proteome Project has produced a blueprint of the human body's protein-based molecular architecture and served as a tool for improving disease detection and therapy by shedding light on biological and molecular processes. Although genes encode functional abilities, proteins are responsible for carrying out the actual function. Consequently, it is crucial to comprehend protein expression levels in both normal and cancerous states. Actually, protein-based techniques (immunohistochemistry) were the first to be authorized by the FDA for use in cancer detection and diagnosis [61, 62]. Protein interactions form the basis of the main pathways involved in cancer development and the signals that transmit information between them, including the receptor kinase route, m-Tor pathway, MAP kinase pathway, apoptosis, EGFR pathway, tyrosine kinase pathway, and Notch pathway [63]. Proteins and signal transduction pathways mediated by enzymes are involved in cancer, even though mutations start the process.

The International Human Epigenome Consortium (IHEC) aims to create reference epigenome maps for humans, covering histone modifications, DNA methylation, transcription start sites, small RNAs, and non-coding RNAs [64, 65]. The IHEC plans to decipher 1,000 epigenomes within seven to ten years to ensure comprehensive coverage of the human epigenome [66]. Researchers will conduct surveys of people, families, and genetic twins to understand genetic and epigenetic variation worldwide. Metabolomics, a relatively recent area of research in personalized medicine, is a relatively recent area of study [67, 68]. Despite promising results, metabolomics faces obstacles such as limited training opportunities, limited expertise, and concerns over cost, intellectual property rights, and economic incentives.

LIMITATIONS OF AVAILABLE ASSAYS FOR MEASURING HYPOXIA FOR PRECISION ONCOLOGY

Tumor oxygen measurement methods should be straightforward, easy to understand, quick, safe, and painless. They should be serially performed during treatment, demonstrating intervention changes in the tumor's oxygen status. The Eppendorf electrode technique is considered the "gold standard" but is not practical due to its complexity, needle range, and operator skill. PET imaging has shown promising results, and agents can identify areas with low oxygen levels or blood flow sensitivity [69]. As an example, there have been effective cases of using 18 F-MISO during treatment [49, 70]. Clinical trials using 18 F-MISO have shown that tumors that were previously severely hypoxic frequently turn euoxic as a result of the treatment [51]. Numerous ^{1}H-magnetic resonance susceptibility imaging (MRS) techniques [71] and blood flow-sensitive ^{1}H-SPECTROScopy [72, 73] have the potential to be used in clinical settings. ^{19}F-MRS can be covalently attached to molecules having large oxygen shifts and operates at frequencies comparable to ^{1}H. The usage of ^{19}F-fluorobenzene in animal models has been documented [74, 75]. Atom spin resonance (ESR) imaging methods can also determine oxygen levels [76].

Near-infrared optical spectroscopic techniques have been developed for routine tumor oxygen assessment, detecting the saturation of capillary hemoglobin, which is indicative of local tissue oxygen level [77]. These technologies can be used to measure brain oxygenation levels and heart bypass surgery with less brain injury. Surrogate oxygen measures, such as blood flow, can be used to identify hypoxic tumors. However, these tests come at a high cost and have not yet been evaluated for clinical benefit. Proton therapy [78] facilities have shown potential for detecting ^{15}O-water blood flow, but the clinical benefit of this treatment has not been evaluated. Dynamic, noninvasive studies of tumor metabolism provide evidence that tumors can endure extremely acidic conditions, a lack of glucose and oxygen, and severe hypoxia, which could select aggressive tumors for harsh treatment settings [79]. How we can overcome the limitations in precision oncology is shown in Table 14.2.

TABLE 14.2
To Overwhelmed Limitations: Functional Precision Medicine of Hypoxic Tumor

Strategy	Description
Functional precision medicine: the role of patient-derived organoids (PDOs) and patient-derived xenografts in a personalized approach	• There is hope that functional precision cancer treatment can supplement existing genetic methods. • Accurate validation of precision medicine has been impeded by the limits of preclinical models now utilized for medication selection and the small relevance of genetic profiling in predicting response to targeted therapies [80]. • Recently, functional analysis for therapeutic efficacy in solid tumors has been made easier with the use of 3D culture (also known as organoids) and xenograft models obtained from patients. • One way that translational medicine has been put into practice is by using patient-derived xenograft (PDX) models [14]. • These models are created by transferring tumor cells from patients into mice that lack an immune system. • The original tumor features, including heterogeneity, are preserved by PDXs. • Drug sensitivity and resistance predictions for various tumor types could be aided by PDXs, making them a useful tool for improving tailored approaches [81, 82]. • Organoids are a better alternative to the more prevalent monolayer cell cultures for preserving tissue biological properties; they are derived from tumor cells of patients. • An important step toward a tailored strategy is the potential to conduct tests directly on a patient's tumor.
Dynamic evaluation of tumors: the role of liquid biopsy	• Liquid biopsy analysis of plasma cell-free DNA (cfDNA) has significantly improved the dynamic evaluation of solid tumors. • Despite the lack of precise targetable biomarkers, cfDNA can detect molecular processes of acquired resistance, allowing for accurate assessment of tumor heterogeneity [14]. • This technique allows for precise assessment of genomes and molecular modifications at a precise moment, enabling the identification of distinct tumor sub-clones with their own resistance mechanisms [14]. • However, the variability of cancer cell populations influenced by target therapy's selective forces may be too great for single-biopsy methods to capture. • Using cfDNA can detect numerous contemporaneous heterogeneous resistance mechanisms [14, 83].
Molecular tumor board: why do we need it?	• Advancements in molecular tumor diagnosis and genetically matched targeted treatments have significantly improved cancer treatment outcomes. • Precision medicine began with antiestrogens for breast cancer treatment, and genetic testing is increasingly important due to expanding genetic knowledge and drug development. • However, there is an excess of genetic tests and data, and other genetic abnormalities may go unnoticed. • Accurately interpreting molecular tumor profiles is crucial for providing the best possible cancer treatment. • Expert evaluation is necessary to translate molecular profiles into clinical benefit.

CONCLUSIONS

Hypoxia is one of the most important prognostic indicators and moderators of treatment response. Many signaling pathways are driven by hypoxia; these pathways are also targets of cancer therapy. Unfortunately, there is currently no reliable way to measure hypoxia, which is a major problem because hypoxia is at the heart of many harmful aspects of tumor physiology, cancer progression, treatment resistance, and the many opportunities to counteract its harmful effects. More and more options for measuring oxygen or a proxy are becoming available. The ability to serially photograph tumors deep within the body, together with simplicity, precision, reproducibility, and economy, is essential for developing an optimum approach. Neither the mechanical Clark-type electrodes nor direct measurements of oxyhemoglobin saturation are suitable for frequent usage at this time, but these are the only approaches that are currently accessible. Direct or indirect measurement of tumor oxygenation could be possible in the future with the use of biological markers that are either endogenously expressed (such as cytokines) or given to patients just before a biopsy. Potentially useful in the future are molecular imaging techniques for assessing metabolic rate or blood flow, such as near-infrared reflectance/oximetry (NIRO), PET, MRI/MRS, and similar approaches. Personalized medicine has come a long way in the last several years, especially for patients with solid tumor diagnoses. One promising area of research in cancer treatment is the development of molecularly based tailored approaches for individual patients. Improving our knowledge of molecular biology is essential if we are to make any meaningful progress toward bettering therapeutic outcomes. A multi-omic strategy that can incorporate proteomics, metabolomics, DNA and RNA modifications, and other similar fields is required for progress. To identify resistance mechanisms and potentially new combination treatments, translational studies using organoids or xenografts in conjunction with liquid biopsy could assess molecular alterations brought on by clonal pressure from target agents or tumor heterogeneity. Immediate additional study is required to enhance accuracy.

CONSENT FOR PUBLICATION

Not applicable.

FUNDING

None.

CONFLICT OF INTEREST

The authors declare no conflict of interest, financial or otherwise.

ACKNOWLEDGMENTS

Declared none.

REFERENCES

1. Krzyszczyk P, Acevedo A, Davidoff EJ, Timmins LM, Marrero-Berrios I, Patel M, White C, Lowe C, Sherba JJ, Hartmanshenn C, O'Neill KM, Balter ML, Fritz ZR, Androulakis IP, Schloss RS, Yarmush ML. The growing role of precision and personalized medicine for cancer treatment. Technology (Singap World Sci). 2018 Sep-Dec;6(3–4):79–100. doi: 10.1142/S2339547818300020.
2. Housman G, Byler S, Heerboth S, Lapinska K, Longacre M, Snyder N, Sarkar S. Drug resistance in cancer: An overview. Cancers (Basel). 2014 Sep 5;6(3):1769–1792. doi: 10.3390/cancers6031769.
3. Patel A, Unni N, Peng Y. The changing paradigm for the treatment of HER2-positive breast cancer. Cancers (Basel). 2020 Jul 28;12(8):2081. doi: 10.3390/cancers12082081.
4. Perez EA, Reinholz MM, Hillman DW, Tenner KS, Schroeder MJ, Davidson NE, Martino S, Sledge GW, Harris LN, Gralow JR, Dueck AC, Ketterling RP, Ingle JN, Lingle WL, Kaufman PA, Visscher DW, Jenkins RB. HER2 and chromosome 17 effect on patient outcome in the N9831 adjuvant trastuzumab trial. J Clin Oncol. 2010 Oct 1;28(28):4307–4315. doi: 10.1200/JCO.2009.26.2154.
5. Godet I, Doctorman S, Wu F, Gilkes DM. Detection of hypoxia in cancer models: Significance, challenges, and advances. Cells. 2022 Feb 16;11(4):686. doi: 10.3390/cells11040686.

6. Mehta S, Shelling A, Muthukaruppan A, Lasham A, Blenkiron C, Laking G, Print C. Predictive and prognostic molecular markers for cancer medicine. Ther Adv Med Oncol. 2010 Mar;2(2):125–148. doi: 10.1177/1758834009360519.
7. Rosenzweig MQ, Gardner D, Griffith B. The history and physical in cancer care: A primer for the oncology advanced practitioner. J Adv Pract Oncol. 2014 Jul-Aug;5(4):262–268. doi: 10.6004/jadpro.2014.5.4.3.
8. Das S, Dey MK, Devireddy R, Gartia MR. Biomarkers in cancer detection, diagnosis, and prognosis. Sensors (Basel). 2023 Dec 20;24(1):37. doi: 10.3390/s24010037.
9. Dwivedi S, Purohit P, Misra R, Pareek P, Goel A, Khattri S, Pant KK, Misra S, Sharma P. Diseases and molecular diagnostics: A step closer to precision medicine. Indian J Clin Biochem. 2017 Oct;32(4): 374–398. doi: 10.1007/s12291-017-0688-8.
10. Ray SK, Mukherjee S. Starring role of biomarkers and anticancer agents as a major driver in precision medicine of cancer therapy. Curr Mol Med. 2023;23(2):111–126.
11. Berger MF, Mardis ER. The emerging clinical relevance of genomics in cancer medicine. Nat Rev Clin Oncol. 2018 Jun;15(6):353–365. doi: 10.1038/s41571-018-0002-6.
12. Lambert AW, Pattabiraman DR, Weinberg RA. Emerging biological principles of metastasis. Cell. 2017 Feb 9;168(4):670–691. doi: 10.1016/j.cell.2016.11.037.
13. Martí C, Sánchez-Méndez JI. Neoadjuvant endocrine therapy for luminal breast cancer treatment: A first-choice alternative in times of crisis such as the COVID-19 pandemic. Ecancermedicalscience. 2020 Apr 27;14:1027. doi: 10.3332/ecancer.2020.1027.
14. Gambardella V, Tarazona N, Cejalvo JM, Lombardi P, Huerta M, Roselló S, Fleitas T, Roda D, Cervantes A. Personalized medicine: Recent progress in cancer therapy. Cancers (Basel). 2020 Apr 19;12(4):1009. doi: 10.3390/cancers12041009.
15. André F, Ciruelos E, Rubovszky G, Campone M, Loibl S, Rugo HS, Iwata H, Conte P, Mayer IA, Kaufman B, Yamashita T, Lu YS, Inoue K, Takahashi M, Pápai Z, Longin AS, Mills D, Wilke C, Hirawat S, Juric D, SOLAR-1 Study Group. Alpelisib for PIK3CA-mutated, hormone receptor-positive advanced breast cancer. N Engl J Med. 2019 May 16;380(20):1929–1940. doi: 10.1056/NEJMoa1813904.
16. Krop IE, Kim SB, González-Martín A, LoRusso PM, Ferrero JM, Smitt M, Yu R, Leung AC, Wildiers H, TH3RESA study collaborators. Trastuzumab emtansine versus treatment of physician's choice for pretreated HER2-positive advanced breast cancer (TH3RESA): A randomised, open-label, phase 3 trial. Lancet Oncol. 2014 Jun;15(7):689–699. doi: 10.1016/S1470-2045(14)70178-0.
17. Paez JG, Jänne PA, Lee JC, Tracy S, Greulich H, Gabriel S, Herman P, Kaye FJ, Lindeman N, Boggon TJ, Naoki K, Sasaki H, Fujii Y, Eck MJ, Sellers WR, Johnson BE, Meyerson M. EGFR mutations in lung cancer: Correlation with clinical response to gefitinib therapy. Science. 2004 Jun 4;304(5676): 1497–1500. doi: 10.1126/science.1099314.
18. Soda M, Choi YL, Enomoto M, Takada S, Yamashita Y, Ishikawa S, Fujiwara S, Watanabe H, Kurashina K, Hatanaka H, Bando M, Ohno S, Ishikawa Y, Aburatani H, Niki T, Sohara Y, Sugiyama Y, Mano H. Identification of the transforming EML4-ALK fusion gene in non-small-cell lung cancer. Nature. 2007 Aug 2;448(7153):561–566. doi: 10.1038/nature05945.
19. Flaherty KT, Puzanov I, Kim KB, Ribas A, McArthur GA, Sosman JA, O'Dwyer PJ, Lee RJ, Grippo JF, Nolop K, Chapman PB. Inhibition of mutated, activated BRAF in metastatic melanoma. N Engl J Med. 2010 Aug 26;363(9):809–819. doi: 10.1056/NEJMoa1002011.
20. Borger DR, Tanabe KK, Fan KC, Lopez HU, Fantin VR, Straley KS, Schenkein DP, Hezel AF, Ancukiewicz M, Liebman HM, Kwak EL, Clark JW, Ryan DP, Deshpande V, Dias-Santagata D, Ellisen LW, Zhu AX, Iafrate AJ. Frequent mutation of isocitrate dehydrogenase (IDH)1 and IDH2 in cholangiocarcinoma identified through broad-based tumor genotyping. Oncologist. 2012;17(1):72–79. doi: 10.1634/theoncologist.2011-0386.
21. Dienstmann R, Rodon J, Prat A, Perez-Garcia J, Adamo B, Felip E, Cortes J, Iafrate AJ, Nuciforo P, Tabernero J. Genomic aberrations in the FGFR pathway: Opportunities for targeted therapies in solid tumors. Ann Oncol. 2014 Mar;25(3):552–563. doi: 10.1093/annonc/mdt419.
22. Kimmelman J, Tannock I. The paradox of precision medicine. Nat Rev Clin Oncol. 2018 Jun;15(6): 341–342. doi: 10.1038/s41571-018-0016-0.
23. Rodriguez H, Pennington SR. Revolutionizing precision oncology through collaborative proteogenomics and data sharing. Cell. 2018 Apr 19;173(3):535–539. doi: 10.1016/j.cell.2018.04.008.
24. Puchades-Carrasco L, Pineda-Lucena A. Metabolomics applications in precision medicine: An oncological perspective. Curr Top Med Chem. 2017;17(24):2740–2751. doi: 10.2174/1568026617666170707120034.
25. Clayton TA, Lindon JC, Cloarec O, Antti H, Charuel C, Hanton G, Provost JP, Le Net JL, Baker D, Walley RJ, Everett JR, Nicholson JK. Pharmaco-metabonomic phenotyping and personalized drug treatment. Nature. 2006 Apr 20;440(7087):1073–1077. doi: 10.1038/nature04648.

26. Gambardella V, Gimeno-Valiente F, Tarazona N, Martinez-Ciarpaglini C, Roda D, Fleitas T, Tolosa P, Cejalvo JM, Huerta M, Roselló S, Castillo J, Cervantes A. NRF2 through RPS6 activation is related to anti-HER2 drug resistance in HER2-amplified gastric cancer. Clin Cancer Res. 2019 Mar 1;25(5): 1639–1649. doi: 10.1158/1078-0432.CCR-18-2421.
27. Rojo de la Vega M, Chapman E, Zhang DD. NRF2 and the hallmarks of cancer. Cancer Cell. 2018 Jul 9;34(1):21–43. doi: 10.1016/j.ccell.2018.03.022.
28. Garralda E, Dienstmann R, Piris-Giménez A, Braña I, Rodon J, Tabernero J. New clinical trial designs in the era of precision medicine. Mol Oncol. 2019 Mar;13(3):549–557. doi: 10.1002/1878-0261. 12465.
29. Tarca AL, Romero R, Draghici S. Analysis of microarray experiments of gene expression profiling. Am J Obstet Gynecol. 2006 Aug;195(2):373–388. doi: 10.1016/j.ajog.2006.07.001.
30. Offit K. Personalized medicine: New genomics, old lessons. Hum Genet. 2011 Jul;130(1):3–14. doi: 10.1007/s00439-011-1028-3.
31. Stefanicka-Wojtas D, Kurpas D. Personalised medicine-implementation to the healthcare system in Europe (Focus group discussions). J Pers Med. 2023 Feb 21;13(3):380. doi: 10.3390/jpm13030380.
32. Gajria D, Chandarlapaty S. HER2 amplified breast cancer: Mechanisms of trastuzumab resistance and novel targeted therapies. Expert Rev Anticancer Ther. 2011 Feb;11(2):263–375. doi: 10.1586/era.10.226.
33. Tolomeo M, Dieli F, Gebbia N, Simoni D. Tyrosine kinase inhibitors for the treatment of chronic myeloid leukemia. Anticancer Agents Med Chem. 2009 Oct;9(8):853–863. doi: 10.2174/187152009789124637.
34. Amarante-Mendes GP, Rana A, Datoguia TS, Hamerschlak N, Brumatti G. BCR-ABL1 tyrosine kinase complex signaling transduction: Challenges to overcome resistance in chronic myeloid leukemia. Pharmaceutics. 2022 Jan 17;14(1):215. doi: 10.3390/pharmaceutics14010215.
35. Valle I, Tramalloni D, Bragazzi NL. Cancer prevention: State of the art and future prospects. J Prev Med Hyg. 2015 Jun 10;56(1):E21–E27.
36. Hughes VS, Wiggins JM, Siemann DW. Tumor oxygenation and cancer therapy-then and now. Br J Radiol. 2019 Jan;92(1093):20170955. doi: 10.1259/bjr.20170955.
37. Hall EJ, Giaccia AJ. Radiobiology for the radiologist, 6th edn. Lippincott Williams & Wilkins, Philadelphia. 2006. 85–105.
38. Zhuang Y, Liu K, He Q, Gu X, Jiang C, Wu J. Hypoxia signaling in cancer: Implications for therapeutic interventions. MedComm (2020). 2023 Jan 23;4(1):e203. doi: 10.1002/mco2.203.
39. Bui BP, Nguyen PL, Lee K, Cho J. Hypoxia-inducible factor-1: A novel therapeutic target for the management of cancer, drug resistance, and cancer-related pain. Cancers (Basel). 2022 Dec 8;14(24):6054. doi: 10.3390/cancers14246054.
40. Graeber TG, Osmanian C, Jacks T, Housman DE, Koch CJ, Lowe SW, Giaccia AJ. Hypoxia-mediated selection of cells with diminished apoptotic potential in solid tumours. Nature. 1996 Jan 4;379(6560): 88–91. doi: 10.1038/379088a0.
41. Zhang C, Liu J, Wang J, Zhang T, Xu D, Hu W, Feng Z. The interplay between tumor suppressor p53 and hypoxia signaling pathways in cancer. Front Cell Dev Biol. 2021 Feb 18;9:648808. doi: 10.3389/ fcell.2021.648808.
42. Vaupel P, Mayer A. Hypoxia in cancer: Significance and impact on clinical outcome. Cancer Metastasis Rev. 2007 Jun;26(2):225–239. doi: 10.1007/s10555-007-9055-1.
43. Vaupel P, Briest S, Höckel M. Hypoxia in breast cancer: Pathogenesis, characterization and biological/ therapeutic implications. Wien Med Wochenschr. 2002;152(13–14):334–342. doi: 10.1046/j.1563-258x. 2002.02032.x.
44. Nordsmark M, Bentzen SM, Rudat V, Brizel D, Lartigau E, Stadler P, Becker A, Adam M, Molls M, Dunst J, Terris DJ, Overgaard J. Prognostic value of tumor oxygenation in 397 head and neck tumors after primary radiation therapy. An international multi-center study. Radiother Oncol. 2005 Oct;77(1):18–24. doi: 10.1016/j.radonc.2005.06.038.
45. Nordsmark M, Alsner J, Keller J et al. Hypoxia in human soft tissue sarcomas: Adverse impact on survival and no association with p53 mutations. Br J Cancer. 2001;84:1070–1075.
46. Hockel M, Schlenger K, Aral B et al. Association between tumor hypoxia and malignant progression in advanced cancer of the uterine cervix. Cancer Res. 1996;56:4509–4515.
47. Wang JZ, Li XA, Mayr NA. Dose escalation to combat hypoxia in prostate cancer: A radiobiological study on clinical data. Br J Radiol. 2006;79:905–911.
48. Movsas B, Chapman JD, Hanlon AL et al. Hypoxic prostate/muscle pO_2 ratio predicts for biochemical failure in patients with prostate cancer: Preliminary findings. Urology. 2002;60:634–639.
49. Eschmann S-M, Paulsen F, Reimold M et al. Prognostic impact of hypoxia imaging with 18F-misonidazole PET in non-small cell lung cancer and head and neck cancer before radiotherapy. J Nucl Med. 2005;46:253–260.

50. Koh WJ, Rasey JS, Evans ML et al. Imaging of hypoxia in human tumors with [F-18]fluoromisonidazole. Int J Radiat Oncol Biol Phys. 1992;22:199–212.
51. Mortensen LS, Buus S, Nordsmark M et al. Identifying hypoxia in human tumors: A correlation study between 18 F-FMISO PET and the Eppendorf oxygen-sensitive electrode. Acta Onco. 2010;l49:934–940.
52. Varia MA, Calkins-Adams DP, Rinker LH et al. Pimonidazole: A novel hypoxia marker for complementary study of tumor hypoxia and cell proliferation in cervical carcinoma. Gynecol Oncol. 1998;71:270–277.
53. Chou L-W, Wang J, Chang P-L et al. Hyaluronan modulates accumulation of hypoxiainducible factor-1 alpha, inducible nitric oxide synthase, and matrix metalloproteinase-3 in the synovium of rat adjuvant-induced arthritis model. Arthritis Res Ther. 2011;13:R90.
54. Said HM, Supuran CT, Hageman C et al. Modulation of carbonic anhydrase 9 (CA9) in human brain cancer. Curr Pharm Des. 2010;6:3288–3299.
55. Ding I, Okunieff P, Salnikow K et al. A new intrinsic hypoxia marker in esophageal cancer. Adv Exp Med Biol. 2003;540:227–233.
56. Cangul H. Hypoxia upregulates the expression of the NDRG1 gene leading to its overexpression in various human cancers. BMC Genet. 2004;5:27.
57. Chakravarthi BV, Nepal S, Varambally S. Genomic and epigenomic alterations in cancer. Am J Pathol. 2016 Jul;186(7):1724–1735. doi: 10.1016/j.ajpath.2016.02.023.
58. Ray SK, Mukherjee S. Epigenetic reprogramming and landscape of transcriptomic interactions: Impending therapeutic interference of triple-negative breast cancer in molecular medicine. Curr Mol Med. 2022;22(10):835–850.
59. Das SK, Menezes ME, Bhatia S, Wang XY, Emdad L, Sarkar D, Fisher PB. Gene therapies for cancer: Strategies, challenges and successes. J Cell Physiol. 2015 Feb;230(2):259–271. doi: 10.1002/jcp.24791.
60. Su M, Zhang Z, Zhou L, Han C, Huang C, Nice EC. Proteomics, personalized medicine and cancer. Cancers (Basel). 2021 May 21;13(11):2512. doi: 10.3390/cancers13112512.
61. Passaro A, Al Bakir M, Hamilton EG, Diehn M, André F, Roy-Chowdhuri S, Mountzios G, Wistuba II, Swanton C, Peters S. Cancer biomarkers: Emerging trends and clinical implications for personalized treatment. Cell. 2024 Mar 28;187(7):1617–1635. doi: 10.1016/j.cell.2024.02.041.
62. Narrandes S, Xu W. Gene expression detection assay for cancer clinical use. J Cancer. 2018 Jun 5;9(13):2249–2265. doi: 10.7150/jca.24744.
63. Bou Antoun N, Chioni AM. Dysregulated signalling pathways driving anticancer drug resistance. Int J Mol Sci. 2023 Jul 30;24(15):12222. doi: 10.3390/ijms241512222.
64. Rivera CM, Ren B. Mapping human epigenomes. Cell. 2013 Sep 26;155(1):39–55. doi: 10.1016/j.cell.2013.09.011.
65. Stunnenberg HG, International Human Epigenome Consortium, Hirst M. The International Human Epigenome Consortium: A blueprint for scientific collaboration and discovery. Cell. 2016 Nov 17;167(5):1145–1149. doi: 10.1016/j.cell.2016.11.007.
66. Shakya K, O'Connell MJ, Ruskin HJ. The landscape for epigenetic/epigenomic biomedical resources. Epigenetics. 2012 Sep;7(9):982–986. doi: 10.4161/epi.21493.
67. Clish CB. Metabolomics: An emerging but powerful tool for precision medicine. Cold Spring Harb Mol Case Stud. 2015 Oct;1(1):a000588. doi: 10.1101/mcs.a000588.
68. Trifonova OP, Maslov DL, Balashova EE, Lokhov PG. Current state and future perspectives on personalized metabolomics. Metabolites. 2023 Jan 1;13(1):67. doi: 10.3390/metabo13010067.
69. Anand SS, Singh H, Dash AK. Clinical applications of PET and PET-CT. Med J Armed Forces India. 2009 Oct;65(4):353–358. doi: 10.1016/S0377-1237(09)80099-3.
70. Rischin D, Hicks RJ, Fisher R et al. Prognostic significance of [18F]-misonidazole positron emission tomography-detected tumor hypoxia in patients with advanced head and neck cancer randomly assigned to chemoradiation with or without tirapazamine: A substudy of Trans-Tasman Radiation Oncology Group Study 98.02. J Clin Oncol. 2006;24:2098–2104.
71. Pacheco-Torres J, López-Larrubia P, Ballesteros P et al. Imaging tumor hypoxia by magnetic resonance methods. NMR Biomed. 2011;24:1–16.
72. Kotas M, Schmitt P, Jakob PM et al. Monitoring of tumor oxygenation changes in headand-neck carcinoma patients breathing a hyperoxic hypercapnic gas mixture with a noninvasive MRI technique. Strahlenther Onkol. 2009;185:19–26.
73. Fan B, Wang X-Y, Yang X-D et al. Blood oxygen level-dependent MRI for the monitoring of neoadjuvant chemotherapy in breast carcinoma: Initial experience. Magn Reson Imaging. 2011;29:153–159.
74. Diepart C, Magat J, Jordan BF et al. In vivo mapping of tumor oxygen consumption using (19)F MRI relaxometry. NMR Biomed. 2011;24:458–463.

75. Salmon HW, Siemann DW. Utility of 19F MRS detection of the hypoxic cell marker EF5 to assess cellular hypoxia in solid tumors. Radiother Oncol. 2004;73:359–366.
76. Epel B, Haney CR, Hleihel D et al. Electron paramagnetic resonance oxygen imaging of a rabbit tumor using localized spin probe delivery. Med Phys. 2010;37:2553–2559.
77. Scheeren TW, Schober P, Schwarte LA. Monitoring tissue oxygenation by near infrared spectroscopy (NIRS): Background and current applications. J Clin Monit Comput. 2012 Aug;26(4):279–287. doi: 10.1007/s10877-012-9348-y.
78. Liu H, Chang JY. Proton therapy in clinical practice. Chin J Cancer. 2011 May;30(5):315–326. doi: 10.5732/cjc.010.10529.
79. Paredes F, Williams HC, San Martin A. Metabolic adaptation in hypoxia and cancer. Cancer Lett. 2021 Apr 1;502:133–142. doi: 10.1016/j.canlet.2020.12.020.
80. Letai A. Functional precision cancer medicine-moving beyond pure genomics. Nat Med. 2017 Sep 8; 23(9):1028–1035. doi: 10.1038/nm.4389.
81. Okada S, Vaeteewoottacharn K, Kariya R. Establishment of a patient-derived tumor xenograft model and application for precision cancer medicine. Chem Pharm Bull (Tokyo). 2018;66(3):225–230. doi: 10.1248/cpb.c17-00789.
82. Bhimani J, Ball K, Stebbing J. Patient-derived xenograft models-the future of personalised cancer treatment. Br J Cancer. 2020 Mar;122(5):601–602. doi: 10.1038/s41416-019-0678-0.
83. Ray SK, Mukherjee S. Cell free DNA as an evolving liquid biopsy biomarker for initial diagnosis and therapeutic nursing in cancer – An evolving aspect in medical biotechnology. Curr Pharm Biotechnol. 2022;23(1):112–122.

Index

M

N

O

P

R

S

T

U

V

W

X